Practical Orthopedics
Biological Options and Simpler Techniques for Common Disorders
(With an Atlas of Rare Conditions)

Practical Orthopedics
Biological Options and Simpler Techniques for Common Disorders
(With an Atlas of Rare Conditions)

Third Edition

SM Tuli MBBS MS PhD FAMS
Senior Consultant, Spinal Diseases and Orthopedics
Vidyasagar Institute of Mental Health and Neurosciences (VIMHANS),
and Moolchand hospital
New Delhi, India

Formerly
Chairman, Department of Orthopedics
Banaras Hindu University
Varanasi, Uttar Pradesh, India
Professor and Head
Department of Orthopedics
University College of Medical Sciences
New Delhi, India

Foreword
Apurv Mehra

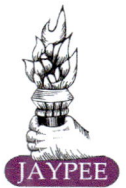

JAYPEE BROTHERS MEDICAL PUBLISHERS
The Health Sciences Publisher
New Delhi | London

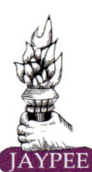 **Jaypee Brothers Medical Publishers (P) Ltd**

Headquarters

EMCA House
23/23-B, Ansari Road, Daryaganj
New Delhi 110 002, India
Landline: +91-11-23272143, +91-11-23272703
+91-11-23282021, +91-11-23245672
E-mail: jaypee@jaypeebrothers.com

Corporate Office

Jaypee Brothers Medical Publishers (P) Ltd.
4838/24, Ansari Road, Daryaganj
New Delhi 110 002, India
Phone: +91-11-43574357
Fax: +91-11-43574314
E-mail: jaypee@jaypeebrothers.com

Overseas Office

JP Medical Ltd.
83, Victoria Street, London
SW1H 0HW (UK)
Phone: +44-20 3170 8910
Fax: +44(0)20 3008 6180
E-mail: info@jpmedpub.com

Website: www.jaypeebrothers.com

Website: www.jaypeedigital.com

© 2024, Jaypee Brothers Medical Publishers

The views and opinions expressed in this book are solely those of the original contributor(s)/author(s) and do not necessarily represent those of editor(s) or publisher of the book.

All rights reserved. No part of this publication may be reproduced, stored or transmitted in any form or by any means, electronic, mechanical, photocopying, recording or otherwise, without the prior permission in writing of the publishers.

All brand names and product names used in this book are trade names, service marks, trademarks or registered trademarks of their respective owners. The publisher is not associated with any product or vendor mentioned in this book.

Medical knowledge and practice change constantly. This book is designed to provide accurate, authoritative information about the subject matter in question. However, readers are advised to check the most current information available on procedures included and check information from the manufacturer of each product to be administered, to verify the recommended dose, formula, method and duration of administration, adverse effects and contraindications. It is the responsibility of the practitioner to take all appropriate safety precautions. Neither the publisher nor the author(s)/editor(s) assume any liability for any injury and/or damage to persons or property arising from or related to use of material in this book.

This book is sold on the understanding that the publisher is not engaged in providing professional medical services. If such advice or services are required, the services of a competent medical professional should be sought.

Every effort has been made where necessary to contact holders of copyright to obtain permission to reproduce copyright material. If any have been inadvertently overlooked, the publisher will be pleased to make the necessary arrangements at the first opportunity.

Inquiries for bulk sales may be solicited at: jaypee@jaypeebrothers.com

Practical Orthopedics—Biological Options and Simpler Techniques for Common Disorders / SM Tuli

First Edition: 2015

Third Edition: **2024**

ISBN: 978-93-5696-433-4

Printed at: Replika Press Pvt. Ltd.

Dedicated to

*My teachers Professor KS Grewal, Professor PK Duraiswami and
Professor Balu Sankaran, the great orthopedic educators of their time,
My enquiring students who induced me to continue as
"student of orthopedics"
and
My ungrudging patients who could understand and accept
a balance between their expectations and constraints or
limitations of clinical medicine.*

Foreword

Professor Dr SM Tuli, a name that gets smile on face of every Orthopedic Surgeon, due to his academic and surgical excellence. Standing true to the lines "The Learning Never Ends" for the author in professor Tuli has enriched this book with Basics, Evidence and Experience, to create this class apart masterpiece titled as "Practical Orthopedics".

The book talks about Biological Options and Simpler Techniques for Common Disorders for the entire spectrum of Orthopedics, the compilation is carefully drafted, keeping in mind that our branch Orthopedics lays its foundation on the biological options, understanding and utilizing them to enhance healing. The strongest feature of this book is its simple flowing language that will leave an everlasting impression in the brains of the students. My favourite line from the book is "The injury itself triggers the cascade of healing process". This describes the author's in-depth analysis of not only the disease, the subject but also the life in broader perspective.

This wonderful book also has an Atlas of rare disorders with key features for the students to identify as they keep evolving as an orthopedic surgeon, these are carefully curated out of the vast collection of professor Tuli sir over last 6 decades of his orthopedics experience.

For **Professor SM Tuli Sir**, the lines from poem "Invictus" are enough to describe the legend sitting at the top of the mountain which only mortals are trying to climb.

"I am the Master of my Fate"

"I am the Captain of my Soul"

Enjoy the Ride and remember "The Learning Never Ends"

Apurv Mehra
MBBS MS (Orthopedics) DNB (Orthopedics)
Author, Motivational Speaker
Founder "Conceptual Orthopedics"
Vidya Jeevan Orthopedic Centre
Max Hospital, New Delhi, India

Preface to the Third Edition

The best clinical learning even today in through ancestral or traditional mantra of listening, looking, feeling, moving, measuring, and comparing for reaching a rational diagnosis, suggesting appropriate investigations, and offering the patient the most efficacious and cost-effective therapeutics. Despite the availability of imaging modalities, artificial intelligence (AI), navigational facilities and robotics, we must optimize our clinical acumen to offer the best to the people. Let us try what John Hunter wrote "Civilized men who get by stratagem what an armed savage would get by force."

The author has the privilege of having learnt from the great teachers of orthopedics. The present days, AI technologies can provide us most of the information contained in textbooks and an exhaustive list of references. The aim of this handbook, however, is to offer a write-up to the students and practicing orthopedists, based upon personal experience of learning, teaching, and practicing clinical orthopedics for nearly 65 years in teaching hospitals.

During post-COVID period there has been a drastic change in the publications of scientific and medical journals. One can pay for "publication" or you pay for "editing". Replication of information in many current publications has been observed to be about 35%, naturally this induces a crises in confidence especially for clinical applications. In this book exhaustive list of references has been avoided. Most of the references included in this text show where the thought process started, how it evolved over the years and what are the current thoughts for future development.

Dr Dattatreya Mohapatra collated many new, rare, and educative illustrations which have been added in Chapter 19 the ATLAS. These figures would help orthopedic specialists and the evolving new generation to reach at correct diagnosis and seek help for optimum therapeutics. Images and illustrations at, presentation and at follow-up help us develop visual dimensions to understand the natural history of disease, response to therapeutics and complications in untreated (and treated) patient. Many new images have been added in all the 19 Chapters. I hope this write-up would provide credible, accessible, and affordable options for common orthopedic disorders, useful for family physicians, orthopedists, physical therapists, and medical care personnel. Problems such as complex and rare disorders, repeat spinal surgeries, repeat joint replacements and care of malignant disease would however, need the help of dedicated specialized facilities.

The readers of this book are requested and encouraged to communicate their thoughts to us suggesting deletions, corrections, and additions. Hopefully, this spirit of cooperation may help us transmission of more balanced knowledge of Orthopedics for today and tomorrow.

SM Tuli

Preface to the First Edition

There are many books on orthopedics but most of these are written by authors working in resource-rich countries. One must, however, realize that nearly 70 percent of people worldwide are living in resource-compromised environment far away from the modern facilities of metropolitan cities. The world is not made of New York, Paris, or Tokyo, and similarly Indian subcontinent is not made of Delhi, Mumbai or Chennai. Seventy percent of orthopedic problems are being managed in areas, which barely have moderate infrastructure facilities available. One should appreciate the skill, and ingenuity of these specialists, who show responsiveness to the needs of people who do not have access to the metropolitan facilities. Despite intentions of upgradation of infrastructure facilities worldwide, at all times there would be differences of economic inequalities and such differences are not likely to disappear in future as well. Due to perpetual man-made conflicts and natural disasters, there would always be pockets of deprivation, crowding, malnutrition and inaccessibilities.

The experience and observations of orthopedic surgeons in resource-limited environments, related published material in national and international literature, and personal observations of over 60 years in the management of common orthopedic disorders in moderate facilities form the basis of this book. The readers of this book are requested and encouraged to communicate their thoughts for corrections, deletions and additions. I seek their cooperation for help to continually improve orthopedic education and related health care.

The guidelines suggested here are based upon the observations of the natural course of common conditions and the observed efficacy of biological options and simpler techniques. The suggestions made here are not limited to geographic boundries, but are generally applicable to the patients who would prefer modalities in environments where they reside, options, which do not require major changes in their lifestyle or entail frequent medical or operative intervention, and are cost effective.

I hope this write-up would provide credibility to the efforts and techniques for development of accessible, affordable and effective options for many orthopedic disorders. Sound advice would be available for the family physicians, physical therapists, nursing care personnel and concerned orthopedic specialists. Some problems, like complex spine operations, repeat surgeries for joint replacement and the care of the malignant disease, would, however, need to be referred to dedicated specialized hospitals.

SM Tuli

Acknowledgments

Any attempt at writing a book on a clinical subject is a complex and interactive process. Between the second and third edition of this book, many orthopedic colleagues working in VIMHANS Hospital, Nehru Nagar, New Delhi and Moolchand Hospital, Lajpat Nagar, New Delhi, helped me to collate clinical, radiological, and follow-up data to be included in third edition. I gratefully acknowledge the help provided by Dr Varun Kapoor, Dr Dattatreya Mohapatra, Dr Deepak Thakur, Dr Vaibhav Jain and Dr Vipin Khatkar. My family indirectly participated in this great endeavor. My wife Swarn, and the next generation Dr VB Bhasin, Dr Neena Bhasin, Dr Gagan Joshi, Dr Varuna Joshi offered their suggestions, inspired me, and tolerated my eccentricities for many years.

We would like to extend our special thanks to Shri Jitendar P Vij (Group Chairman), Mr Ankit Vij (Managing Director), and Mr MS Mani (Group President) of M/s Jaypee Brothers Medical Publishers (P) Ltd, New Delhi, India, for publishing the book in the same format as wanted, well in time.

We would like to offer a huge appreciation to the wonderful work done by Ms Chetna Malhotra (Senior Director—Professional Publishing, Marketing and Business Development), Ms Pooja Bhandari (Director—Production), Mr Ajay Kumar Sharma (DGM—Production), Mr Anirban Mukherjee (Development Editor), Mr Shubham Kumar (Typesetter), and Mr Armaan Ali (Graphic Designer) of M/s Jaypee Brothers Medical Publishers (P) Ltd, New Delhi, India.

SM Tuli

Contents

SECTION 1: General Orthopedic Conditions

1. **Regeneration and Repair of Osseous Tissues**   3
   Healing of Fractures and Osseous Tissues   3
   Biology of Natural Fracture Healing (Secondary Healing)   5
   Time Table of Fracture Union   6
   Fracture Stabilization—Options   8
   Rigid Internal Fixation   8
   Osteotomies in Orthopedics   9
   Ilizarov's (1950s) Technique of Corticotomy, Distraction Histogenesis and Deformity Correction   10
   Bone Grafts and Graft Substitutes   11

2. **Infections of Bones and Joints**   17
   Acute Hematogenous Osteomyelitis   17
   Functional Position of Joints   20
   Septic Arthritis   20
   Chronic Osteomyelitis   21
   Iatrogenic Infections in Orthopedics   24
   Tuberculosis of Bones and Joints   26
   Principles of Management   30
   Tuberculosis of the Spine (Pott's Disease)   34

3. **Inflammatory Rheumatoid Disorders**   38
   Monoarticular Presentation   39
   Treatment   40
   Role of Operative Intervention   40
   Prognosis   41
   Seronegative Spondyloarthropathies   41
   Ankylosing Spondylitis   41
   Reiter's Syndrome and Reactive Arthritis   43
   Psoriatic Arthritis   43
   Enteropathic Arthropathy   43
   Juvenile Rheumatoid (Idiopathic) Arthritis (JRA or JIA)   43
   Connective Tissue Rheumatoid Like Diseases   44
   Basic Treatment of Inflammatory Rheumatoid Disorders   44
   Diffuse Idiopathic Skeletal Hyperostosis   45
   Gout   47

4. **Osteoarthrosis**   48
   Treatment   *50*

5. **Avascular Necrosis of Bone or Osteonecrosis**   52
   Pathology   *52*
   Diagnosis   *53*
   Treatment   *54*
   Osteonecrosis Other than Femoral Head   *59*

6. **Common Metabolic Bone Disorders**   60
   Normal Age-related Changes in Bones   *60*
   Rickets in Children and Osteomalacia in Adults   *61*
   Correction of Deformities   *64*
   Growth Plate (Physis) Modulations   *66*
   Osteoporosis   *67*

7. **Common Generalized Congenital Deformities and Dysplasias in Orthopedics**   71
   Clinical Diagnosis   *71*
   Congenital Connective Tissue Disorders   *73*
   Generalized Skeletal Dysplasias   *73*
   Basic Principles of Deformity Correction   *78*
   Common Soft Tissue Procedures   *79*
   Dyschondroplasia, Enchondromatosis (Ollier's Disease) and Enchondroma   *79*

8. **Localized Congenital Deformities (Anomalies) of Limbs**   81
   Radial Deficiency   *81*
   Developmental Dysplasia of the Hip (Congenital Dislocation of Hip Joint)   *83*
   Congenital ClubFoot   *88*
   Operative Correction   *89*
   Local congenital Defects   *91*

9. **Common Orthopedic Tumors**   95
   Clinical Features   *96*
   Investigations   *96*
   Benign "Tumor-like" Lesions   *99*
   Benign Bone Tumors   *101*
   Malignant Bone Tumors   *107*
   Reticulum-cell Sarcoma of Bone (Non-Hodgkin's Lymphoma)   *111*
   Neoplasms: Pitfalls are in Plenty   *112*

10. **Common Neuromuscular Disorders**   114
    Poliomyelitis   *114*
    Muscular Dystrophies   *116*
    Arthrogryposis Multiplex Congenita (Amyoplasia)   *117*
    Cerebral Palsy (Little's Disease)   *117*
    Leprosy (Hansen's Disease)   *120*
    Peripheral Nerves   *122*

Contents xvii

SECTION 2: Regional Orthopedic Conditions

11. Disorders Related to Neck   127
- Cleidocranial Dysostosis *127*
- Torticollis *127*
- Brachialgia *127*
- Cervical Spine Disc Prolapse *128*
- Cervical Canal Stenosis and Myelopathy *129*
- Congenital Torticollis due to the Contracture of Sternocleidomastoid Muscle *130*

12. Shoulder   133
- Painful Shoulder: Common Pathologies *133*
- Painful Shoulder Common Pathologies *134*
- Instability of Shoulder *136*

13. Elbow and Forearm   140
- Tennis Elbow (Lateral Epicondylitis) *140*
- Golfer's Elbow *140*
- Congenital Slipping of Ulnar Nerve *141*
- Cubitus Valgus *141*
- Cubitus Varus (Gunstock) Deformity *142*
- Distal Humeral Osteotomy *142*
- Olecranon Bursitis *144*
- Stiff Elbow *144*
- Congenital Radioulnar Synostosis *145*
- Congenital Absence of Radius *146*
- Myositis Ossificans (Heterotopic Ossification) *147*

14. Wrist and Hand   149
- Wrist Drop *149*
- Claw Hand *149*
- Carpal Tunnel Syndrome *150*
- Carpal Tunnel Release *151*
- Ganglion *151*
- Deformities in Wrist and Hand *151*
- Gross Deformities *152*
- Constrictive Tenosynovitis *152*
- Kienböck's Disease *155*
- Sudeck's Dystrophy [Currently Addressed as Complex Regional Pain Syndrome (CRPS)], or Reflex Pain Syndrome (RPS) *155*

15. Back Pain and Spine   157
- Scoliosis *158*
- Kyphosis *160*
- Spondylolysis and Spondylolisthesis *160*

Spina Bifida *161*
Ankylosing Spondylitis and Rheumatoid Spondylitis *161*

16. Hip — 171

Walking and Standing *171*
Movements *171*
Perthes Disease (Legg–Calvé–Perthes Disease) *174*
Classification of Perthes Disease *175*
Slipped Capital Femoral Epiphysis (Adolescent Coxa Vara) *178*
Osteotomies of Proximal Femur *179*
Innominate Osteotomies *187*
Pemberton's (1965) Acetabuloplasty *194*

17. Knee and Leg — 196

Deformities of the Knee *197*
High Tibial Osteotomy *202*
Operative Techniques *205*

18. Ankle and Foot — 208

Ankle *208*
Foot *208*

19. Atlas of Rare Conditions (One may Encounter through the Journey in Orthopedics) — 215

X-rays of Pelvis Reflect General Health of the Skeleton *215*

Index — **243**

SECTION 1

GENERAL ORTHOPEDIC CONDITIONS

Section Outline

1. Regeneration and Repair of Osseous Tissues
2. Infections of Bones and Joints
3. Inflammatory Rheumatoid Disorders
4. Osteoarthrosis
5. Avascular Necrosis of Bone or Osteonecrosis
6. Common Metabolic Bone Disorders
7. Common Generalized Congenital Deformities and Dysplasias in Orthopedics
8. Localized Congenital Deformities (Anomalies) of Limbs
9. Common Orthopedic Tumors
10. Common Neuromuscular Disorders

CHAPTER 1

Regeneration and Repair of Osseous Tissues

HEALING OF FRACTURES AND OSSEOUS TISSUES

Most of the fractures would unite whether splinted or not due to an in-built mechanism of healing. Land-animals afterall have been walking after such fractures. Any damaged bone has the biological potential of repairing by "bone formation".

In clinical practice, fractures require stable immobilization to alleviate pain, ensuring adequate contact of fracture ends in near anatomical position, preventing excessive movements at fracture site, however, permitting early axial loading of the limb. Axial physiological loading permits healing by natural way by formation of external callus. Visible external callus will not form if the fracture is fixed rigidly. The progress of healing process by rigid fixation cannot be easily appreciated. The bones under rigid implants due to stress shielding become osteoporotic, fracture at the weakened bone is not uncommon after the implant removal.

An outline of "natural healing" of a fracture is described below. All the structures, periosteum, endosteum, cells contained within the broken bones and muscles and soft tissues contribute to the process of fracture healing. The injury itself triggers the cascade of healing process. The cascade of fracture or bone healing starts after traumatic fracture, osteotomies (controlled fractures), pathological fractures (except due to malignancies), or any operation on bone.

Throughout the process of fracture healing (from fracture hematoma **(Fig. 1.1)**

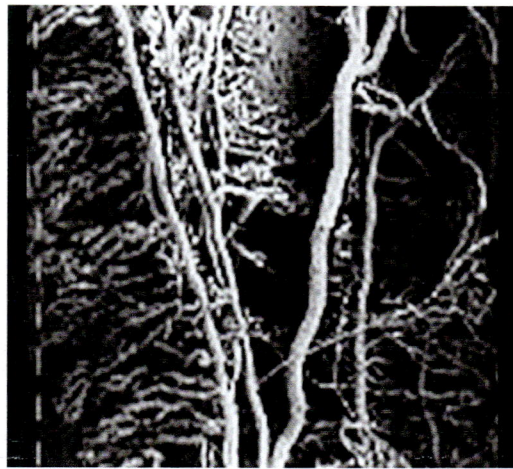

Fig. 1.1: Bone is essentially a vascular tree surrounded by mineralized tissue, thus maintaining it's viscoelasticity. This is the appearance of 'bone' after removal of all mineralized tissues.

till the end of remodeling), many growth factors like bone morphogenic proteins, cytokines and other growth factors continuously play a role in cascadal fashion. The cellular and molecular responses are practically uniform up to the stage of soft callus formation, further behavior of growth factors and cellular response would, however, depend upon the environments provided for the healing process. The pluripotent reparative mesenchymal cells under variable conditions may induce woven bone (fiber bone), chondrogenesis, endochondral ossification, lamellar bone; or fibrous tissue when environments are unfavorable **(Figs. 1.2 and 1.3)**.

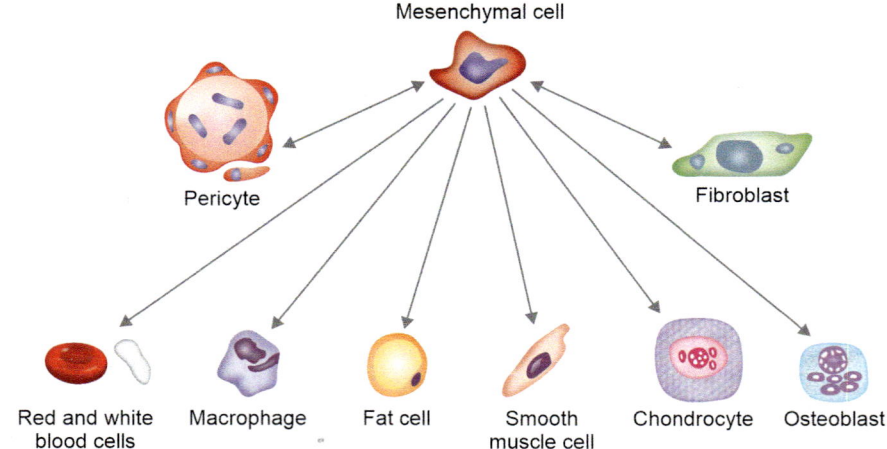

Fig. 1.2: Reparative mesenchymal cells can be induced to form any mesenchymal tissue depending upon the environments.

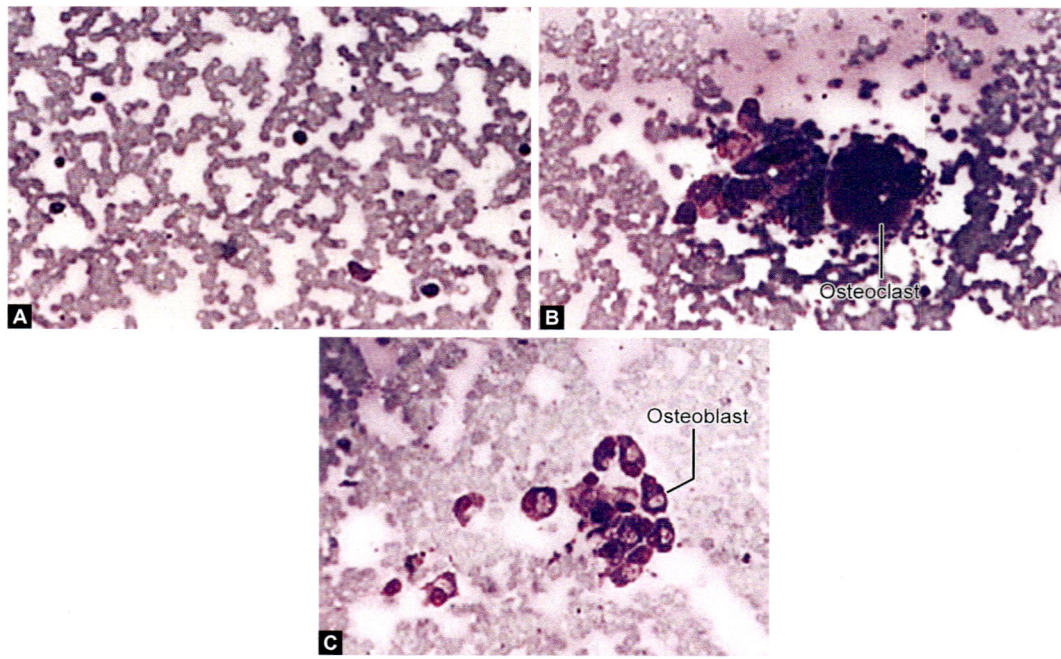

Figs. 1.3A to C: Cellular response in early stages of repair. (A) During first week—nonspecific inflammatory cells; (B) Between 2–4th week—osteoclasts and osteoblasts; (C) Between 3–5th week—clump of osteoblastic cells.

Immediately after a fracture, in addition to the formation of fracture hematoma, there is intense vascular response in the injured area (not unlike in the Ilizarov's process). The vascularity increases at every level, medullary vessels, periosteal vessels, from capillaries to nutrient arteries. With healing, the continuity of endosteal, periosteal and extra-osseous vasculature is re-established across the site of fractured area.

BIOLOGY OF NATURAL FRACTURE HEALING (SECONDARY HEALING)

The fractures heal by various biological stages in a cascadal fashion. The stages generally described are for convenience and possible understanding. Fracture or any injury to the bone triggers following biological cascade of repair **(Fig. 1.4)**.

Stage I—Fracture Hematoma: Blood collects around the broken bones, because there is rupture of endosteal and periosteal blood vessels and the vessels in the disrupted soft tissues around the site of broken bones. At the fracture ends, 1–2 mm of bone dies because of disruption of its blood supply.

Stage II—Soft Callus: Within about 8 hours of the fracture, the hematoma gets organized (formation of granulation tissues) and invaded by neocapillaries accompanied by endothelial and perithelial cells under the influence of many growth factors and cytokines **(Figs. 1.5A and B)**.

Stage III—Mineralization of Callus: Calcium starts getting deposited around the neocapillaries (neo-osteogenesis), peripheral parts earlier than deeper parts.

The pluripotent mesenchymal cells of the granulation tissue, under the influence of bone morphogenetic agents and growth factors, differentiate into osteogenic, chondrogenic and osteoclastic cells. Osteoclasts

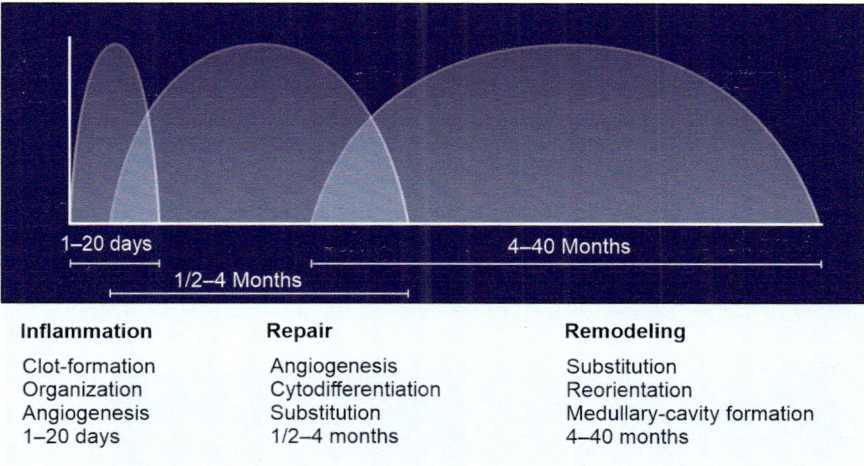

Fig. 1.4: Biological cascade of repair and regeneration of bone.
Source: Adapted from literature.

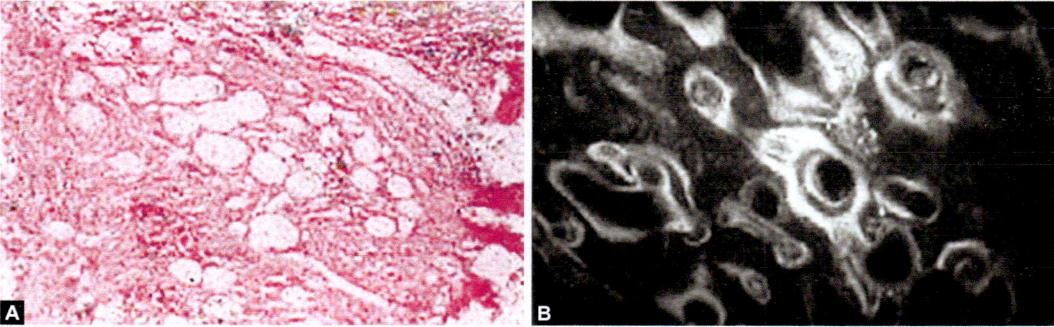

Figs. 1.5A and B: (A) Abundant neocapillaries formed at early stages of repair; (B) Neo-osteogenesis seen by tetracycline fluorescence around neoangiogenesis. Newly mineralized bone is seen as fluorescent band (labeled by tetracycline) in ultraviolet light microscopy.

remove the dead bone and dead tissues, thus, creating channels (cutter heads) for neocapillaries to spread across the fracture site. Earliest neo-osteogenesis is observed around the neocapillaries and vascular spaces **(Figs. 1.5 and 1.6)**. Mineralization of callus is a diffuse process, external callus is radiologically visible, however, internal callus (medullary callus) is not easily discernable.

Stage IV—Callus Consolidation: The whole of callus is now mineralized spreading astride the fractured site. The fracture lines do not remain visible in the X-rays. The outer surface of callus is irregular (rough).

Stage V—Callus Remodeling: The bone laid down in the initial stages is as woven bone (fiber bone) or as endochondral bone. The restoration of the normal architecture occurs by the process of remodeling according to the Wolff's law (function determines the form of bone). The geometry, thickness and trabecular pattern of callus and bone are dependent upon the functional loading (probably the most important physical or mechanical factor) and muscular action of the limb. Ultimately the trabeculae are laid (reorganized) in the direction of functional loading, woven bone or endochondral bone gets replaced by trabecular lamellar bone, the external callus gets resorbed (decreases in size), the medullary canal and medullary vessels get re-established. Radiologically the callus has normal mineralization and there is smoothening of the external surfaces **(Fig. 1.7)**.

TIME TABLE OF FRACTURE UNION

How long does a fracture take to unite and consolidate? No precise answer is possible because age, general health, status of soft tissue cover, blood supply, nature of fracture (closed or compound), the site of fracture and type of treatment, all influence the time taken. Approximate prediction may be possible for fractures of major bones in an adult (with optimum health) according to Perkin's timetable. A spiral fracture in the upper limb unites in three weeks, for consolidation (time to permit all activities without protection) multiply by 2; for lower limb, multiply all figures by 2; for transverse fractures, multiply all figures again by 2.

With optimum health and nutrition of the patient, having been offered a biologically

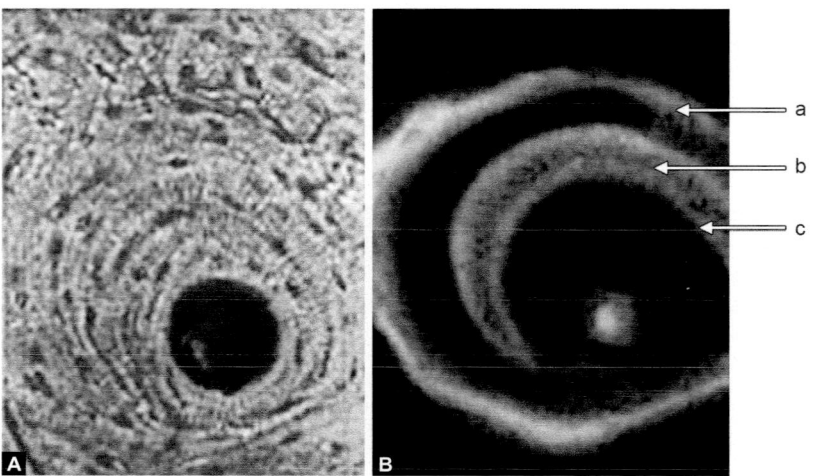

Figs. 1.6A and B: Outer most layer of bone was laid about one month before harvesting this tissue, around a large vascular space. Successive layers of bone formed (as seen by tetracycline-fluorescence) in 1 month's time reducing the size of the vascular space to form an osteon. New bone forming 30 ± days before harvesting this specimen (a), 20 ± days before (b), and 10 ± days before harvesting (c).

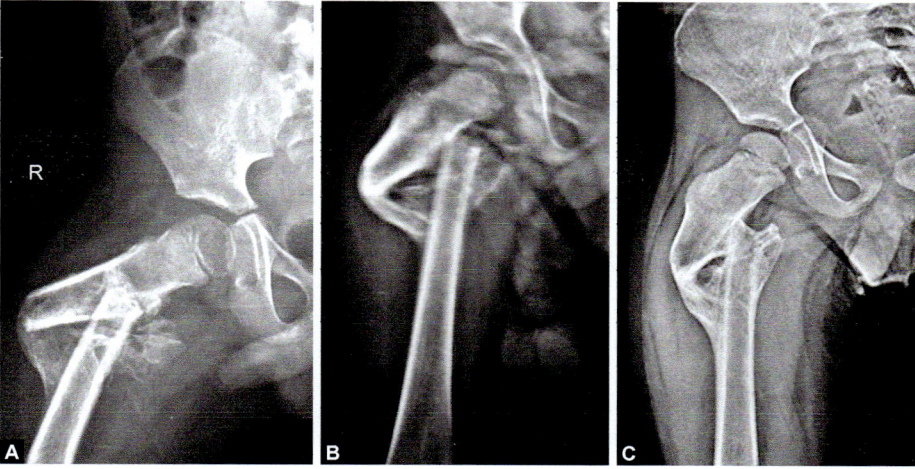

Figs. 1.7A to C: Remodeling of uniting fractures: During growing age even gross deformities may remodel with time. Angular deformities near the joint remodel completely. The remodeling become less active as we grow with age, especially rotation deformities rarely get corrected (A to C = 2 years).

sound treatment most of the fractures heal with optimum biological process. However, 5–10 % of fractures undergo delayed union and non-union, many due to poorly understood causes. Optimization or enhancement of the healing process of such patients is being debated and tried.

We may not completely understand methods for enhancement of the process of fracture healing, however, causes of nonunion or delayed unions are fairly well known.

Nonunions

If a fracture does not unite in double the expected time of union for that fracture, it is accepted to be called nonunion. Common causes of nonunion are:
1. Distraction of fracture fragments, either as a result of interposition of soft tissues, or failure of soft tissues to hold the fragments in contact, or as a result of fixation of fragments in distraction (bipolar interlocking, plating).
2. Excessive movements at fracture site.
3. Severe damage to soft tissues (extent of trauma or iatrogenic).
4. Poor local blood supply of bone.
5. Infection (infected nonunions are most difficult to treat).
6. **Iatrogenic:** Surgical intervention leading to excessive soft tissue stripping (damage), fixing the fracture with a gap between the fragments.
7. **Intracapsular fractures:** Fracture line within the synovial fluid (fractures of femoral neck, scaphoid, talus).

Fracture line remains visible in X-rays after many months of treatment. Some operative intervention is indicated when a particular fracture is not expected to unite: The X-rays may show a gap of more than 3 mm, the bone ends are sclerosed, there is thinning of bone ends or the medullary canal is closed. Nonunions are classified as hypertrophic or atrophic or a mixed variety. In cases of difficulty or when the fragments are already fixed with implants, "stress X-rays" in various planes may help to reach the decision. Some nonunions especially in the elderly and located in upper limb may be managed by a suitable orthosis, which permits the patient function and ambulation without much pain. However, in general, the principles of open reduction, freshening of edges, internal fixation and barrel-stieve like copious autogenous bone grafting is mandatory. Postoperatively encourage active exercises and loading of the operated limb. When in doubt about the stability provided by the implant do not hesitate to use additional cast or orthosis. A few cm of shortening to achieve union is not much of a price to ensure union.

FRACTURE STABILIZATION—OPTIONS

Despite all the technological advances made in the operative treatment of fractures (open reduction and internal fixation–ORIF), surgical intervention is not free of complications, and many a time a second operation (reoperation) is indicated for implant removal. Nonoperative management is a sound method of treating many fractures especially in places with moderate or compromised infrastructure available. Most of the fractures of upper end of humerus, humeral shaft, lower end of radius, fractures of forearm bones, fractures of tibia, fractures around the ankles, clavicle, carpal and tarsal bones, metacarpals and metatarsals can be effectively managed by nonoperative (less aggressive) treatment. Multiple Kirschner wires (K-wires) fixation percutaneously with biplanar and bicortical engagement under C-arm guidance can improve the stability around osteochondral fracture sites. Many fresh osteochondral fractures (>10 days duration) can be managed by closed reduction (functional reduction) and insertion of K-wires under C-arm.

Other methods of achieving stability at the fracture site are plates, screws, external fixations, bridging plates, intramedullary fixations. Rigid-internal fixation was advocated by AO–school in the second half of 20th century; however, at present, the preference and consensus is for stable fixations. Ideally one should prefer a fixation which permits early axial physiological loading, as during walking and while doing active muscle exercises.

Intramedullary nails with many of its modifications are used as a standard option for most of the diaphyseal fractures of bones. Reaming of the medullary canal for insertion of the nail is still controversial and debated. There are proponents for reaming to permit insertion of nails with larger diameter, we prefer minimal reaming to open the isthmic areas to permit a snug fitting nail, and there are some surgeons who insert nails without reaming especially while operating on a polytraumatized patient. Do not attempt extensive operations (to achieve "anatomical" reduction) which may lead to devascularization of bone. Basic goals of fracture treatment should be aimed at stable fixation (by any means) with least disruption of endosteal and periosteal circulation, respect to and restoration of soft tissue coverage with provision for relatively pain free movements of the adjacent joints. Micromotions do not impede the healing process. Prolonged non-weight-bearing can lead to local osteoporosis, soft tissue dystrophy and loss of articular cartilage nutrition. Some known substances that have inhibitory effect on bone healing are nonsteroidal anti-inflammatory drugs (NSAIDs), tobacco (nicotine), steroids, diabetic state, rheumatoid disorders, malnutrition, osteoporosis, cytotoxic drugs and irradiation.

RIGID INTERNAL FIXATION

With rigid fixation, medullary circulation may get re-established early, the "cutter heads" may cross the fracture site, however, the so called "primary healing" or "osteon by osteon" healing takes place very slowly and means to accurately determine the progress (extent) of primary healing are unreliable. For early ambulation, casts or orthosis are still required to protect the limb during full weight-bearing. Rigid fixation with plates results in stress shielding under the implant leading to cortical thinning (bone loss), which may cause fracture at the ends of plate (site of stress concentration), or at the site of thinning of cortex. The reported incidence of such fractures is 10–15% **(Table 1.1)**. The

TABLE 1.1: Healing of bone.	
Natural/by callus (since antiquity)—SECONDARY HEALING	***"Osteonal" (1965–1985±)—PRIMARY HEALING***
Stable immobilization by POP or ORIF	Rigid internal fixation (RIF) in every fracture
Micromotion and axial loading encouraged	Aim: No motion at site of fixation
Micromotion → Stimulus for callus	No micromotion → No stimulus for callus
Union judged by visible callus	Judgment of union uncertain
Refracture through callus extremely rare	Refracture not uncommon at implant—bone interface
Load/Stress sharing	Load/Stress shielding
(ORIF: open reduction and internal fixation; POP: plaster of Paris)	

likelihood of refracture of bones that heal with external callus (natural healing) is extremely rare.

The classical diaphyseal fractures which are stable (transverse, or short oblique) can be managed by intramedullary nails without interlocking. However, unstable diaphyseal fractures, very oblique, long spiral, grossly comminuted segmental fractures, or fractures with loss of bone fragments, are candidates for interlocking (with screws). Early loading in cases of interlocking is inadvisable because the stress would be on screws, which are likely to bend or break. When one is using bipolar interlocking, dynamization must be done to avoid nonunion. On an average dynamization for upper limb in recommended after 6 weeks, for the lower limb after about 9 weeks.

OSTEOTOMIES IN ORTHOPEDICS

Our ancestors in orthopedics evolved many osteotomies for a variety of orthopedic affections (conditions). These are essentially low technology but high biology procedures. If our patient selection is appropriate and the procedure is performed following the principles advocated by the exponents one can get a satisfactory result in a number of disorders for many years.

Ideally any corrective osteotomy should be done nearest to the deformity. For genu varum, select proximal tibial osteotomy; for genu valgum, select distal femoral osteotomy; for cubitus varum or cubitus valgum, select distal humeral osteotomies proximal to olecranon fossa. Proximal femoral osteotomies are generally indicated for fixed hip deformities or certain problematic fractures. Innominate osteotomies help provide 'shelf' for stability of hip joint. There are many methods of obtaining correction of deformities. It can be close-wedge osteotomy, it does not need bone grafting, however, the bone-wedge which one removes may be used as a bone graft to place over the osteotomy site before wound closure. If one opts for an open wedge osteotomy, one has to secure the correction by a suitable implant, most surgeons consider filling of the open wedge with bone grafts. Another method of achieving correction is by a dome-shaped (ball and socket) osteotomy. The convexity of the dome is generally towards the joint or broader end of the bone. After completion of the ball and socket osteotomy, the correction can be achieved in any direction—abduction, adduction, external rotation and internal rotation in isolation or in combination.

Once any of the above corrective osteotomies are completed, it is wise to correct all deformities, as planned preoperatively. The contralateral normal limb should be easily accessible for comparison of the achieved correction during surgery. The site of osteotomy can be fixed by any of the methods, plaster cast only, K-wires and plaster cast, tubular plates, screws and wires (like French osteotomy), angled blade plates, or external fixators. While providing stability one should minimize further stripping of soft tissue coverage of bones. Depending upon the growth potential of the bone, one may do over-correction of the deformity by 5-10 degrees to negate the recurrence of deformity with growth. Basic priniciples of fracture healing must be observed during operation, fixation, postoperative immobilization, loading and rehabilitation.

Osteotomy performed by a surgeon should be considered a controlled fracture. While doing osteotomy if soft tissues are respected, while achieving correction bone ends are not treated roughly, raw surfaces at the osteotomy site are held in good apposition for at least 70% of the circumference, implants when used provide a stable fixation (without distraction) to permit axial loading in the lower limbs or active exercises (in the upper limb) 3-6 weeks after the osteotomy, non-union at the osteotomy site should be a rare complication. While using rigid implants for fixation of osteotomy, the surgeon must ensure the best desired position on the operating table. If one is using a semirigid implant (K-wires), the correction can be improved to the best desired at the time of stitch removal and application of definitive plaster around 2-3 weeks after the osteotomy. Most of the corrective osteotomies for joint problems provide adequate relief of pain, maintain functional mobility, retain natural bone stock and articular cartilage, provide proprioception and permit fairly high degree of activity for 10-15 years. Juxta-articular osteotomies may improve the blood supply and nutrition of the articular cartilage and do not necessarily compromise the later arthroplasty procedure.

ILIZAROV'S (1950s) TECHNIQUE OF CORTICOTOMY, DISTRACTION HISTOGENESIS AND DEFORMITY CORRECTION

Distraction osteogenesis is a form of tissue engineering founded on the principle of generation of new tissues in response to gradual increase in tension. The basis of the technique is to produce a careful fracture of bone or corticotomy, followed by a short wait (5-10 days) for young callus to form at the site of 'fracture'. Distraction is now applied gradually via a circular or unilateral external fixator device **(Fig. 1.8)**.

In *corticotomy*, the bony cortex is partially divided in a circumferential manner using sharp narrow osteotomes through small skin incisions. The break is completed by gentle manual force (*osteoclasis*), thus, leaving endosteal and periosteal blood supply intact. Alternatively, the site of osteotomy is exposed subperiosteally, multiple drill holes are made all around the site of bone division in the cortex without going across the endosteum and medullary canal. The osteotomy is completed using a sharp narrow osteotome.

One can understand the biological principles, however, mastery of the technique has a long learning curve. The operative technique is got to be tailored to each patient. Probably this method is best indicated in patients who have concomitant complex deformities such as angulation, rotation, translation and shortening. The corticotomy or osteotomy must be completed by low energy technique (sharp, narrow osteotomes) to minimize necrosis and

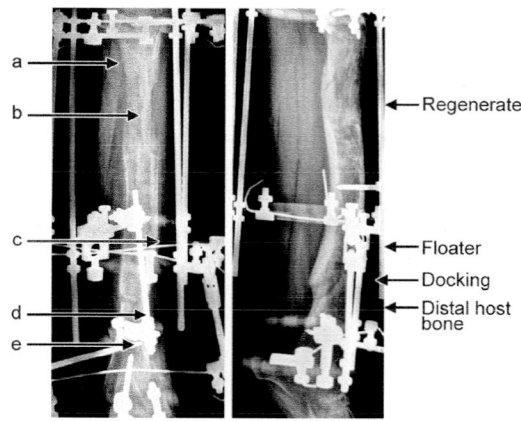

Fig. 1.8: Ilizarov's technique for neohistogenesis by slow distraction (axial and transverse). (a) Proximal host bone; (b) Regenerate (neo-histogenesis); (c) Floater; (d) Docking site (e) Distal host bone.

damage to endosteal and periosteal blood supply. Distraction osteogenesis has the best potential of "regeneration" at metaphyseal or metaphysio-diaphyseal junctional areas as compared to diaphyseal sites. A nearly tenfold spatial increase in blood flow through neoangiogenesis following corticotomy (and possibly following osteotomy) has been observed. Neoangiogenesis is the precursor to neo-osteogenesis. Distraction is recommended at 0.25 mm four times a day. Distraction at this rate causes neovascularization, neo-osteogenesis, generalized cellular proliferation almost in all the tissues, skin, muscles, nerves and vessels (most appropriately termed distraction histogenesis) under the effect of tension distraction. Ilizarov's corticotomy can be successfully used even in the presence of moderate active infection and local scarring of soft tissues.

Distraction is usually applied through a circular or unilateral or bilateral external fixator. Depending upon the age of the patient and the health of the concerned bone, after 5–10 days of waiting period of osteotomy, graduated distraction generally forms a soft callus (regenerate) at the site of distraction in about 3–4 weeks. If distraction is too fast, the regenerate may be thin (poor) and has hourglass appearance. If distraction is too slow, the regenerate shows a bulbous appearance and may undergo premature rapid consolidation defeating the purpose of the whole procedure. Ilizarov's principle of distraction histogenesis has also been used for distraction of the growth plate (chondrodiastasis), preferably in children close to the closure of the physis. Growth plate generally closes or gets sealed after this procedure.

Ilizarov's principle has also been used for correction of soft tissue contractures, like Volkmann's ischemic contracture in upper or lower limbs, and resistant clubfoot deformities. Another indication for this technique is for filling of segmental defects in bone (bone-transport). Probably bone loss of more than double the diameter of tibia or femur would need the help of bone transport techniques. The gap is gradually filled by creating a "floating segment" of bone by performing a corticotomy (or osteotomy) proximal or distal (or bifocal corticotomy) to the site of bone gap. Ilizarov's technique offers a reliable method to correct complex deformities, overcome shortening, and bridge bone gaps. However, the complications in the hands of a general orthopedist remain high, therefore, for the best results, Ilizarov's technique should remain in the domain of especially trained and committed surgeons with adequately resourced infrastructure.

BONE GRAFTS AND GRAFT SUBSTITUTES

Bone grafts are needed in clinical orthopedics mostly for treatment of nonunion of fractures, for filling large cystic lesions of bone and for reconstruction of large osteoperiosteal bone defects **(Table 1.2)**. The best bone graft is autogenous, because it provides: (i) osteogenesis by the osteoinduction property of the graft inducing the reparative mesenchymal cells (from the host) into osteoprogenitor cells, (ii) it provides an ideal

TABLE 1.2: Rough biological behavior of bone-grafts and substitutes.

	Osteogenicity	Osteo-induction	Osteo-conduction	Antigenicity	Speed of incorporation
Autogenous	+	++++	++++	0	++++
Allogenous	0	+++	+++	+	+++
Xenogenous	0	+	++	++	+
Graft substitutes	0	0	++	0	+

porous scaffold for penetration of vessels and cells, upon which the new bone can form, (iii) structural (mechanical) stability is provided minimally by cancellous, moderately by corticocancellous grafts and predominately by tubular bones, (iv) osteogenesis may also be brought about by a few surviving surface cells of autogenous grafts. Bone cells have a potential of survival up to 12–24 hours of anoxia. Neoangiogenesis or vascularization of the graft is the essence of success of any (bone) grafting procedure. The grafted bone is resorbed, replaced, remodeled (process of creeping substitution) to become the mature bone needed by the functional requirements of the body.

Donor area morbidity is recorded, however, any orthopedic surgeon with moderate training would learn to obtain adequate amount of cancellous bone from the thickest part of iliac crest without serious complications. After subperiosteal exposure of the iliac crest and outer surface of the "harvest area," one can remove adequate amount of cancellous bone as slivers. If one leaves the inner table intact and does a meticulous closure of muscles and skin, as a rule no complication is encountered. The most disturbing complication observed by us has been a sliding hernia through a major defect in the full thickness of iliac bone, this is, however, avoidable. The iliac bone provides a rich source of cancellous bone. Tricortical bone harvested from the thickest part of iliac crest constituted by the upper border, medial and lateral cortices of the bone can provide about 6 cm × 1.5 cm × 1.5 cm segment of bone for use as a structural graft. Cancellous autogenous bone grafts are best suited for nonunions, and for filling of "Cavitary lesions". For structural integrity, tricortical bone from iliac crest or a segment from distal half of fibula, or ribs when one is operating on spine would serve the purpose. One may sometimes need to use both the structural grafts combined with cancellous bone. The limitation of autogenous bone grafts is the availability of sufficient quantity required especially in children. Cortical bones provide mechanical stability, however these are very slow regarding incorporation. Part of fibular grafts may still be radiologically visible 7–10 years after operation (implantation). Cancellous bone grafts provide poor mechanical stability however, these get completely incorporated within 2–5 years after implantation.

Allografts: Earlier than 1965, fresh allografts generally donated by 'mother' of a child were used when no other material was available. Such grafts have no surviving cells, however, these cells have illicit antigenicity and induce an inflammatory response, which may lead to failure of the grafts. Slow penetration of neocapillaries in the transplanted fresh allogenic bone did not create a sudden surge of antigen-antibody reactions. Thus, the immune reaction was mild. However, since mid-sixties clinical use of untreated allografts is not permitted.

When adequate amount of autogenous bone graft is not available to fill or bridge large defects, one has to depend upon allogenic bone. Currently the allografts are harvested under sterile conditions, the donor is cleared for malignancy, infection, and viruses (including HIV). The harvested bones are stored or preserved by deep freezing (at –70°C), freeze-drying or ionizing radiation. Osteoinductive potential of such grafts is, however, markedly reduced.

Demineralization (according to the principles of Urist, 1965) is another way of reducing antigenicity, and increasing the porosity for better osteoconduction. Decalcified bone matrix retains sufficient osteoinductive agents (BMPs, growth factors) inducing the host mesenchymal cells to osteoprogenitor cells. The author has used such allogenic grafts between 1972 and 2020 for cavitory lesions, spinal fusions (in children) and for structural defects with impressive success comparable with the grafts from more sophisticated banking facilities **(Figs. 1.9A and B)**. Preparation and maintenance of decalbone banks is simpler, less expensive and can be practised in

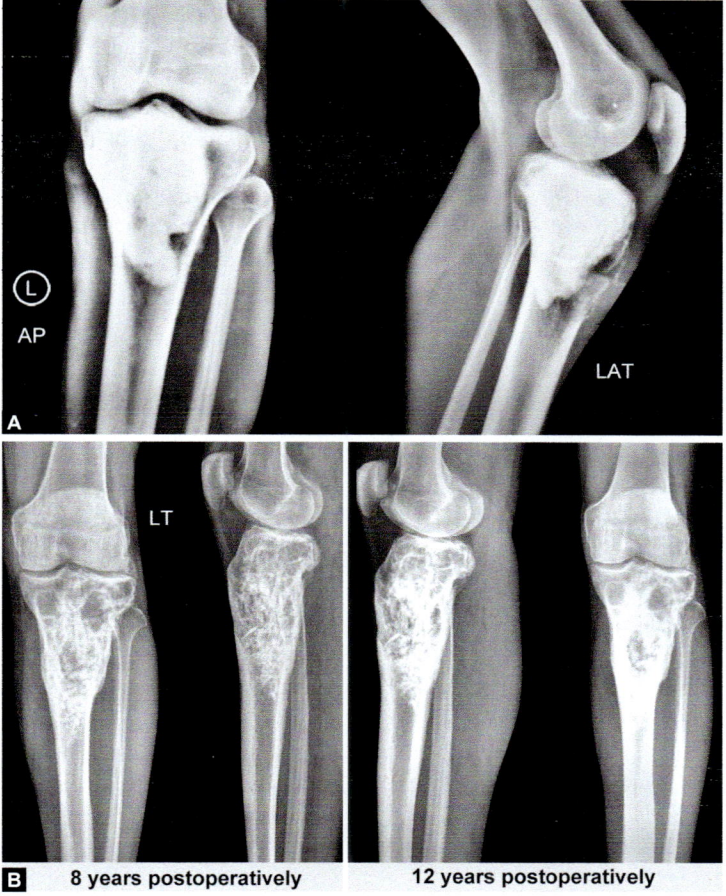

Figs. 1.9A and B: After curettage of giant-cell-tumor of proximal tibia, the cavity was filled with (A) cementation. The tumor recurred within 18 months after the operation; The cement was removed, intralesional curettage of the tumor was performed and the cavity was compactly filled with allogenic bone graft. The biological activity of the host bone and the graft helped heal the osseous cavity (B).

hospitals with moderate facilities **(Figs. 1.10A and B)**. Allografts are ideal for conditions like polyostotic fibrous dysplasia, generalized enchondromatosis, neurofibromatosis with pseudarthrosis and osteogenesis imperfecta. In such cases, the autogenous bone per se is inherently defective.

Allografts or bone graft substitutes can also be used as autogenous bone grafts expander. The process of incorporation of allografts is similar to that of autogenous grafts but slower. Deficient bone stock is a major challenge in any limb salvage procedure or revision of joint replacements

Bone Graft Substitutes (Synthetics)

Synthetically produced graft substitutes are prepared from calcium phosphate, hydroxyapatite and calcium carbonate in various combinations. These graft substitutes, biomimetic or porous scaffolds, act as osteoconductive agents for osteoprogenitor cells (accompanying neocapillaries) to penetrate in their pores and lay down bone. Mechanical strength and rate of resorpotion (1–2 years) vary with different combinations.

Bone cement: Cementation may be used for filling-up benign cavities in bone if bone grafts or substitutes are not available. Cementation leads to exothermal reaction on the recipient wall. Probably the reaction eliminates the reparative potential from the host-bed **(Figs. 1.9A and B)**. Once infected the infection persists.

Metal implants at best provide stability to damaged bones. If the underlying damaged bone does not stabilize in the "critical" time the implant would break due to the accumulation of "metal-fatigue" **(Figs. 1.11A and B)**. Stainless steel implants probably provide us the longest duration before these undergo fatigue and fracture. Sometimes, metal implants may lead to osteolysis.

Bone Morphogenetic Proteins (BMPs)

These bone inducing agents were earlier extracted from allogenic bones. The process was too complicated and the yield was too small (probably one mg from one kg of bone). At present, BMP-2 and BMP-7 are commercially prepared by recombinant techniques, these are available for clinical use, however, the cost is prohibitive (e.g., $ 400 for a single level disc fusion) for widespread use.

Fibula as a Bone Graft

Fibula is another source of autogenous bone graft especially for structural integrity. It provides an excellent mechanical stability, but has scanty cellular contents. The compact structure of fibula makes permeation by repairing mesenchymal cells and neocapillaries a slower process, delaying complete incorporation. The deepest part

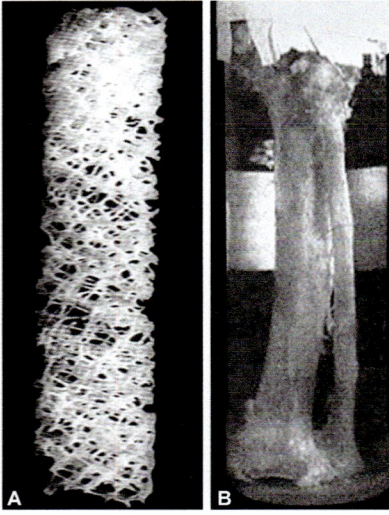

Figs. 1.10A and B: (A) Synthetic bone graft substitute; (B) Decal-bone preserved in ethanol (prepared according to Urist's technique).

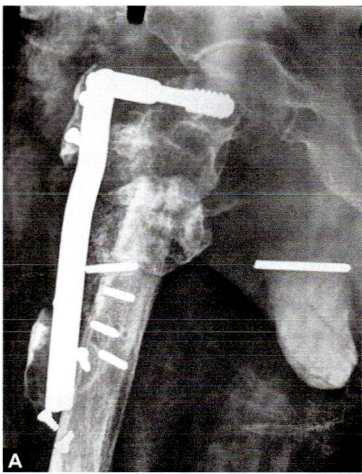
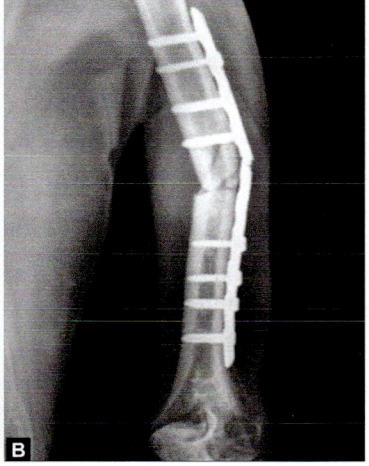

Figs. 1.11A and B: Any metal-implant would fail due to accumulation of metal fatigue unless the underlying bone gets stabilized before implant failure (within critical time): (A) In the femur; (B) In the humerus. Stainless steel probably provides us the longest duration before it's fatigue and fracture.

of fibular grafts may not get completely incorporated even after many years.

One can safely harvest about 15–20 cm of fibula. The distal cut should be at least one cm proximal to the inferior tibio-fibular joint. If one is impelled to obtain the upper end of fibula (as for reconstruction of distal end of radius), one must ensure the safety of the common peroneal nerve winding around the neck of fibula.

Transfer of Vascularized Bone Graft (Taylor, 1975)

The commonest free vascularized bone graft used in clinical practice has been the fibula. This procedure, however, requires microvascular expertise and sound orthopedic principle with two operating teams working simultaneously at the donor-site and the recipient area. Besides the highly specialized expertise, the other limiting factors are scarring at the recipient area due to infection, soft tissue damage or radiation necrosis. This option may be considered only when simpler techniques have failed or judged to fail. Nearly 50% of such grafts have been observed to incorporate like a nonvascularized graft.

Muscle Pedicle-based Bone Grafts (Huntington, 1905)

Muscle pedicle-based bone grafts can be performed by most of the orthopedic surgeons, however, the limitation in this procedure is that the "pedicled bone" has a limited radius of excursion. The most popular (and successful) graft has been the transfer of muscle pedicled vascularized fibula to repair or replace large defects in the ipsilateral tibia. The author has used this technique (tibialization of fibula) successfully for repair of large tibial defects due to traumatic extrusion, extensive sequestration, oncological resection and congenital defects **(Figs. 1.12A to C)**.

Many other muscle pedicled bone grafts have been innovated by orthopedic surgeons, a few examples are sartorius and tensor fascia lata based bone from anterior part of iliac crest, for neglected or nonunion of femoral

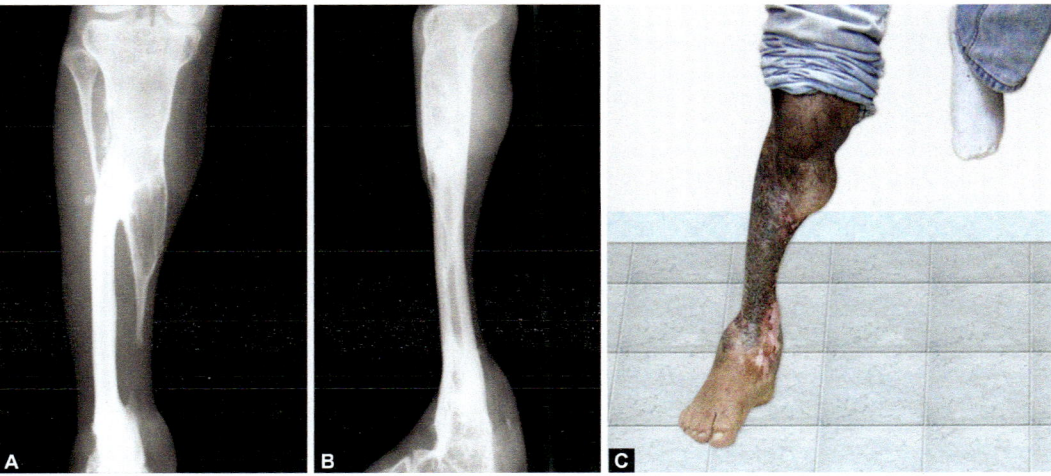

Figs. 1.12A to C: Ipsilateral fibula is one of the most vital grafts available to reconstruct any large defect in the tibia. Distal half of tibia was lost after an open injury of this leg (A and B). Ipsilateral fibula was "tibialized" to bridge the gap with fusion of the ankle joint (C). Note hypertrophy and remodeling of the fibular graft, according to the Wolff's law; the proximal non-weight-bearing fibula has not hypertrophied

neck fractures, and for avascular necrosis of femoral head in young patients. This would delay the need for total joint replacement by 10–15 years. Lumbosacral paravertebral muscle based bone from posterior part of iliac crest, for posterior or posterolateral fusion of lumbar or lumbosacral spine, and quadratus femoris based bone graft from ischeal tuberosity are other examples. Pedicled bone grafts provide the benefit of osteogenesis as of living bone, irrespective of the length of bone defect and condition of the recipient bed. These grafts are tolerant to moderate infection and are capable of hypertrophy according to the Wolff's law. For success, adherence to sound orthopedic principles for repair and regeneration of bone is mandatory.

SUGGESTED READINGS

1. Huntington TW. Case of bone transference. Ann Surg. 1944;26:455.
2. Urist MR. Bone formation by autoinduction. Science. 1965;150:893-99.
3. Companacci M, Zaanoli S. Double tibio fibular synostosis (fibula pro tibia) for non-union and delayed union of the tibia: End results review of one hundred seventy-one cases. J Bone Joint Surg. 1966;48A:44-56.
4. Tuli SM. Traumatic extrusion of the diaphyses of the radius and ulna successfully treated by replacement. J Bone Joint Surg. 1967;49(A):745-9.
5. Gupta DK, Tuli SM. Osteoinductivity of partially decalcified alloimplants in healing of large osteoperiosteal defects. Acta Orthop Scand. 1982;53:857-65.
6. Tuli SM, Srivastava TP, Sharma SV, Goel SC, Gupta D, Khanna S. The bridging of large osteoperiosteal gaps using 'Decalbone'. Int Orthop. 1988;12(2): 119-24.
7. Ilizarov GA. The tension-stress effect on the genesis and growth of tissues. Part II. The influence of the rate and frequency of distraction. Clin Orthop Relat Res. 1989;239:263-85.
8. Ilizarov GA. Clinical application of the tension-stress effect for limb lengthening. Clin Orthop. 1990;250:8-26.
9. Paley D, Chaudhry M, Pirone AM, Lentz P, Kautz D. Treatment of malunions and mal-nonunions of the femur and tibia by detailed preoperative planning and the Ilizarov techniques. Orthop Clin North Am. 1990;21:667-91.
10. Tiedeman JJ. Healing of a large nonossifying fibroma after grafting with bone matrix and marrow. Clin Orthop Rel Res. 1991;265:302-5.
11. Perren SM. Evolution of the internal fixation of long bone fractures. The scientific basis of biological internal fixation: choosing a new balance between stability and biology. J Bone Joint Surg. 2002;84B: 1093-110.
12. Tuli SM. Tibialization of the fibula: A viable option to salvage limbs with extensive scarring and gap nonunions of the tibia. Clin Orthop Relat Res. 2005;431:80-4.
13. Sarmiento A, Latta L. The evolution of functional bracing of fractures. J Bone Joint Surg. 2006;88B: 141-8.
14. De Long WG, Einhorn TA, Koval K, McKee M, Smith W, Sanders R, et al. Bone grafts and bone graft substitutes in trauma surgery. A critical analysis. J Bone Joint Surg. 2007;89A:649-58.
15. Kelly MP, Savage JW, Bentzen SM, Hsu WK, Ellison SA, Anderson PA. Cancer Risk from Bone Morphogenetic Protein Exposure in Spinal Arthrodesis. J Bone Joint Surg. 2014; 96A:1417-22.
16. Yadav SS. The use of a free fibular strut as a "Biological Intramedullary Nail" for treatment of complex nonunion of long bones. J Bone Joint Surg Open Access. 2018:e0050.
17. Rex C. K-wiring: Principles and Techniques. Thieme Medical and Scientific Publishers Pvt Ltd. 2022.

CHAPTER 2

Infections of Bones and Joints

INTRODUCTION

Infection of any bone caused by infective organisms is addressed as osteomyelitis. Commonly the infective organisms may be *Staphylococcus*, *Streptococcus*, typhoid and para-typhoid bacilli, pneumococci and *Haemophilus influenzae*. Granulomatous infections are a result of infection by *Mycobacterium tuberculosis* or syphilitic osteomyetitis. Mycetoma (fungal) infections may produce 'actinomycosis' or 'maduramycosis'. Rarely parasitic infestation may cause hydatid disease of bone or spine. Clinically the patient may present as acute osteomyelitis, subacute osteomyelitis, chronic osteomyelitis and an acute exacerbation of a pre-existing chronic osteomyelitis. Due to many factors there is a looming pandemic of "superbugs" of pyogenic, mycobacterial and viral organisms. We need affordable and widely available drugs for clinical use. The maximum threat for infection by superbugs is to immune compromised populations, critically ill patients, postoperative conditions, and geriatric population.

ACUTE HEMATOGENOUS OSTEOMYELITIS

This is a disease of childhood and adolescence generally occurring in under nourished children with poor defensive immune system. The commonest source of infection is due to hematogenous spread from a distant infected site such as ear, nose, mouth, respiratory tract, the bowel or genitourinary tract. The infecting organisms are carried to all parts of the skeleton, however, the bacteria get localized in the highly vascular and fast growing metaphyseal region of bones. A mild trauma near the bone ends may create a hematoma in the metaphyseal area which would act as a nidus for bacterial localization and infection. In the operating rooms and hospital environments, the most common source of infection is by nosocomial transmission. The commonest cause of osteomyelitis in the affluent societies is an open fracture or operative reduction with internal fixation of fractures.

Pathology

The pathological picture varies considerably depending upon the virulence of the organisms and host immunity. The initial focus of infection is usually the metaphyseal region of bone. The rich vascular pattern of this region favors the localization of infection. The initial focus of infection, if not treated, spreads outwards, penetrates the cortex and forms a subperiosteal abscess, which may burst to present as a subcutaneous abscess or pus discharging through sinuses. The pus can also spread subperiosteally or through medullary canal toward the diaphyseal area. In very young children, the infection may penetrate the physis, infect the epiphysis and spread to the joints. The joints get readily infected even if a part of metaphyseal area is intracapsular as in hip, elbow, and shoulder joints.

Exuberant periosteal reaction is seen between 2 to 7 years of age because the periosteum is very tough. Stripping of the periosteum, thrombosis of the vessels and increased intraosseous tension may result in ischemia of cortex of bone. Nonviable cortex becomes a "cortical sequestrum". When the infection is fulminant, varying extent of diaphysis may become necrosed and form a "diaphyseal sequestrum" and result in a pathological fracture.

The healing response of bone to infection (or any injury) is new bone formation under the raised periosteum. The new bone formed around an area of infected cavity would lead to the thickening of cortex; the new bone that forms around a sequestrum is called the involucrum. The involucrum generally has holes in it for discharge of pus and small sequestra, the holes or gaps are called 'cloacae'. Sequestrum is defined as a dead piece of bone surrounded by infected granulations and/or pus. The sequestrum gets separated from the parent bone by granulation tissue. Its surface is smooth, however, the margins and areas in contact with granulation tissue may have serrated edges and rough surfaces. In fulminating infections, sometimes, the periosteum may undergo necrosis, the involucrum is incomplete or deficient in such areas. Pus will continue to discharge through sinuses or ulcers, till spontaneous extrusion of sequestra or its surgical removal. In young children, once the infection is controlled, the 'sterile' sequestrum may undergo resorption and incorporation not unlike a bone graft (Fig. 2.1A to C).

Clinical Presentation

The patient is usually a child or an adolescent presenting with history of fever, pain, toxemia, swelling and difficulty in the function of limb. Any bone can be involved, however, the commoner areas presenting with infection are upper end of tibia and lower end of femur. Examination would reveal a swollen, warm and tender area. The adjacent joints may also show swelling, which may be a 'sympathetic' effusion due to synovial irritation or actual involvement by infection. All the signs and symptoms may be subdued if the patient had already received antibiotics prior to your examination. Septic arthritis, rheumatic arthritis, bleeding disorder, and cellulitis are commoner conditions in differential diagnosis.

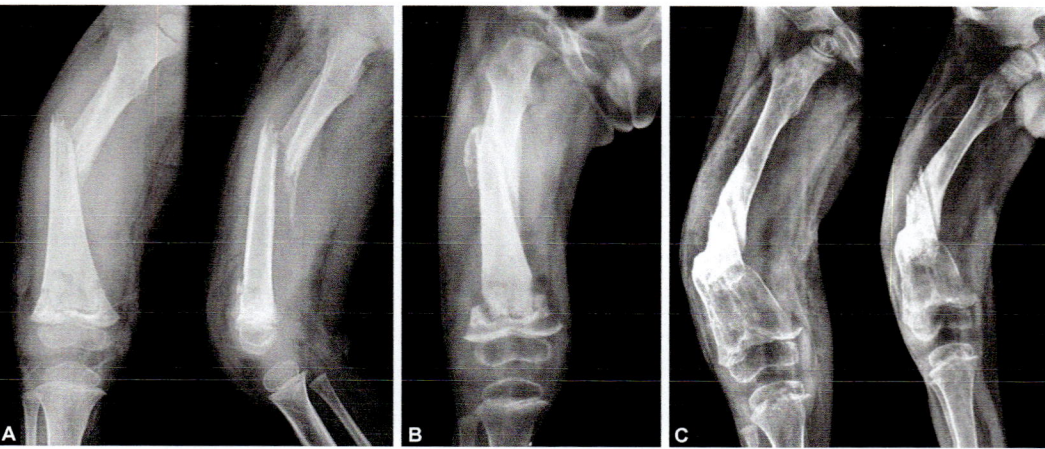

Figs. 2.1A to C: A neglected case of acute osteomyelitis of femur in a child. Distal half of femur has sequestrated, there is a pathological fracture in the distal metaphyseal region and in the middle of femur. The involucrum formation was incomplete, probably the periosteum was necrosed due to fulminating infection. Proximal part of uncovered sequestrum was exised, the distal part got incorporated (C). The follow-up revealed an excellent remodeling.

Radiological Features

X-rays may not show any changes in the bone for 10-14 days except a soft tissue swelling. After about 2 weeks, X-rays may show patchy areas of destruction in the bone, elevation of periosteum with subperiosteal new bone formation **(Figs. 2.2A and B)**. In later stages, a cortical sequestrum or a diaphyseal sequestrum may be seen. In chronic stage, bone becomes more thick, there is more obvious patchy rarefaction (cavitations) with different shapes and sizes of sequestra. The living bone (metabolically active) will show osteoporosis in early stages because of reactive hyperemia which will ultimately show thickening due to formation and deposition of subperiosteal new bone. The dead bone (metabolically inactive) or sequestrum does not show any reaction except at the edges being separated from the living bone by granulation tissues. There is a natural biologic tendency to "wall off" foreign material or a sequestrum by encapsulating layers of inflammatory fibrous tissue.

While examining X-rays in early stages of acute infection, soft tissue signs should not be forgotten. Edema of muscles is seen as soft tissue swelling, the fat planes in between the muscles get obliterated. Ultrasonography is a good investigation to show soft tissue changes. MRIs may help distinction between living and dead bone, and show the extent of soft tissue involvement.

Treatment

Without any delay, rest the limb with a suitable splint in the best functional position. The splint must permit periodic inspection of the infected area. Ideally before starting parenteral antibiotics, aspirate pus or tissue fluids from the depth of suspected area, and obtain a blood sample. Send the material for microbiological examination. Start with "best guess" antibiotics by intravenous route. Blood cultures are usually positive in 40-50%, and aspirate from the infected area positive in 50-60%.

Unfortunately, a large number of infective organisms are resistant to first line antibiotics like penicillin and many other commonly used antibiotics. As a rule, more than one antibiotic should be started, ideally by intravenous route as soon as the samples have been obtained for microbiological investigations and major bleeding disorders excluded. Parenteral antibiotics therapy for 2-4 weeks should be followed by oral antibiotics for another 4-6 weeks.

Patients with acute osteomyelitis or acute septic arthritis must be hospitalized and kept under close observation while on intravenous antibiotics. If rapid subsidence of local and

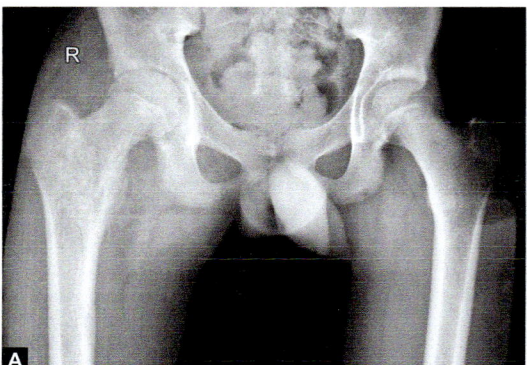 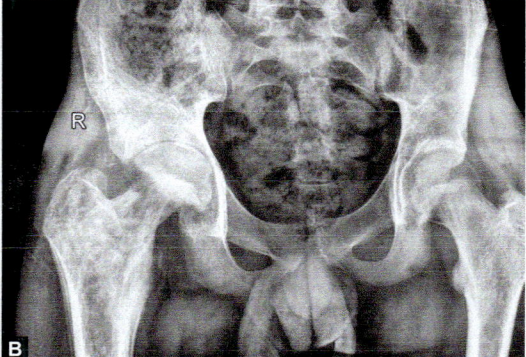

Figs. 2.2A and B: (A) Early radiological features of osteomyelitis of right femur. The comparison with contralateral femur shows irregular patchy areas of osteoporosis, faint periosteal reaction and soft tissue swelling. The limb at this stage must be splinted to prevent a pathological fracture; (B) About 1 month after the onset, more changes are visible with subperiosteal new bone formation.

systemic signs of infection and inflammation does not occur, operative intervention is needed.

Operative Intervention for Acute Osteomyelitis

Make a standard incision at the site of maximum involvement of bone, up to the periosteum, evacuate all abscess and infected soft tissues. There is generally a debate regarding making multiple drill holes at the site of osteomyelitis. If no pus wells out, making drill holes is mandatory. It is wise to make holes in the longitudinal axis of bone. There are more chances of a pathological fracture if the holes are made right angle to the long-axis. Having exposed the infected area, obtain a few pieces of bone, infected soft tissues for histological examination. Infected granulation tissues and pus must be sent for microbiological investigations. Close the wound loosely over a drain. Ideally, two drains should be put in, one in the medullary canal and one in the soft tissues around the bones. Avoid negative suction on the intramedullary drain lest it may suck out too much of blood from the medullary vessels. If lymph nodes are available, send those also for histological studies. Splint the limb for about 6–8 weeks, you may permit nonweight-bearing ambulation (for lower limb infections) after 4–6 weeks of operation and initiation of antibiotic therapy. There is a real danger of a pathological fracture of the bone having acute osteomyelitis, because initial X-rays up to 2–4 weeks may practically "look normal".

FUNCTIONAL POSITION OF JOINTS

When a joint requires to be given rest for acute inflammation or a chronic condition, a plaster splint or an orthotic appliance should hold the joint in the best functional position as outlined below.

Hip: About 10–30 degrees of flexion almost related to age, neutral between adduction and abduction and 5 degrees of external rotation.

Knee: About 5–10 degrees of flexion to help foot to clear the ground while walking, and 5 degrees external rotation. Some flexion at knee joint helps sitting on chair.

Ankle: At right angle (plantigrade) and in 5 degrees external rotation.

Wrist: about 10 degrees of dorsiflexion to allow a firm grip.

Elbow: About 90 degrees of flexion and in mid-pronation.

Shoulder: "Saluting position"—about 60 degrees abduction, 40 degrees flexion and 40 degrees internal rotation.

SEPTIC ARTHRITIS (FIG. 2.3)

Septic arthritis is most common in children with 1–5 years of age. Typically the patient presents with pain, fever and inability to bear weight (lower extremity joints) or inability to use the limb (pseudoparalysis). In young children, the distinction between transient synovitis of hip and septic arthritis of hip can be difficult, however, four easily obtainable predictors like fever, inability to bear weight, erythrocyte sedimentation rate (ESR) 40 mm or greater, and serum white blood cell count (WBC) $12,000/mm^3$ or greater can be used to establish the possibility of septic arthritis.

In neonates, it is difficult to clinically distinguish between septic arthritis of hip and septic arthritis associated with osteomyelitis of upper end of femur (upper end of femur is intracapsular). Similar difficulty would arise in other joints like shoulder and elbow. Antibiotic policy is same as for acute osteomyelitis.

Surgical Management

Arthrotomy of the infected hip and shoulder is mandatory for adequate decompression. Superficial joints like knee, ankle and elbow can be repeatedly aspirated with instillation of antibiotics, if desired. Aspiration should be done using 16G or 18G needles. The aspirate may be serosanguinous (earliest), cloudy or turbid, or frankly purulent (later).

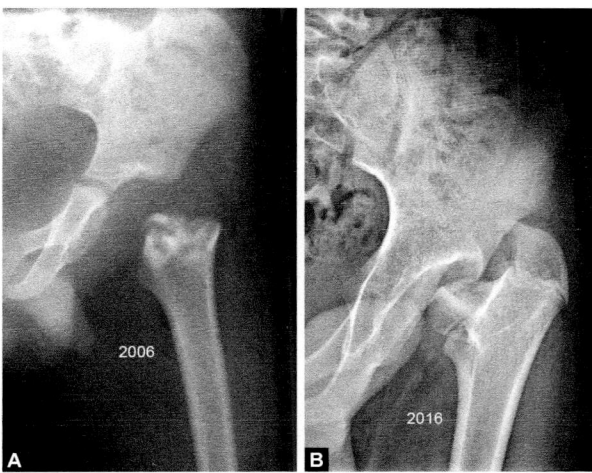

Figs. 2.3A to B: Functional treatment for articular infections can heal the disease with retention of functional range of motion. X-rays at presentation (A), regeniration on healing of disease (B) and follow-up.

If aspiration and instillation with antibiotics does not control the infection an arthrotomy is mandatory.

Arthrotomy should be done as early as possible, open the joint through a standard incision in the capsule, collect the infected material from the joint for microbiological and histological investigations. Irrigate joint with normal saline. Only close the skin after inserting a suction drain in the depth of wound. Either apply a traction for postoperation observation and management, or apply a plaster cast in the best functional position. The suction drain is removed after 2–4 days. If hip is dislocated, it is reduced and immobilized in hip spica, one may use 1 or 2 stout Kirschner's wire(s) to hold it in good position. Same principle is applicable for acute septic arthritis of any joint in children.

CHRONIC OSTEOMYELITIS

If treated well in time and adequately, the acute infection of bone would heal; swelling, pain, tenderness and toxemia would resolve or disappear and laboratory investigations would be normal. The infected bone may, however, show thickening in the X-rays for a long time. Depending upon the age of patient, the thickened area with growth would move away from the metaphyseal area and undergo gradual remodeling to near normal shape. To avoid reactivation of infection, one must maintain good nutritional status.

Some of the patients of acute osteomyelitis develop chronic osteomyelitis. The main factors are poor nutritional status, delayed or inadequate drainage of pus or infected cavities, ineffective or inadequate use of antibiotics, presence of sequestra, or foreign bodies (metallic or nonmetallic) in cases of infection following open injuries or operations. In addition to pyogenic infection, chronic osteomyelitis may also be caused by tuberculosis, fungal or syphilitic microbes.

The patient presents with one or more sinuses over the involved bone. There may be multiple scars due to old infection or operative incisions. The sinuses or scars may be adherent to the underlying bone, pouting/protruding granulation tissue may be seen through the sinuses. The involved bone is thick and tender, there would be a history of periodic acute "flare-ups" of pain, swelling and fever. The "flare-up" is generally associated with closure of sinuses, collection of pus in the tissues or a history of trauma. The flare-up symptoms would subside when the sinuses burst open, discharge pus and/

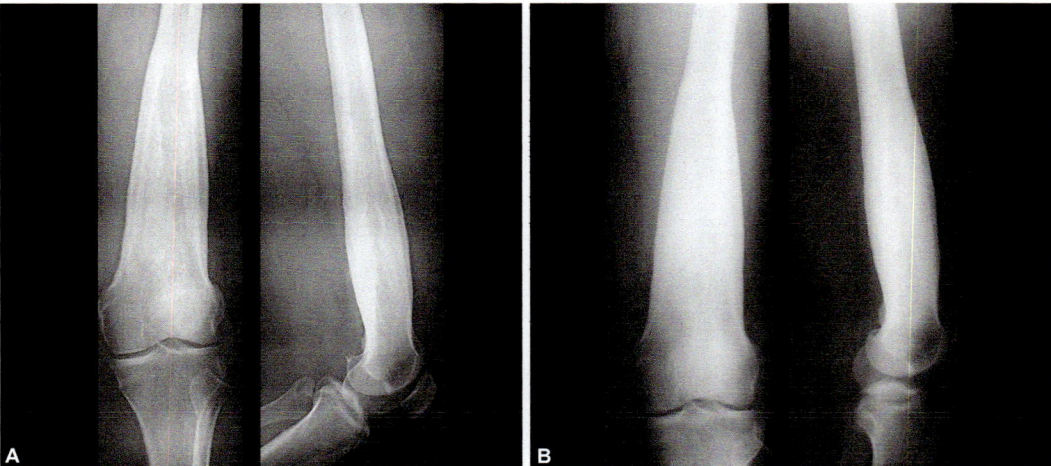

Figs. 2.4A and B: Healed status of chronic osteomyelitis of distal femur. (A) Note thickening of bone, small patchy cavitations within the bone and periosteal reaction; (B) X-rays of the same patient after a gap of 2 years, clinically there has been no evidence of active infection, however, the bone thickening persists.

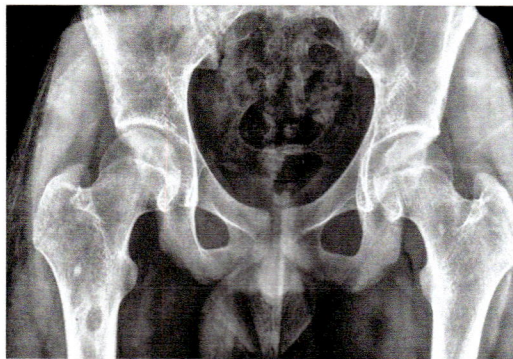

Fig. 2.5: A typical Brodie's abscess in right upper femur.

or small sequestra. X-rays would reveal the thickened bone with infected cavities, with or without sequestra, and involucrum **(Figs. 2.2 to 2.5)**. Involucrum formation suggests the presence of a viable periosteal sleeve around the sequestrum.

Sequestrum and Involucrum

Sequestrum is a dead piece of bone surrounded by infected granulations or frank pus. A bone may become necrosed or dead due to devascularization as a result of hematogenous osteomyelitis or due to extensive loss or stripping of soft tissues and periosteum because of trauma or rough iatrogenic handling.

A free bone graft, say harvested from iliac bone transplanted around nonunion of tibia, is practically a dead bone. Carefully performed (aseptic technique and gentle tissue handling) procedure would permit healthy granulations to surround the grafted bone ultimately leading to successful incorporation. If, however, there is infection and the free bone graft gets surrounded by infected granulations or frank pus, it is now a sequestrum.

Fate of Sequestrum

Sequestrum initiates a reaction in the surrounding bone and periosteum. Subperiosteal bone formation around the sequestrum forms an involucrum as a reparative process. In young children, sometimes, under the influence of effective antibiotics and supportive therapy the infected granulations surrounding a sequestrum become sterile, the healthy granulations would then invade the dead bone resulting in resorption of the sequestrum or reincorporation as a grafted bone. If sequestrum persists despite supportive therapy and antibiotics, the involucrum would grow around the sequestrum.

Behavior of Involucrum

Formation of involucrum is the activity of the surrounding healthy periosteum. If periosteum is necrosed, the involucrum will not form. If the exposed bone is dead and not covered by periosteum, again involucrum will not form. The activity of the formation of involucrum can be judged by X-rays of the limb at 4–6 weeks intervals. If its outer surface is rough, the size of involucrum is likely to increase. If the outer surface of involucrum has become smooth, further increase of its size in unlikely.

Sequestrectomy

It is wise to wait till the formation of sufficient involucrum. Sequestrum should be carefully removed without jeopardizing the stability of the infected bone. The window in the involucrum should not be >1/3 of the diameter of the bone. Overzealous removal of involucrum or premature operation may lead to an iatrogenic fracture of bone. In case of loss of integrity of the parent bone, the infected cavity should be filled up with copious fresh autogenous bone grafts and the limb should be protected in a suitable plaster cast. Mechanical protection may be achieved by inserting an intramedullary device without reaming, or the use of an external fixation. Success is achieved by adequate debridement, however removal of dead bone through the cortical "window" must be compatible with mechanical stability of the parent bone **(Figs. 2.6A to C)**.

Papineau's Procedure, Open Bone Grafting

If the cavity left behind after sequestrectomy is large or you are dealing with infected nonunion or symptomatic infected large cavities in bone, Papineau's principles are a rational option. Remove grossly infected tissues, leave behind bleeding recipient surfaces. Harvest adequate amount of autologous cancellous bone grafts, fill up the cavity with copious bone grafts, or in case of infected nonunion place the slivers of bone around the site of nonunion. Cover the operated area by loosely stitching the soft tissues over it. If one cannot achieve a satisfactory soft tissue cover, which may be the situation due to scarring of long standing in chronic osteomyelitis or infected nonunions, cover the cancellous bone grafts with sterile vaseline gauze. The dressing would require a change 2 to 3 times a week. Mechanical stability in cases of infected fractures may be provided by the use of an external fixation or by intramedullary elastic rods or plaster cast.

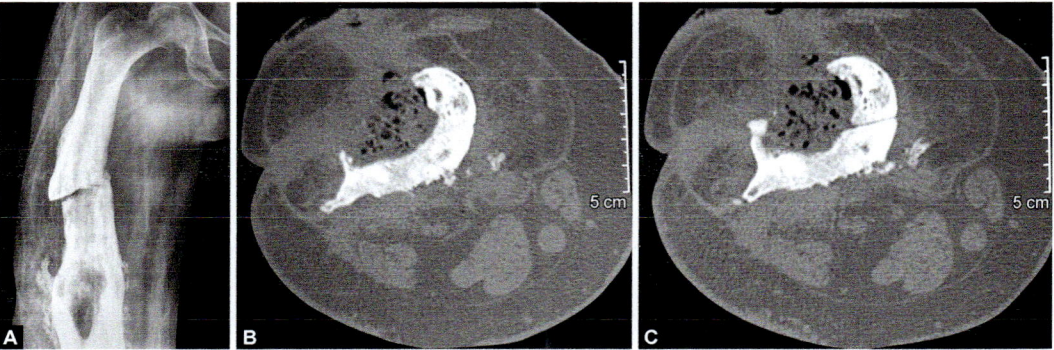

Figs. 2.6A to C: A window to perform sequestrectomy must be made carefully. Overzealous window has created an iatrogenic pathological fracture of femur through the infected bone, an extremely difficult problem to treat.

Papineau's technique can also be used for infected area through a window in plaster cast. While changing the vaseline gauze dressing, some superficial pieces of cancellous graft may become discolored (grayish) and fall off as loose pieces. Within 3–6 weeks, most of the graft gets covered with healthy granulations, which may epithelize on its own or may be covered by split skin graft. We have successfully used this technique for large infected cavities and infected nonunions with inadequacy of soft tissue covering.

Alternative methods: Alternative methods that are available entail plastic surgery procedures to replace the scarred tissue prior to bone grafting. This would increase the number of days in the hospital and the resultant financial burden.

Some workers have tried evacuation of the infected cavities followed by continuous antibiotic instillation and suction (ingress–egress) or use of antibiotic-impregnated cement beads with the aim of continuation of high concentration of local antibiotics. Simpler and cost-effective treatments, however, are preferred because many studies have shown adequate concentrations of antibiotics at the site of chronic osteomyelitis even when the patient was only on systemic parenteral or oral antibiotics.

'Curing' chronic osteomyelitis is an illusion; at best one can achieve a lasting healed status. Some cases of chronic osteomyelitis may show no activity of infection despite the persistence of radiological evidence of infection. Such cases may be called **"dry chronic osteomyelitis"**, other cases keep on showing occasional activity of infection (local pain, swelling, collection of pus and spontaneous discharge) and may be called **"wet chronic osteomyelitis"**. Poor nutritional status, diabetes, prolonged use of steroids and immunosuppressive drugs and local trauma increase the chances of recrudescence of infections. Persistance of sequestra (necrotic bone), infected intraosseous cavities, cicatrix (scarring) formation in skin and soft tissues, poor body resistance (immunity), and diabetic state are generally responsible for persistance of chronic osteomyelitis. An unhealing ulcer associated with chronic osteomyelitis may rarely undergo malignant change after 15–20 years. The author encountered five such patients during 50 years of orthopedic outpatient services, one related to infection in humerus, three associated with infection of tibia, and one related to chronic infection after cementation of a cystic lesion in proximal tibia.

IATROGENIC INFECTIONS IN ORTHOPEDICS

One of the most dreaded complications of operative procedures in orthopedics is operation-induced (iatrogenic) infection **(Figs. 2.7 and 2.8)**. The commonest organisms related to such infections are aerobic or anaerobic pyogenic bacteria, however, in countries where tuberculosis is almost endemic, tuberculous infection after implant surgery or operative intervention must also be considered. The author has observed tuberculous infection after joint replacements around knee, hip and shoulder joints. Tuberculous infection was also seen around the implants used for open-reduction and internal fixation in general, and after arthroscopic exploration of the joints. The ubiquitous mycobacteria are capable of implantation or impregnation at the site of operative trauma, especially in patients with immune compromise.

Any practicing orthopedic surgeon should be cognizant to this type of infection. Strict aseptic precautions are mandatory for any physician and healthcare workers. Proper handwashing is one of the most important means of controlling nosocomial transmission during any operative intervention or an invasive procedure. The most effective method of sterilization of operative instruments, is still considered to be high pressure autoclaving. The endoscopic equipments, are not autoclaved and most

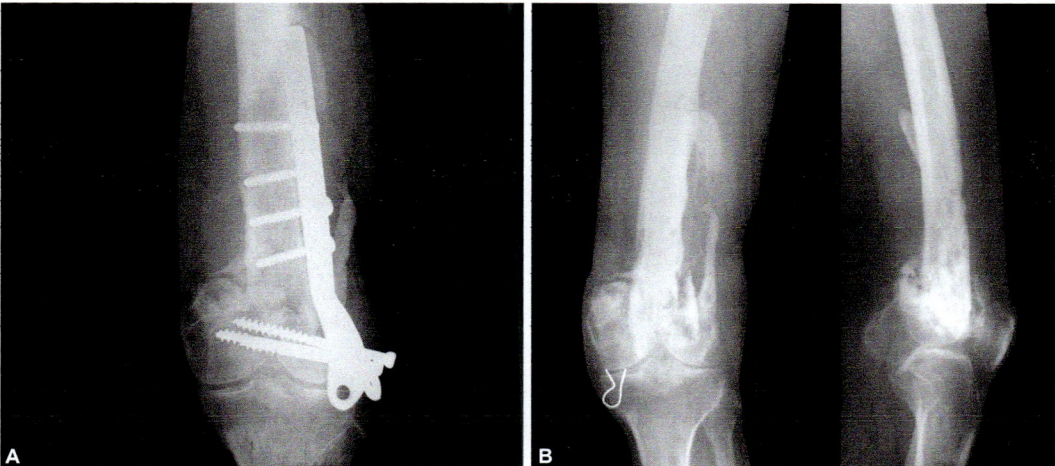

Figs. 2.7A and B: Osteomyelitis of the femur as a sequel of fixation of femoral fracture. Distal half of the femoral shaft is sequestrated. Attempt at formation of involucrum is incomplete probably because the periosteum had undergone necrosis.

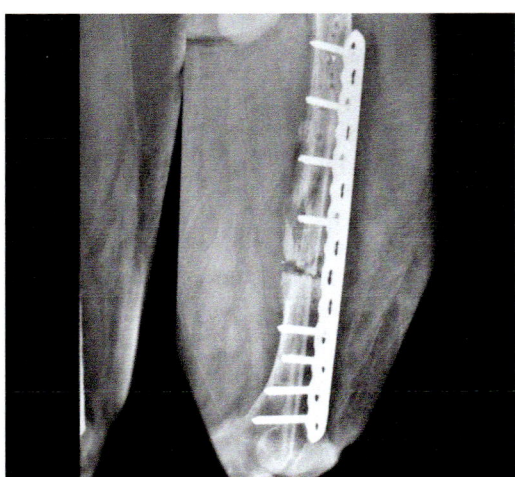

Fig. 2.8: An example of infected nonunion: Note a huge soft tissue swelling of whole of thigh, site of fracture fixed with a gap, an extra long plate probably resulted in extensive soft tissue stripping disturbing the osseous blood supply, a few sequestra are present around the site of nonunion.

of them are sterilized by Glutaraldehyde 2.45% formalin chamber, ethylene oxide vapors, or gas sterilization. It is wise to be reminded that postoperative discitis after open operation on the spine is 1%, whereas the incidence after endoscopic procedures is about 3%. Cannulated instruments have been implicated as potential source of contamination.

Diagnosis

A high suspicion index plays a crucial role in diagnosis at an early stage of infection. Clinical examination of the operated area must observe the degree of inflammation, the margins of operative incision; look for undermined edges of ulcers and sinuses, pouting granulations through sinuses and nature of discharge from the wounds. Every effort must be made to obtain material for microbiological investigations. Whenever debridement is done, the tissue must be sent for histological examination for pyogenic, tuberculous and fungal pathologies. Despite X-rays and modern imaging modalities, microbiological and histological investigations, the clinician may be confronted with final diagnosis as "chronic/subacute/acute inflammation/infection". Assessment by repeated clinical or interval assessment is supreme to help make therapeutic choices.

Patients at risk of iatrogenic infections are immunocompromised due to conditions like hemoglobinopathy, diabetes, liver disease, alcohol abuse, substance abuse, rheumatoid disorder, immune-suppressive and antimitotic drugs. Local tissue damage caused by operative intervention or injury provides a nidus for seeding for the microbacteria.

Therapeutic Options

Remove all stitches of the operative incision preferably up to the deepest layer. Do adequate debridement of infected area and ensure drainage or postural dependent drainage, possible active exercises of the limb would help pump out the collection from deeper parts.

Having sent the material for microbiological and histological (when possible) studies, start a combination of at least 2 drugs of 'best guess' of broad spectrum antibiotics by parenteral route for about 2 weeks. The antibiotics may then be modified according to the available microbiological (and histological) reports; and appropriate oral antibiotic therapy must be continued for 6–8 weeks. Supportive therapy and improvement of nutritional status is equally important.

If the infection is coming under control, the implant may not be removed, however, if the infection is not coming under control or it is a case of fulminating infection, it is wise to remove the implant, and splint or rest the joint or limb in the best functional position. If one is impelled to try a second implant replacement, it may be wise to use an inert "spacer" during the waiting period till the infection is controlled and the tissues are ready for the next surgery.

TUBERCULOSIS OF BONES AND JOINTS

General Clinical Picture

World-wise nearly one million lives are lost each year because of tuberculous infection.

Skeletal tuberculosis mostly occurs during first three decades of life; no age, however, is immune. With increasing longevity, the disease is being reported now in the elderly as well. The characteristics are insidious onset, monoarticular or mono-osseous involvement and the constitutional symptoms like low-grade fever and lassitude (especially in the afternoon), anorexia, loss of weight, "night cries", painful limitation of movements, muscle wasting, and regional lymph nodes enlargement. During active stage, the protective muscle spasm is severe holding the diseased area immobilized. During sleep, the muscle spasm relaxes and permits movement between the inflamed surfaces resulting in pain causing the typical night cries (especially in children). Commonly involved joints in descending order are vertebral column, hip, knee, ankle-foot, wrist-hand, elbow and shoulder.

Diagnosis

In resources constrained countries, in general, diagnosis of tuberculosis of bones and joints can be reliably made on clinical and radiological examination. However, in early stages and whenever in doubt a positive proof of the disease must be obtained employing semi-invasive or invasive investigations. In the affluent societies, corticosteroids, alcoholism, prolonged illness, diabetic state, immunosuppressive drugs, and old age are the probable predisposing factors. Skeletal tuberculosis must be included in differential diagnosis of chronic/subacute mono-articular arthritis, chronic abscess, draining sinus, chronic swelling or osteomyelitis; tuberculous infection is a great mimic even today **(Figs. 2.9 to 2.11)**.

Roentgenograms and Images

Anteroposterior and lateral views of the part, and an X-ray of the chest are required. Localized osteoporosis is the first radiological sign of active disease. The articular margins and bony cortices become hazy, (giving a "washed out" appearance), there may be development of areas of trabecular or bony destruction and osteolysis. The synovial fluid, thickened synovium, capsule and pericapsular tissues may cause a soft tissue

CHAPTER 2: Infections of Bones and Joints

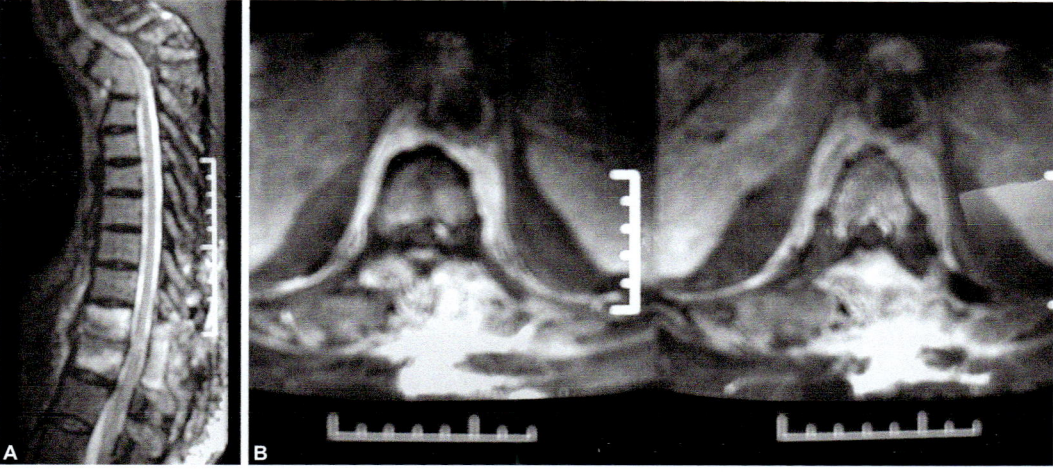

Figs. 2.9A and B: (A) In skeletal tuberculosis, one can at best achieve a lasting healed status. This case shows a healed tuberculosis at cervico-dorsal lesion in childhood. Patient now reported with a fresh active infection in lower dorsal spine after 2 years of the first lesion; (B) MRI-T2 shadows show bright signals (pus collection) in the vertebral bodies, perivertebral region and posterior elements of the lower dorsal spine.

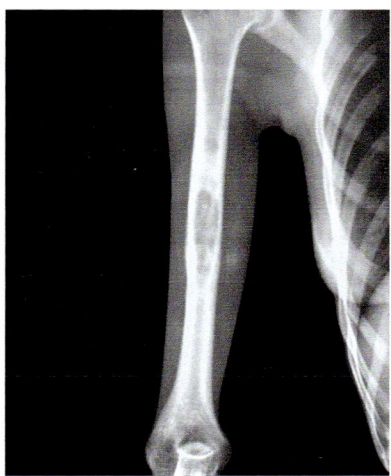

Fig. 2.10: Tuberculous infection is a great mimic. Multiple lytic lesions in the humerus in this lady are due to tuberculosis. The soft tissue swelling around the lesion was a cold abscess, patient had concomitant active tuberculous lesions in the lungs and vertebral column.

swelling. With the involvement of articular cartilage, the joint space (articular cartilage space) shows diminution in the X-rays. As the destructive process advances, there may be collapse of bone, subluxation/dislocation, migration and deformity of the joints. In a typical paradiscal spinal tuberculosis earliest radiological signs are diminution of the disc space with erosion of paradiscal margins of vertebrae. MRIs would show bright signal in T2 and dark singal in T1 images in the paradiscal region, during the active phase of infection.

MRIs now available almost in all countries, it is the most useful investigation for disorders of the skeletal system, it does not expose the patient to radiations.

Mnemonic may help remember MRI images:
- T2 water white: T1 water black (dark); T1 and T2 fat white; T1 and T2, ligaments capsule, desiccated disc or scars are black (dark) "Water" = inflammatory fluid.

Blood

A relative lymphocytosis, low hemoglobin, and raised ESR are often found in the active stage of disease. ESR, however, is not necessarily a proof of activity of the infection.

Biopsy

Whenever there is doubt (particularly in early stages), it is mandatory to prove the

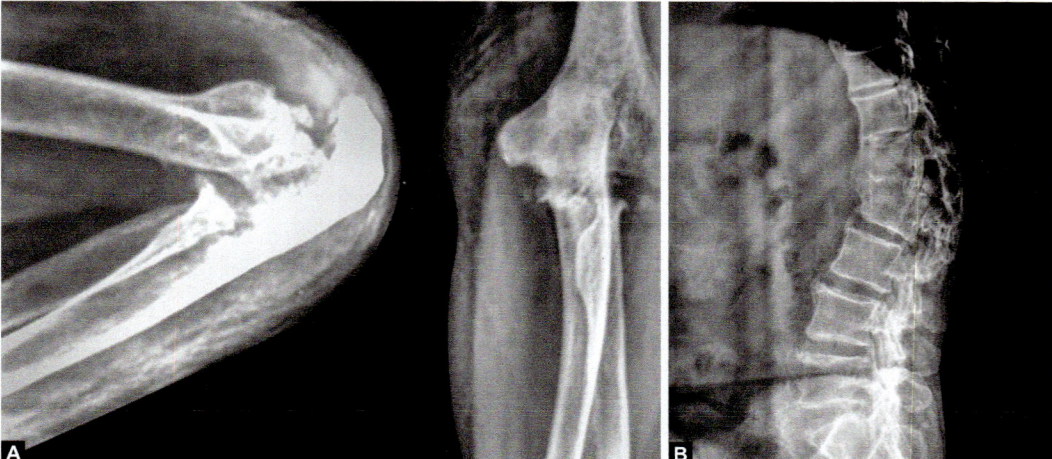

Figs. 2.11A and B: (A) X-rays of advanced tuberculous arthritis of elbow in a 66 years male. Patient was treated by antitubercular drugs, and range of motion exercises (functional treatment). On healing, he could retain flexion-extension arc from 5 to 140 degrees; (B) X-ray of spine of the same patient: He was treated for spinal tuberculosis 15 years ago. The disease remained healed for many years. Patient reported for recurrence of infection in the elbow after developing diabetes.

diagnoses by obtaining the diseased tissue (granulation and/or synovium and/or bone and/or lymph nodes). At the time of open biopsy of a joint or an osseous lesion, a wise orthopedic surgeon would perform synovectomy or curettage as a part of therapeutic measures. The diseased tissue obtained should be submitted for histology, microbiology and serological tests.

Modern Imaging Techniques

MRI would confirm whatever one can see in the plain X-rays and CT scans. However, it also shows the predestructive lesions like edema or inflammation of the bone in active disease, which is more extensive than the areas of radiological destruction in the bones. Once the radiological changes have been established, no great advantage is gained by radioisotope scanning or MRI. Earliest radiological changes are discernable in the standard X-rays 2 to 4 months after the onset of disease whereas MRIs would reveal the changes between 3 and 6 weeks, radioisotope scanning can demonstrate a metabolically active lesion around 5–7 days. Generalized screening of any person presenting with active osteo-articular tuberculosis would reveal another subclinical active lesion in about 40% of patients.

Antitubercular Chemotherapy

The mainstay of treatment is multidrug antitubercular chemotherapy. No local operation can eradicate the disease as most of the patients have many other foci of tuberculous infection. Even when the disease has clinically healed, many tubercle bacilli survive for many years in the lymph nodes and the healed affected tissues. There are several recommended regimens of chemotherapy. At present, we use the following **(Fig. 2.12)**:

Intensive phase—consists of isoniazid 300–400, rifampicin 450–600 mg and fluoro-quinolones 400–600 mg daily for 5–6 months. All replicating sensitive bacteria are likely to be killed by this bactericidal combination.

Continuation phase—is aimed to eliminate the slow-growing persisters, dormant or intracellular mycobacteria. This consists of isoniazid and pyrazinamide 1500 mg daily for 4–5 months followed by isoniazid and rifampicin for another 4–5 months.

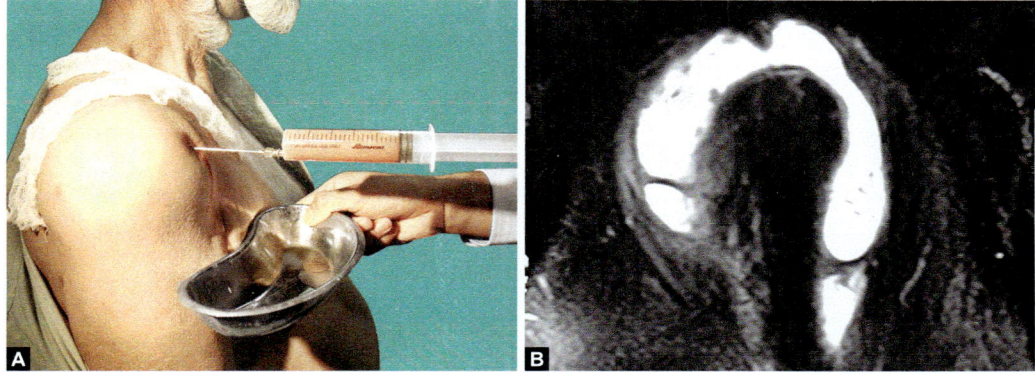

Figs. 2.12A and B: Aspirate from a cold abscess (TB) showing the pinkish color of rifampicin. Most of the anti-TB drugs reach the site of active disease in adequate concentrations. (A) Clinical picture, (B) MRI-T2 showing abscess in the shoulder joint.

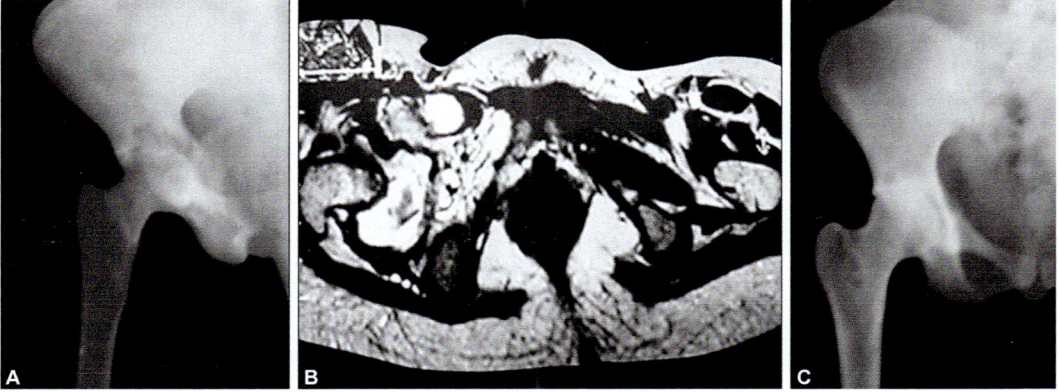

Figs. 2.13A to C: Tuberculosis of right hip joint. (A) Gross destruction of articular margins and diminished joint space; (B) MRI shows collection in the joint and suppurating inguinal lymph node; (C) Antitubercular drugs healed the infection, restored the joint margin and space, and clinical function.

Prophylactic phase—is aimed at protecting the patient who by this time would be back to his environments of work. It consists of isoniazid and ethambutol 1,200 mg/day for a further of 4–5 months.

Prognosis and Course

The use of modern antitubercular drugs has revolutionized the outcome of bone and joints tuberculosis. Death due to uncontrolled disease, meningitis, miliary tuberculosis, amyloidosis, paralysis and crippling seen frequently before the availability of antitubercular drugs is now rare. If a patient is diagnosed early and treated vigorously, healing can be accomplished without residual ankylosis of the joints **(Figs. 2.13 and 2.14)**.

Classification of Articular Tuberculosis

In untreated cases, tuberculous disease of joint passes through the following stages; I—synovitis, II—early arthritis, III—advanced arthritis, IV—advanced arthritis with subluxation/dislocation, V—aftermath of advanced arthritis **(Table 2.1)**.

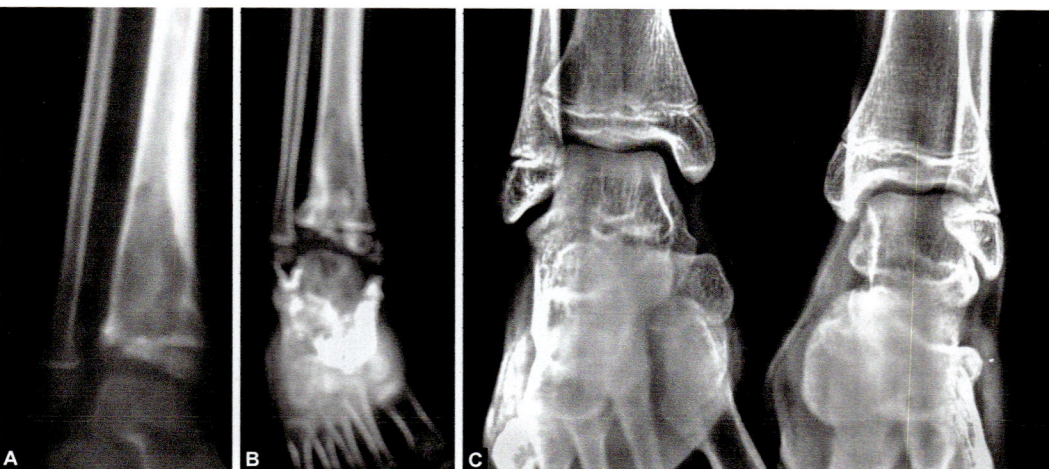

Figs. 2.14A to C: Tuberculosis osteomyelitis: Potential of recovery in children: (A) The cystic cavity in distal metaphyseal area of tibia histologically proved to be tuberculosis; (B) On antitubercular drugs there is healing of the cavitary lesion; (C) After 2 years of follow-up one can appreciate the repair that has occurred as compared to the uninvolved left leg.

TABLE 2.1: Staging of tuberculosis of the joints and its outcome in general.

Stage	Clinical	Radiology	Usual effective treatment	Expected outcome
Synovitis-I	Movements Present >75%	Soft tissue swelling, osteoporosis	Chemotherapy and movements, rarely synovectomy	Retention of near full mobility
Early arthritis-II	Movements present 50–75%	In addition to I, moderate diminution of joint space and marginal erosions	Chemotherapy and movements, rarely synovectomy or debridement	Restoration of 50–70% of mobility
Advanced arthritis-III	Loss of movements of >75% in all directions	In addition to II, marked diminution of joint space and destruction of joint surfaces	Chemotherapy and surgery, generally arthrodesis in lower limbs	Ankylosis*
Advanced arthritis with subluxation/dislocation-IV	Loss of movement of >75% in all direction	In addition to III, joint is disorganized with subluxation/dislocation	Chemotherapy and surgery, generally arthrodesis	Ankylosis*
Aftermath/terminal of gross arthritis-V	Gross deformity and ankylosis	In addition to IV, grossly deformed articular margins + degenerative osteoarthrosis	Chemotherapy and surgery: arthrodesis/corrective osteotomy	Ankylosis*

*After completion of growth of involved bones for elbow and hip, one may, if desired obtain a fairly mobile joint by excision-arthroplasty. Replacement arthroplasty for knee and hip after healed status is considered rational for improvement of function (under *antituberculosis* drugs umbrella).

PRINCIPLES OF MANAGEMENT

General (Fig. 2.15)

The general and systemic treatment is like that of tuberculosis in general, antitubercular multidrug therapy is the mainstay. Any concomitant disease must be treated to build the general body resistance. In active stage of disease, the joints are given rest in the position of function. In the presence

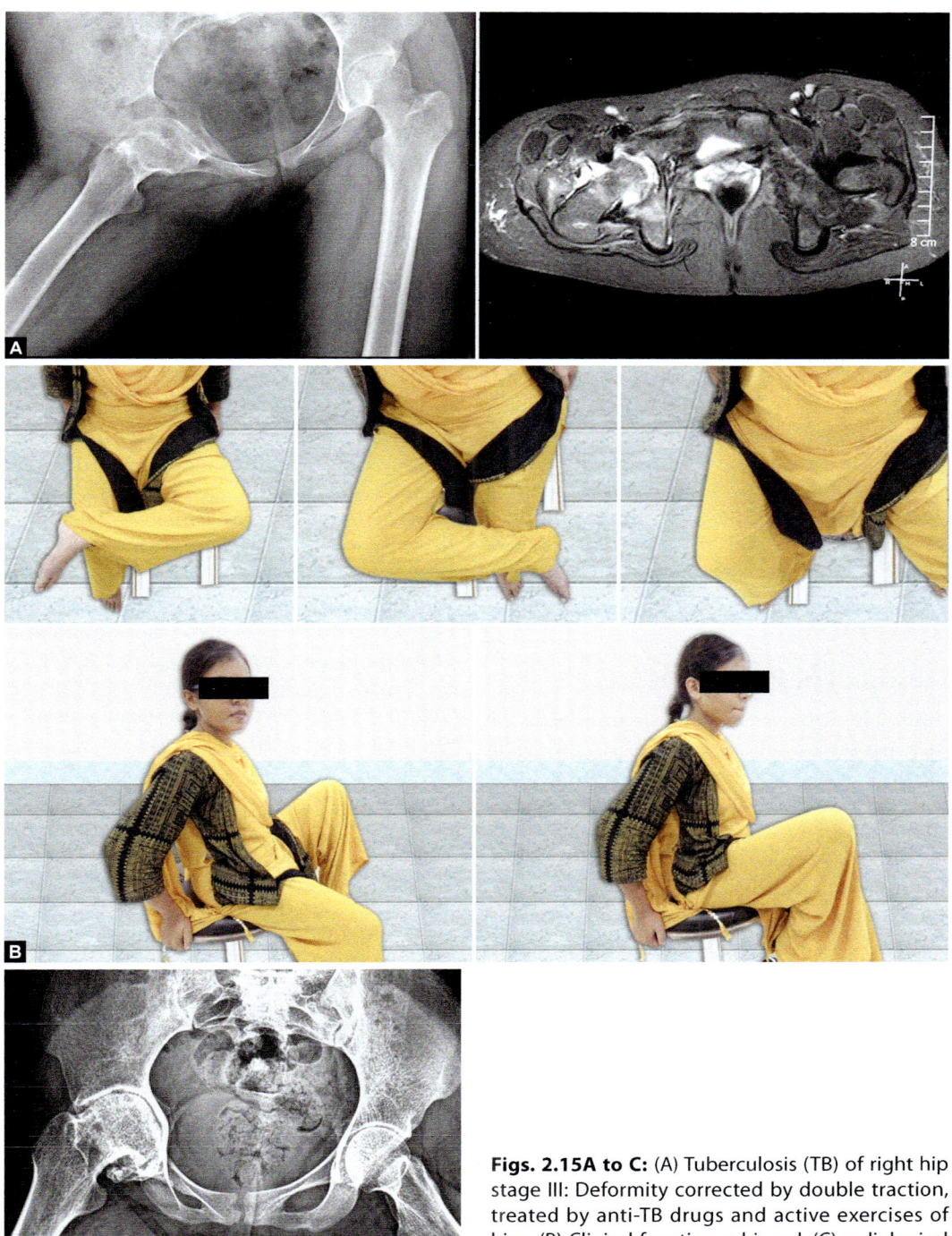

Figs. 2.15A to C: (A) Tuberculosis (TB) of right hip stage III: Deformity corrected by double traction, treated by anti-TB drugs and active exercises of hips. (B) Clinical function achieved, (C) radiological appearance 12 years after the treatment, joint space is present with irregular joint margins.

of gross destruction, continuation of the immobilization may lead to spontaneous sound ankylosis. Cases with early disease with subsidence of pain are put on one hourly intermittent guarded active and assisted exercises under cover of antitubercular drugs, with the aim of retaining a useful range of movements (functional treatment for joint tuberculosis). Traction is one of the best available methods to correct a deformity, maintain the limb in the functional position, offer unhindered observation regarding the local response to treatment, holding the inflamed joint surfaces apart, and permit repetitive active joint motion. This may permit return of reasonable function even in joints damaged by infection, and maintain a lasting healed status of the disease. Guarded weight bearing in the lower limbs is started 3-6 months after the subsidence of signs of activity. The braces/appliances are gradually discarded after its use for about 2 years **(Fig. 2.15)**.

Abscess, Effusion and Sinuses

Palpable abscesses and large joint effusion are aspirated and one gram of streptomycin alone or combined with isoniazid is instilled at each aspiration. Sinuses in a large majority of cases would heal within 6-12 weeks under the influence of systemic antitubercular drugs. A small number (<1%) may require longer treatment and excision of the tract with or without debridement. Sinus ramification is always greater than can be appreciated; complete surgical excision is indeed impracticable, and fortunately unnecessary.

Antitubercular Drugs

In the ever changing scene of more potent and less toxic antitubercular drugs, it may be unrealistic to stick to one particular drug regime; however, it is important to stress to maintain the multidrug therapy for a minimum of 18 months and in some cases for 24 months. In clinical practice, if the activity of tuberculous lesion does not come under control, the cause lies in factors such as acquired or genetic resistance of the infecting organisms to the drugs and the pathological nature of the skeletal lesion, e.g., gross destruction of bones and joints and presence of large sequestra.

After the availability of modern drugs, the incidence of relapse in our patients treated after 1972 seems to be 2% in those followed-up for >10 years. Nearly 50% cases with recurrence of the disease at the first site, or development of tuberculosis in any part of the skeletal system on close questioning revealed inadequate use of drugs. Other precipitating factors for recurrence were use of systemic cortisone therapy, immunosuppressive drugs, malnutrition, development of diabetes, alcoholics or immune deficient state.

The most challenging cause of poor therapeutic response may be multidrug resistance, MDR—microbes resistance to isoniazid and rifampicin, or the microbes may be resistant to INH + RCIN + Fluoroquinolones and one of the three injectables: Amikacin or Capreomycin or Kanamycin (X/MDR-TB). The world-wise resistance at present is about 5% **(Fig. 2.16)**.

Surgery in Tuberculosis of Bones and Joints

Surgery is at best an adjunct to the systemic antitubercular therapy. No surgical resection is a substitute for a prolonged course of drugs. A trial of conservative treatment is justified in most of the cases before surgery is contemplated. Nonoperative treatment is usually adequate in synovial tuberculosis (without articular involvement), low grade or early arthritis of any joint, and even advanced (stage III, IV) arthritis, especially in the upper extremity.

Extent and Type of Surgery

Fusion of a major joint is now rarely indicated as a primary mode of treatment. Reconstruction or reposition of joints, juxta-articular osteotomies, soft tissue release

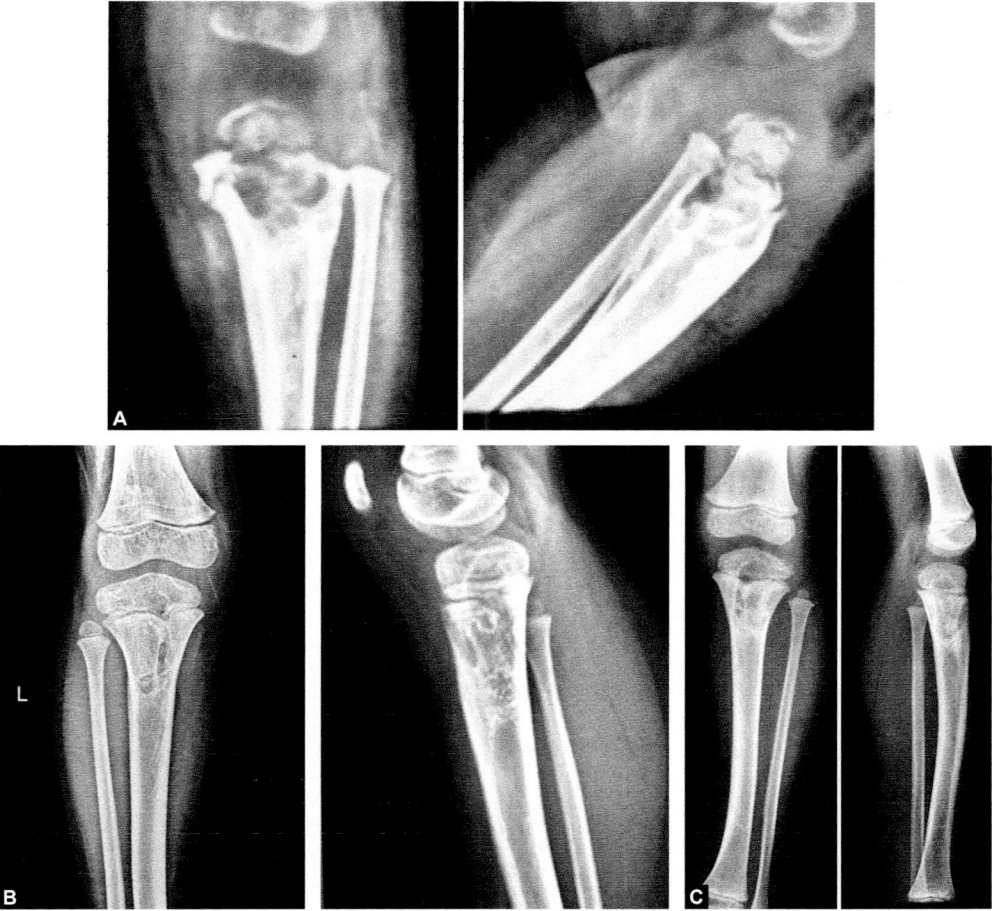

Figs. 2.16A to C: Remarkable potential of repair can be observed in this child. Tuberculosis of upper end of tibia (A) at presentation, (B) during follow-up and (C) about 4 years after treatment, observe remarkable repair and regeneration

and arthroplasty to obtain mobile, stable joints with biological control of disease is considered a rational method. At any stage if a lesion is not responding favorably to effective antitubercular drugs or there is doubt in diagnosis, or it is a case of refractory infection or recrudescence of disease, exploration and appropriate operation is considered mandatory. If a juxta-articular osseous lesion is threatening the joint despite adequate antitubercular drugs, excisional surgery of the focus may be performed. Non-responsive cases of tubercular synovitis and early arthritis may be subjected to subtotal synovectomy and synovectomy combined with joint debridement, respectively. Debridement should be limited to infected synovium, sequestra, pockets/cavities of pus and sinuses. In advanced tubercular arthritis of hip and elbow in adults (nonresponsive cases or cases who did not obtain acceptable range of movements), excision arthroplasty may be tried. Postoperatively all patients, where the aim was mobility, are treated by frequent repetitive active and assisted movements of the operated joint with an aim to obtain a functional arc. If a joint has healed with a painless range of movements in nonfunctional arc, one can do a juxta-articular osteotomy to bring the range of motion to the best functional arc. *Excisional arthroplasty* for hip (Girdlestone) may be considered for no-healing or incapacitating deep infections (pyogenic, tuberculous, iatrogenic) in young adults or the aged or in a patient who desires to avoid repeated surgery. The general outcome of such a procedure is an additional shortening of 2–4 cm, and a fairly mobile and painless hip. The patient should accept a shoe raise by 2–4 cm, a stick in the opposite hand for walking to minimise throwing of body weight over the unstable (operated) hip (Trendelenburg gait). *Low friction arthroplasty* is being tried in patients of tubercular arthritis, which have maintained healed status for 2–3 years. Despite best of selection, reactivation of disease may, however, occur in one-fourth of patients. Arthroplasty performed in patients with active tuberculous disease has proved disastrous. In advanced arthritis of ankle and wrist in adults for gross deformity and pain, compression arthrodesis is a good option. Fusion of hip and knee markedly disturbs the kinematics of locomotion in the long-term. A suitable replacement arthroplasty at an appropriate time is now a preferred treatment. Any surgery even in "healed status" must be done under cover of anti-TB drugs (an umbrella for about 5 months).

TUBERCULOSIS OF THE SPINE (POTT'S DISEASE)

Tuberculosis of the spine constitutes nearly 50% of all cases of skeletal tuberculosis. The localization in the descending order is dorsal, lumbar and cervical spine. The commonest initial lesion is subchondral area of two adjacent vertebrae (paradiscal). The rare locations are central body lesion, anterior surface of vertebrae, posterior appendical type (pedicle, lamina, transverse process, spinous process), and posterior facet joints. If infection is left untreated, the disease destroys the adjacent parts. The commonest presentation is involvement of two adjacent vertebral bodies, however, in the Indian subcontinent some patients may present with disease of more than three vertebrae and gross kyphotic deformities.

Cold Abscess

Formation of a perivertebral cold abscess is a common feature in spinal tuberculosis, however, the size of the cold abscess has no correlation with the extent of destruction. The initial abscess in the cervical spine collects in front of vertebral bodies behind the pharynx and esophagus; in the dorsal spine, it collects behind the mediastinal structures; in the dorsolumbar and lumbar spine, the abscess enters the psoas sheath and tracks down to iliac fossa as iliopsoas abscess. The initial abscess may track downward due to gravity or present far away from the parent lesion following the tracks of nerves and blood vessels.

Diagnosis

Constitutional symptoms are the same as for any active tuberculous lesion. One should suspect the disease at an early stage when there is only persistent local pain, tenderness and rigidity. Kyphotic deformity, a cold abscess and neural signs are features of advanced disease. The earliest radiological signs are diminished disc height, fuzzy paradiscal margins and osteoporosis of the involved vertebrae. With advancing disease, the vertebral bodies may show collapse of varying degrees, soft tissue paravertebral shadows and kyphotic deformity. With the help of MRIs and CT scans, one can diagnose the disease at a predestructive stage and even the disease at difficult sites (craniovertebral junction, cervicodorsal area, sacrum, sacroiliac joints).

Neurological Complications

This is the most dreaded complication of spinal tuberculosis and about 10% of patients present with this problem in the Indian subcontinent. Generally there is spastic (upper motor neuron) type of paraparesis or paraplegia. Highest incidence is due to tuberculosis in the dorsal or cervical spine. In clinical examination, one must always look for early signs of cord compression like unsteady spastic gait, exaggerated knee and ankle jerks, ankle and patellar clonus and extensor plantar response. In a rare case of neural complications due to lumbar disease, the examination would show lower motor neuron type of pattern. For clinical purposes, the severity of paraplegia has been classified as follows **(Table 2.2)**:

- **Stage I:** Patient is unaware of neural involvements, the clinician finds early upper motor signs.
- **Stage II:** Patient is aware of the weakness but is still able to walk with spastic gait.
- **Stage III:** Patient is unable to walk and the lower limbs are paralyzed in extension.
- **Stage IV:** Gross weakness of lower limbs with flexor spasms or paraplegia in flexion or flaccid paralysis with bladder and bowel involvement.

Another classification of paraplegia describes two types: "Early onset" occurring within the first 2 years of the onset of infection. The pressure on the cord is essentially by the inflammatory tissues, e.g., cold abscess, granulation tissues, necrotic debris from vertebrae and discs. These cases have a good prognosis for neural recovery. "Late onset" paraplegia is described if the neural complication occurs >2 years after the onset of disease. Most of these cases are due to mechanical pressure due to the internal kyphosis (salient) or vertebral canal stenosis or rarely due to reactivation of infection. Prognosis for neural recovery is poorer in such patients. Very rarely ischemia of the cord caused by infective thrombosis or endarteritis may cause sudden and complete paralysis. Such cases have very poor prognosis **(Table 2.3)**.

Treatment

Institute the standard treatment for spinal tuberculosis with rest to spine in recumbent

TABLE 2.2: Classification of tuberculous paraplegia/tetraplegia (predominantly based upon motor weakness).

Stage	Clinical features
Negligible	Patient unaware of neural deficit, physician detects plantar extensor and/or ankle clonus
Mild	Patient aware of deficit but manages to walk with support
Moderate	Nonambulatory because of paralysis (in extension), sensory deficit <50%
Severe	III+Flexor spasms/paralysis in flexion/flaccid, sensory deficit >50%, sphincters involved

*Application to compression of cord and not cauda equina.

TABLE 2.3: Clinical factors influencing prognosis in cord involvement.

Cord involvement	Better prognosis	Relatively poor prognosis
Degree	Partial	Complete
Duration	Shorter	Longer (>12 months)
Type	Early onset	Late onset
Speed of onset	Slow	Rapid
Age	Younger	Older
General condition	Good	Poor
Vertebral disease	Active	Healed
Kyphotic deformity	<60	>60
MRI of cord	Healthy cord	Myelomalacia/Syringomyelia
Operative findings	Wet lesion	Dry lesion

position. Progress of neural status is observed closely. With currently available drugs nearly 40% of patients with neural complications would recover completely without operateion. Of the uncomplicated patients of spinal tuberculosis, nearly 95% would heal without operation and without significant increase in the deformity.

Throughout the period of drug treatment modifications may have to be done depending upon the patient's age, drug reaction and response to therapy. For patients who show therapeutic resistance, or recurrence or are immunocompromised second-line drugs and immune modulator may have to be added.

Of all the paralyzed patients operated for absolute indications, the outcome in general, in our hands has been complete recovery with independent walking—85%, ambulatory with walking aid—8% and wheel chair dependent (with return of protective sensations)—7% (Fig. 2.17).

Operative Treatment

Absolute indications for operative treatment are as follows:
 i. Failure to show progressive neural recovery after 4–6 weeks of antitubercular drugs.
 ii. Advanced neural complications, e.g., stage IV paralysis.
 iii. Deterioration of neural status despite anti-tuberculous drugs for 3–4 weeks.
 iv. Failure to show progressive healing in an uncomplicated case of spinal tuberculosis as observed for 3–4 months.
 v. Doubt in diagnosis (despite MRIs, 5–10% patients may have overlapping features of other pathologies).
 vi. In children younger than 10 years whose spine is at risk for severe kyphotic deformity—destruction of more than two vertebral bodies between seventh cervical and first lumbar vertebrae, and radiological deterioration of kyphotic deformity in successive X-rays.
 vii. Drainage of a large cold abscess increasing in size despite attempted aspiration and drugs.

Operations for neural decompression, or debridement of anterior disease are best done through anterior approach with least disturbance to the healthy posterior elements.

In anterolateral extrapleural approach: posterior ends of 2 or 3 ribs and corresponding transverse processes are removed, one reaches the diseased vertebral bodies through the site of costovertebral joint. One can debride the diseased vertebrae, drain the paravertebral abscess, remove the offending parts of bones, discs and infected granulations to decompress the dural tube anteriorly and laterally without violating the thoracic

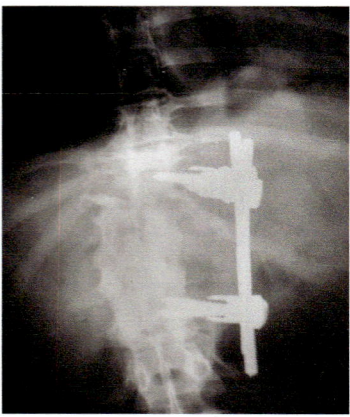
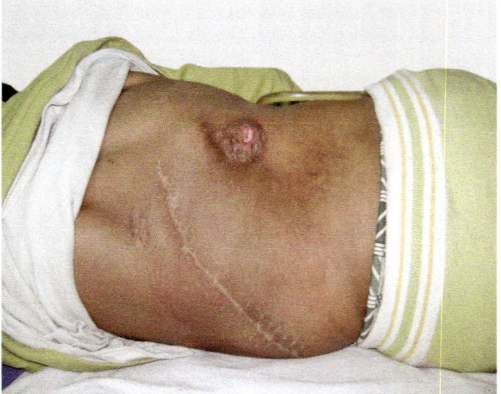

Fig. 2.17: A 23-year-old female now has complete paralysis, indwelling catheter, discharging sinus, despite operative decompression.

cavity. Another operation is *transthoracic, transpleural approach*: Through the left chest, reach the vertebral bodies from left side, after shifting the aorta anteriorly. The excised ribs (in both the procedures) are best used as bone grafts to add stability to the operated area.

Posterior spinal fusion is done: In children where spine is at risk for severe kyphotic deformity (vide supra). One or 2 ribs may be obtained from the patients, in small children one may have to supplement the graft from bank bone. Include in fusion one vertebra above and one below the diseased area.

Laminectomy has no place in the common paradiscal tuberculous lesions. The disease has essentially destroyed the anterior element (vertebral bodies), removing the posterior elements (laminectomy) would make the spine unstable. Besides the offending tissues are located in front of the cord, which cannot be approached from behind. The only indication is a rare symptomatic granuloma causing "tumor syndrome".

While performing anterior decompression in a growing child, remove only the offending segments of the vertebral bodies. The remaining anterior elements due to their growth potential may help negate some kyphotic deformities with growth. Anterolateral approach has a long learning curve, and transthoracic approach requires elaborate infrastructure facilities. Such operations are suitable where specialized facilities are available.

SUGGESTED READINGS

1. Tuli SM. Result of treatment of spinal tuberculosis by "middle-path" regime. J Bone Joint Surg. 1975;57-B:13-23.
2. Cheung WY, Luk KDK. Clinical and radiological outcomes after conservative treatment of TB spondylitis. Is the 15 years follow up in the MRI study long enough? Eur Spine J. 2013;22(Suppl 4): 594-602.
3. Qureshi MA, Afzal W, Khalique AB, Pasha IF, Aebi M. Tuberculosis of the craniovertebral junction. Eur Spine J. 2013;22(Suppl 4):612-7.
4. Jain AK, Kumar J. Tuberculosis of Spine: Neurological deficit. Eur Spine J. 2013;22(Suppl 4):624-33.
5. Panteli M, Puttaswamaiah R, Lowenberg DW, Giannoudis PV. Malignant transformation in chronic osteomyelitis: Recognition and principles of management. J Am Acad Orthop Surg. 2014;22:586-94.
6. Tuli SM. Tuberculosis of the skeletal system, 6th ed. Jaypee Brothers Medical Publishers (P) Ltd, New Delhi; 2016.
7. Kafla G, Garg B, Mehta N, Sharma R, Singh U, Kandasamy D, et al. Diagnostic yield of image-guided biopsy in patients with suspected infectious spondylodiscitis. Bone Joint J. 2022;104-B(1):120-6.

CHAPTER 3

Inflammatory Rheumatoid Disorders

Most of the connective tissue inflammatory disorders have overlapping clinical features. Broadly speaking these are "autoimmune disorders" probably triggered by environmental exposures, viral infections, bacterial antigens, diet, in genetically susceptible population.

INTRODUCTION

Rheumatoid disorders cover a number of diseases from mild localized pains and swelling at tendinous insertions to poly-articular involvement that may be progressive and debilitating. In addition to pain and inflammation around the joints, many patients have associated inflammatory skin rashes, subcutaneous nodules, associated eye problems and irritable bowel symptoms. Approximately, 1% of men and 3% of women worldover suffer from this disorder. It is considered an auto-immune systemic disorder interplaying with genetic predisposition and possible noxious environmental factors. Women are affected more commonly than men, the prevalence increases with advancing age. Severe cases result in high degree of disabilities and shortening of life expectancy due to this disorder; complications associated with prolonged treatment with "anti-rheumatic drugs" may also contribute to short lifespan.

This disease starts as synovitis where-ever synovial sheaths or membrane are present, e.g., tendons and tendinous insertions (tendinosis), small and large joints, sacroiliac joints and the joints of vertebral column. Initially synovitis will cause pain and there may be swelling and tenderness. Persistence of synovitis for some time leads to formation of granulations, which may weaken the tendons, form a lining or sheath of granulations (the pannus formation), which would erode the joint cartilage and bone, clinically producing tender swelling and limitation of joint movements and fibrous ankylosis in advanced stage. Destruction of bone and ligaments (leading to deformities and subluxation of joints), if unabated, the destroyed articular margins may end up as fibrous or bony ankylosis **(Fig. 3.1)**.

The most typical features are morning stiffness, polyarticular pains, tenosynovitis, and elevation of ESR. During acute exacerbations the ESR may be as high as 100 mm/h,

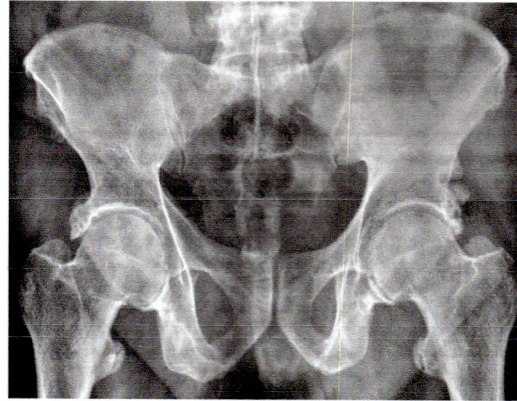

Fig. 3.1: X-ray of pelvis shows generalized enthesopathy around both hip joints and lesser trochanters in a patient suffering from rheumatoid disorder. Note fuzzy bilateral sacroiliac joints.

it may reduce to 30–40 mm with subsidence of symptoms, it becomes normal only when the disease is "burnt out". ESR however is a crude test because it may be elevated in other conditions like infections and malignancies. Auto-antibodies in serum (rheumatoid factor-[RF]) may be positive in about 70% of cases. Rheumatoid factor may also be positive in many (about 5%) normal asymptomatic individuals. Other autoimmune conditions such as systemic lupus erythematosus (SLE) and Sjögren's syndrome are also associated with positive rheumatoid factor. More recently another autoantibody has been identified as a diagnostic aid for rheumatoid disorders. Presence of anti cyclic citrullinated peptide (anti-CCP) antibodies is considered specific for rheumatoid disorder. A positive rheumatoid factor does not necessarily confirm the diagnosis of rheumatoid disorder, nor does a negative test exclude rheumatoid disease.

Diagnosis at early stage: Diagnosis of inflammatory rheumatoid disorders at an early stage is essentially based upon clinical criteria. The gross criteria include, (i) morning joint stiffness lasting for at last one hour, (ii) swelling around 3 or more joints especially around proximal interphalangeal, metacarpophalangeal, or wrist joint, feet and heels, (iii) symmetrical joint involvement. Early stages may be punctuated by spells of quiescence or short duration remissions. In due course of time, there is presence of symmetrical polyarthralgic pains with or without extraskeletal symptoms of fibrofascitis, fibromyelgia, plantar fascitis, tendovaginitis, subcutaneous nodules, cutaneous rashes, inflammation in eyes, urethra, intestines, pleura, lungs, pericardium, etc. **(Figs. 3.2 and 3.3)**.

MONOARTICULAR PRESENTATION

Sometimes, rheumatoid disorder may stay or present confined to one or two large joints such as knees, hips, ankles; enquiry into early history will usually suggest the diagnosis. X-rays in such cases may show significant diminution of joint space without typical changes of osteophytes and sclerosis of subchondral bone characteristic of osteoarthosis. Biopsy from the diseased synovium in such cases is mandatory to distinguish from some common conditions like tuberculosis or low grade pyogenic infection and also from rare conditions

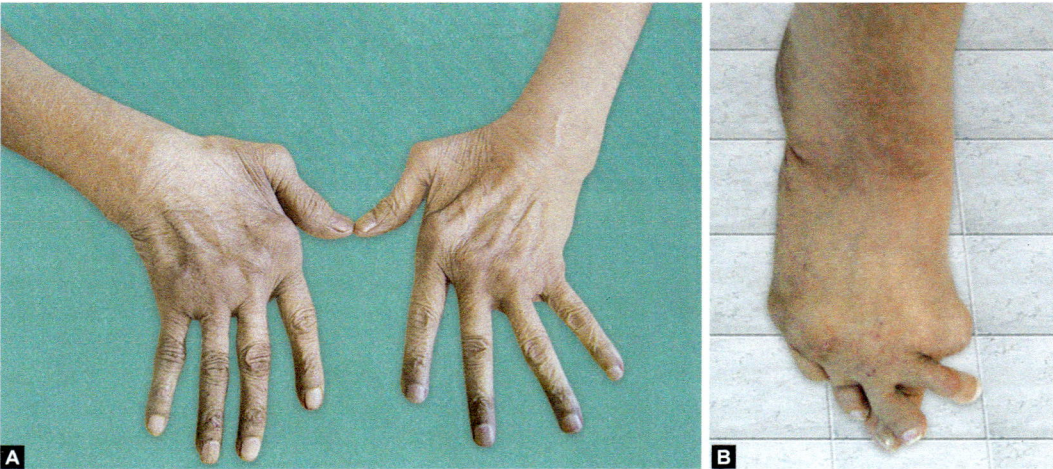

Figs. 3.2A and B: Clinical picture of a case of polyarticular rheumatoid arthritis (RA). (A) Typical deformities of hand showing radial deviation at wrist and ulnar deviation of fingers at metacarpophalangeal joints; (B) Gross deformities of toes with overriding.

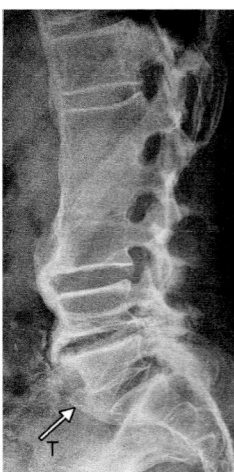

Fig. 3.3: In tuberculosis endemic countries, ankylosing spondylitis may be associated with tuberculous infection: L5-S1 area in this patient.

like rheumatoid arthritis, synovitis due to degenerative changes (loose bodies/floaters) in the joint, villonodular pigmented synovitis, and synovioma.

Generally all the conditions that are grouped under the heading of rheumatoid inflammatory disorders and seronegative spondyloarthropathies have a tendency for some familial aggregation. The author has many a times suspected the possibility of the disorder passed on to the spouse from the affected man. Such a coincidence may, however, be caused by a common environmental exposure.

TREATMENT

There is no cure for rheumatoid disorders. However, multimodal treatment using non-steroidal anti-inflammatory drugs (NSAIDs), supportive therapy to control associated osteoporosis, multidrug therapy with disease modifying anti-rheumatic drugs (DMARDs), active and assisted exercises, corrective splints to avoid deformities, careful use of short course steroids, local heating or use of physiotherapeutic measures, and local instillation of long acting steroids for pauciarticular disease may give relief to a large number of patients. Encourage such patients to continue active exercises and all activities of daily living. If the activity of disease does not come under control by NSAIDs, under supervision add DMARDs such as methotrexate, sulfasalazine, hydrochloroquine, alone or in combination in smaller doses. Leflunomide can be considered if the first-line DMARDs are not tolerated or ineffective. Gold and penicillamine are now used rarely. Biological therapeutics may sometimes be used in patients who are not responding to the above treatment. Biologics that are being tried are infliximab, etanercept, and adalimumab. All biologics are expensive, more toxic, and need close supervision during their use. Cost, dose frequency, and medication tolerance, influence the choice of NSAIDs and other drugs. Any immunosuppressive drug (Methotrexate, Leflunomide, Rituximab-biologics) must be used with great caution. In the Indian-subcontinent, prolonged use may reactivate a tuberculous lesion in the body.

ROLE OF OPERATIVE INTERVENTION

In a case with doubtful diagnosis obtaining a tissue for confirmation of the pathology is mandatory. However, no surgical treatment can provide a cure or lasting relief of symptoms. Patients must be counseled that synovectomy and debridement, or knee or hip joint replacement for a refractory rheumatoid disorder may give relief (for sometime) to symptoms in the operated joint, however, the inflammatory process of the disease would continue in other parts of body and to some extent in the operated joint as well. A persistent and disabling synovial swelling of a tendon-sheath or joint may need synovectomy, a deformity may need a juxta-articular osteotomy, a grossly destroyed and painful joint may benefit by replacement arthroplasty. However even the best performed replacement arthroplasties in active, healthy persons younger than 40 years has limitations. Conditions for which replacement arthroplasty in the young may be considered appropriate are incapacitating stages of polyarticular rheumatoid arthritis or ankylosing spondylitis, multiple epiphyseal dysplasia, mono-articular disease with limited activity/life expectation. In polyarticular disease, fusion of hip or knee is not a good option. In adults hip or knee joint replacement is justified. For a **failed hip joint replacement** or uncontrolled infection excision arthroplasty is still a viable option, as one time procedure. Home environments and lifestyle of the patient must be kept in mind while planning any operative intervention.

PROGNOSIS

Rheumatoid disorders run a variable course. Counseling the patient during early stages to do active exercises and to maintain all the activities of daily living is extremely important. Very high titer of rheumatoid factor and positive family history are bad prognostic signs. *With effective treatment,* (a) about 10% of patients improve markedly and lead a near normal level of activities; (b) nearly 60% have intermittent phases of activity of disease and remissions, (c) about 20% have severe joint involvement within 10 years of the onset of disease, (d) about 10% end up as totally disabled and ultimately confined to wheel chair for ambulation. Life expectancy is reduced by 5–10 years often due to ischemic heart disease with or without chronic renal dysfunction or pulmonary fibrosis.

SERONEGATIVE SPONDYLOARTHROPATHIES (SNSA)

This is a subgroup of rheumatoid disorders. Most of these are generalized disorders with varying degree of involvement of different parts of the skeletal system. In classical rheumatoid arthritis, rheumatoid factor is positive in about 70% of patients; in seronegative spondyloarthropathies; rheumatoid factor is mostly negative; however, HLA-B27 is positive in most of such patients. One should, however, be aware that about 8% of asymptomatic general population may also show prevalence of HLA-B27, and about 5% of asymptomatic people may show positive Rh-factor. Broadly speaking these conditions have a (familial aggregation) positive family history and generalized enthesopathy with preferential involvement of certain parts/regions of the skeletal system. The pathological process involves various joints, sacroiliac joints and vertebral articulations. The inflammation starts at tendinous and ligamentous insertions and synovial linings. In due course, the inflammatory granulation tissues (causing pain and tenderness) are replaced by fibrous tissue (causing restriction of movements) which may undergo calcification (mineralization/ossification) fusing the joints; 'bamboo-spine' as an example. A few relatively common conditions considered as seronegative spondyloarthropathies are mentioned below. Involvement of sacroiliac joints is more common in SNSAs, whereas cervical spine is more commonly involved in RA **(Figs. 3.4 and 3.5)**.

ANKYLOSING SPONDYLITIS

The disease starts as intermittent nonspecific low backache in young adults. Pain and stiffness are more in the morning and after inactivity. The pain may radiate to buttucks and back of thighs. The author has seen such young people having been mistakenly operated as prolapsed intervertebral disc. Over the next few years, the pain and stiffness become continuous and other symptoms of fatigue, tenderness at tendinous insertions (e.g., tendo-Achilles insertions on the calcaneum), development of stiffness of spine and forward stooping posture, restriction of chest expansions become obvious. At every site of involvement, the pathological process passes through stage of inflammation with granulations, fibrosis of the inflamed region and ultimately ossification of the involved segment. Common sites are sacroiliac joints, lumbar spine, costovertebral and

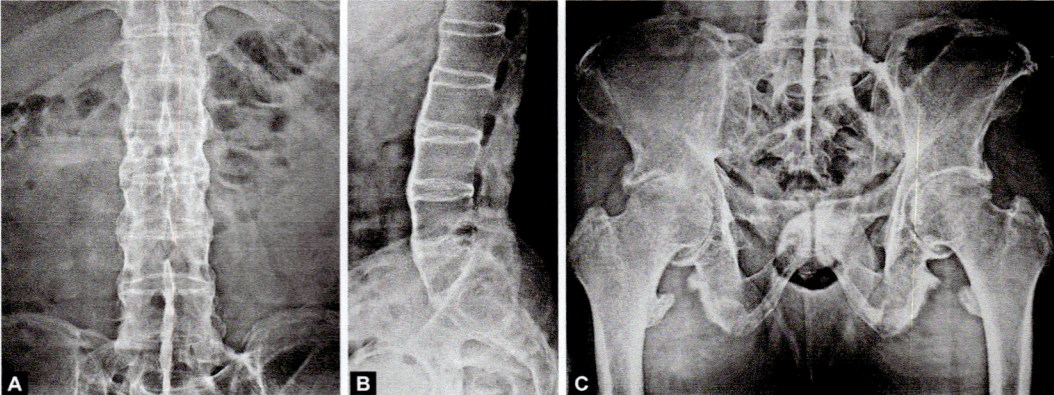

Figs. 3.4A to C: X-rays of an advanced stage of ankylosing spondylitis: Note advanced enthesopathy in pelvis, calcified ligament of sacroiliac joints, and anterior and posterior ligaments of vertebral column, and squaring of a anterior borders of vertebrae.

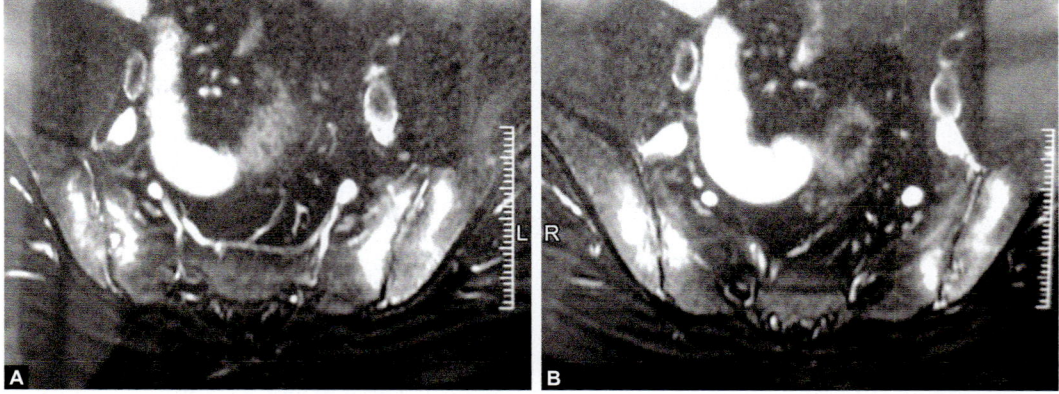

Figs. 3.5A and B: MRI of pelvis: Note inflammatory edema of both sacroiliac joints suggesting spondyloarthropathy.

costochondral articulations, dorsal and cervical spine, and hip joints **(Figs. 3.4 and 3.5)**. Typically if the chest expansion in a young man is <6 cm, one must exclude the diagnosis of ankylosing spondylitis. HLA-B27 may be present in about 70% of such patients, and in about 50% of their first degree relatives.

Treatment

Basic treatment remains the same as that for rheumatoid inflammatory disorders, maintain full activities and active (and assisted) exercises of spine, chest and the whole body. Use of anterior spinal hyperextension (ASH) brace while in upright posture may relieve the pain and minimize kyphotic deformation. Use NSAIDs to counteract pain to permit active exercises and activities of daily living. One may have to use DMARDs, TNF inhibitors for uncontrollable and severe symptoms. Operations to correct deformities of spine and restore mobility of hip joints may be needed. These are, however, difficult and hazardous operations on patients with compromised respiratory functions, and cannot be performed at district hospital level. Though all activities should be encouraged, however, patients should avoid crowded places (like festivals) and rough travels (like pillion riding on motorcycles). These patients can develop complications like fracture of spine, hyperkyphosis causing difficulty in seeing beyond their feet, one may develop neural signs by pressure on spinal cord by deformity or by canal stenosis. In countries where tuberculosis is endemic, one may get pulmonary tuberculosis due to compromised chest excursions and tuberculous infection in the spine.

REITER'S SYNDROME AND REACTIVE ARTHRITIS

It is a clinical triad of arthritis, urethritis and conjunctivitis usually presenting a few weeks after an attack of dysentery and/or genitourinary infection. At present, Reiter's syndrome is considered as a reactive arthritis in response to a recent infection in the bowels or genitourinary passages. Men are affected more than women. Common age is between 20 and 40 years; however, younger people may also be affected. The affected joints (ankle, knee) may show swelling, warmth and tenderness; enthesitis may be present at tendocalcaneal insertion or plantar fascia. Patient may develop clinical features of spondyloarthropathy.

Treatment

Identify the triggering infection and treat it by suitable antibiotics for 4–8 weeks. Like any other inflammatory rheumatoid disorder, symptomatic treatment includes active exercises, and NSAIDs. In nonresponders one may have to use a short course of steroids and/or DMARDs.

PSORIATIC ARTHRITIS

Polyarthritis and psoriasis are often seen together. Skin lesions in most of the cases appear earlier than joint pains and spondyloarthropathies. The skin lesions are generally seen on the extensor surfaces of elbow and knee. In about 7%, the joints show inflammatory disease. The nails may show resorption of the nail tips and transverse ridges on the surface. X-rays of the involved joints may show resorption of articular ends. Joints involvement have many patterns from oligoarthropathy to polyarthropathy, sacroiliatis and spondylo-arthropathy (not dissimilar to ankylosing spondylitis). Rheumatoid factor is negative in most of the cases, HLA-B27 is positive in about 60% cases.

Treatment

In addition to topical application to control skin lesions, the systemic treatment is the same as for rheumatoid inflammatory disorders and for ankylosing spondylitis.

ENTEROPATHIC ARTHROPATHY

Crohn's disease and ulcerative colitis or inflammatory bowel disease may be associated with peripheral arthritis or sacroiliatis and spondyloarthropathic features. This condition has no clear association with rheumatoid factor or HLA-B27. There is also no temporal correlation between the intensity of bowel inflammation and the symptoms of arthritis. Management essentially remains the same as that for rheumatoid inflammation. Inflammatory bowel disease rarely may develop a fistula due to adhesions to the abdominal wall, which may communicate with hip joint or iliopsoas sheath.

JUVENILE RHEUMATOID (IDIOPATHIC) ARTHRITIS (JRA OR JIA)

It is a non-infective inflammatory joint disease in children <16 years of age. The basic cause is of an autoimmune disorder, like rheumatoid disorders, rheumatoid factor is generally absent. The clinical picture is almost like that of rheumatoid arthritis. About 15% have systemic features like low grade fever, anorexia, loss of weight preceding the pain, tenderness, swelling in various joints. Majority of such children (60–70%) have pauciarticular arthritis, about 10% have polyarticular arthritis mostly affecting larger joints, 5–10% present as seronegative spondyloarthropathies. If the disease occurs below the age of 3 years, classically it is called Still's disease. Diagnosis in early stages may be difficult, however, when multiple joints are involved and patient has been clinically observed for a few years the diagnosis is established.

CONNECTIVE TISSUE RHEUMATOID LIKE DISEASES

There are many well known (though rare) conditions closely related to rheumatoid disorder with many overlapping clinical features, and almost all related to auto-immune disorders with possible genetic predisposition. These include SLE, scleroderma, Sjögren's-sicca syndrome, polymyositis, dermatomyositis and post-viral arthropathies (after dengue or chikanguniya fever).

BASIC TREATMENT OF INFLAMMATORY RHEUMATOID DISORDERS

The basic treatment is similar for all varieties of rheumatoid disorders. Antirheumatoid medications are safer to use in a ladder form.

First-line Treatment

First-line treatment includes sympathetic counseling of the patients, parents and the family explaining to them the difficulties of treatment and maintenance of prolonged therapy. Emphasize the importance of active exercises and use of splints to prevent and correct the deformities. Encourage the patients to continue their activities like education, training, and working. Use NSAIDs in various combinations to help the patient cope up with pains, swelling and to permit exercises and activities.

Second-line Treatment

In case of inadequate outcome of first-line drugs, one may start the use of DMAs, in isolation or various combinations such as methotrexate, sulfasalazine, hydrochloroquine.

Third-line Treatment

One may have to use steroids in pulse-mode (aim at short course, if possible) systemically if the response to above therapy does not help the patient. Severe nonresponding inflammation of large joints may be helped by the use of local intra-articular instillation of steroids; maximum of three in 3–6 months duration is the safe limit **(Figs. 3.6 and 3.7)**.

Fourth-line Treatment

Fourth-line of treatment (biologic response modifiers) leflunomide, infliximab, etanercept and adalimumab are potentially useful agent, however, their side effects mitigate against their routine usage.

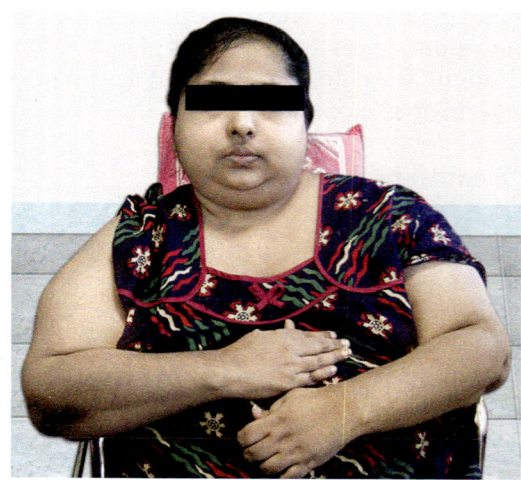

Fig. 3.6: Clinical picture of a young lady with "moon face" and trunkal obesity exhibiting "Cushing syndrome". She was treated for rheumatoid disorder using systemic steroids for many months, she also developed osteonecrosis of both hip joints.

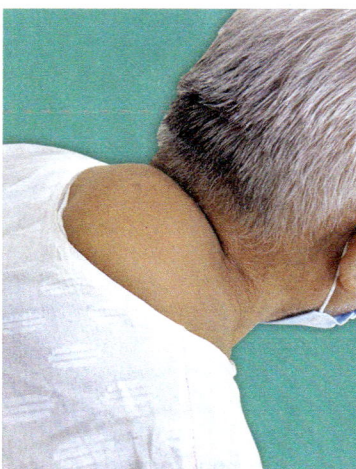

Fig. 3.7: In rheumatoid arthritis prolonged use of steroids may produce a buffalo hump, a manifestation of drug induced "Cushing's syndrome".

"Step-down" philosophy is considered rational during pharmacological treatment of rheumatoid disease: Treat aggressively in the beginning and once the control of acute inflammation has been achieved, continue with least toxic drugs combination.

Fifth-line Treatment

Fifth-line of treatment: Operative intervention. If nonoperative treatment has not been able to prevent gross deformities and maintain function, operative treatment is indicated. The aim is to correct gross deformities by synovectomy and capsulotomies (arthrolysis) or by juxta-articular corrective osteotomy to maintain function and activities. There is no place of doing major surgeries to improve the anatomy and cosmetics in such patients. To improve the function, arthrodesis of wrist and ankle may be justified; however, fusion of other major joints is not justified in a polyarticular disorder. Juxta-articular osteotomies for hip and knee may be indicated in some patients to correct deformities and improve function. With the availability of modern joint-replacement technology, fusion (arthrodesis) for a disease in hip or knee may be considered as obsolete procedures.

In countries where tuberculosis is endemic, prolonged use of immunosuppressive drugs, e.g., methotrexate, leflunomide, steroids, biologics having anti-TNF may induce a clinically manifest tuberculous infection or reactivate an old healed tuberculous lesion. The author has observed both these complications. Another serious complication as a result of prolonged use of steroids has been avascular necrosis of femoral heads. These agents modify the immune response by blocking the cytokines and cells involved in immunopathogenesis of rheumatoid inflammation. There are numerous biologics being tried in clinical settings; the commonly used are infliximab, etanercept, adalimumab. In general for ladies during child bearing age biologics (TNF) and DMARDs are not prescribed because of their teratogenic potential. One should stop steroids, DMAs, biologics-TNF inhibitors for 5–10 days before any major operative intervention.

DIFFUSE IDIOPATHIC SKELETAL HYPEROSTOSIS (DISH)

This disorder generally affects older men, characterized by widespread ossification of anterior longitudinal ligament mostly on the right side of the dorsal and dorsolumbar vertebrae. It is neither a rheumatoid disorder nor an osteoarthrosis. When it occurs by itself, it is usually asymptomatic, back pain and stiffness are seldom seen, sacroiliac joints are not involved and the ESR is normal. More recently many workers have observed that DISH may be associated with ossification of anterior longitudinal ligaments and all axial bones and pelvis may show enthesopathic changes.

Intra-articular Aspiration and Instillation

Aspiration of a joint is a useful outpatient procedure to obtain the joint fluid for diagnostic purposes or for instillation of antibiotics for infective conditions and local steroids for rheumatoid inflammatory lesions. The procedure however must be performed with standard aseptic precautions. All superficial joints can be easily approached with the help of bony landmarks. **Hip joint is the deepest** joint for aspiration and/or instillation, with experience one can succeed using a spinal needle. In case of difficulty (obesity or deformity) the procedure is recommended to be performed under C-arm guidance.

Joint aspirate may be of help in establishing the diagnosis in early stages of any arthritides, such as degenerative disease, rheumatoid disorder, infections, hemarthrosis (traumatic or bleeding disorder), villonodular synovitis or tumorous conditions. The aspirate may be serous, purulent, sanguineous or a mixed appearance, and it may contain some debris. The aspirated material must be submitted for diagnostic purpose: biochemical, microbiological, serological, and histological (if joint debris is available). The joint aspirate may show urate crystals or pyrophosphate crystals. The cell count in synovial fluid may be helpful: normal joint <5, rheumatoid disorders and infection the cell count may be >25,000. During instillation of corticosteroids avoid leaving steroids in subcutaneous tissues lest it may cause depigmentation of the skin color. Intra-articular medications do relieve the pain but rarely slow the progress of disease.

The shoulder (glenohumeral joint) may be entered anteriorly or posteriorly, with the patient sitting or lying down palpate the medial aspect of the humeral head and enter the joint just medial to this. The entry point for posterior approach is 1.5–2 cm distal and one cm medial to the posterior corner of the acromion. The needle is inserted keeping it parallel to the ground in sitting posture or perpendicular to the posterior chest wall. Slight rotation of the shoulder is used to confirm that needle is in the joint space versus stuck in the humeral head, minor changes may be needed for correct relocation of the needle. Through the same entry point the needle may be placed in the subacromial space. After entry through the skin direct the needle about 30 degrees cephalad, if it hits the acromion slight relocation is needed to stay in the subacromial space.

Elbow joint: The soft spot for entry is located at the center of a triangle formed by the lateral humeral epicondyle, the radial head and the lateral corner of the alecranon. This is probably the best approach for aspiration of intra-articular fluid collection.

The second approach is immediately proximal to the superior margin of olecranon. Keep the elbow in about 90 degrees of flexion. Through the transtendinous approach one can reach each side of the olecranon and the olecranon fossa. This is the ideal approach to inject steroids into the posterior capsule and the joint cavity to improve the flexion range of movements. **For tennis elbow** injection is made into the most tender point of origin of extensor carpi radialis brevis. As a last part of the procedure do multiple hits at the lateral supracondylar ridge to agitate the origion of common extensors which may promote healing and pain relief.

The hip: Intra-articular injections into hip are best done with fluoroscopic (C-arm) guidance. For anterior approach the femoral pulse must be palpated and marked to understand the location of neurovascular bundle at the base of femoral triangle. Spinal needles are used to reach the intra-capsular space because the hip joint is deeply placed. Here are a few approaches.

- *Anterolateral*: Draw a line from the most prominent part of greater trochanter on it's lateral surface to join the middle of inguinal ligament. The entry point is at the junction of lateral one third with the middle one third of this line. The spinal needle is directed 45 degrees medially and 45 degree cephalad.
- *The lateral approach*: The needle is inserted just above the tip of greater trochanter aiming straight medially to reach the femoral head-neck junction intracapsularly. One may angle the needle

anteriorly by about 10 degrees to adjust for femoral anteversion. An alternative for this correction is to place the hip joint in internal rotation by 10–15 degrees.

The **greater trochanter bursa** may need to be aspirated for trochanteric bursitis due to tuberculosis or rheumatoid disorder or any other pathology. The needle is inserted at the most prominent or most painful area of the trochanteric bursa.

Knee joint: If the patient has a moderate to large effusion in the joint, a space is created between the patella and femur due to anterior translation of patella. The easiest approach is to enter into the knee joint from the lateral side through the palpable space between the patella and femur. The fluid can be aspirated and the residual contents can be squeezed out by exerting parapatellar pressure medially, superiorly and inferiorly. If there is not much of effusion the entry into the joint space can be difficult.

Keep the knee nearly fully extended, the needle should be inserted either from near the superolateral angle of patella or near the lateral border of patella. The needle should be aimed towards the middle of articular surface of patella. The operator must ensure no damage to the articular surfaces of patella and of femur, this can be easily avoided by adjusting/moving the needle-tip forwards, backwards, anterior or posterior until the injection can be performed without resistance.

GOUT

Gout is a crystal deposition disorder caused by deposition of monosodium urate crystals secondary to hyperuricemia. Often classified as "Primary" and "Secondary" form. The secondary form may be due to rare hereditary conditions or acquired disorders such as myeloproliferative disease, excessive use of diuretics or renal failure. Under excretion of urates through urine results in hyperuricemia, in symptomatic people the serum uric acid levels are >7 mg/dL. Approximately 2% of adults are affected, generally men in fifth decade and women after menopause. Hyperuricemia leads to deposition of monosodium urate crystals in synovium, cartilage, tendons and soft tissues (mostly para-articular). Common sites are first metatarsophalangeal joint, foot, ankle, knee, elbow, wrist and in the pinna of ears. The affected part is extremely painful, swollen, red, hot and tender. The crystal deposition may present as rounded swellings (tophi). X-rays may show a soft tissue swelling and erosive lesions in periarticular area. The confirmation of diagnosis is by the presence of urate crystals in the aspirate. In differential diagnosis any inflammatory disorder may be considered, however septic arthritis remains most important. NSAIDs, colchicine allopurinol, indomethacin in various combinations are recommended with careful monitoring of side effects.

SUGGESTED READINGS

1. Furst DE, Breedveld FC, Kalden JR, Smolen JS, Burmester GR, Dougados M, et al. Updated consensus statement on biological agents for the treatment of rheumatoid arthritis and other immune mediated inflammatory disease. Ann Rheum Dis. 2003;62(Suppl 2):112-9.
2. Shieman JM, Frendick AM. Summing the risk of NSAID therapy. Lancet. 2007;369:1580-1.
3. Sidiropoulos PI, Hatemi G, Song IH, Avouac J, Collantes E, Hamuryudan V, et al. Evidence-based recommendations for the management of ankylosing spondylitis: systematic literature search of the 3E Initiative in Rheumatology involving a broad panel of experts and practising rheumatologists. Rheumatology. 2008:47: 355-61.
4. Handa R, Sharma A, Naidu G. Rheumatology clinic: Spondyloarthritis. Evangel Publishing, New Delhi, 2021.

CHAPTER 4

Osteoarthrosis

INTRODUCTION

Osteoarthrosis or osteoarthritis is primarily a degenerative condition of joints, any inflammatory process in such joints is a reaction to the degenerative changes. Osteoarthrosis may be divided as 'primary' or 'secondary' osteoarthrosis. Primary condition is essentially due to age-related changes, and the secondary osteoarthrosis is caused by mechanical incongruity of the articular surfaces or due to juxta-articular deformity, or even due to a distant pathology leading to disturbed kinematics of locomotion and work. Primary osteoarthrosis is common in weight-bearing joints like hip and knee, obesity hastens the onset of this condition. It is rare in nonweight-bearing joints, like shoulder and elbow; however, even small joints of hands may be affected in some patients. In the Indian subcontinent, primary osteoarthrosis of the hip is much less common than the Western countries; however, osteoarthrosis of the knee joints is met with more frequently. The lower incidence of hip involvement may be attributed to the social habit of floor activities such as squatting and sitting cross-legged. Full range physiological movement, during these activities probably distributes the stresses to the whole of articular surfaces and optimizes its nutrition.

Primary or secondary osteoarthrosis is a progressive process of degeneration in which the articular cartilage undergoes surface fibrillations, fragmentation, focal and general degeneration. Once the cushioning effect of articular cartilage is disturbed, the subchondral bone starts showing sclerosis (eburnation), subchondral small cysts formation, and marginal peri-articular reactive osteophyte formation. With progressive changes, the synovial membrane undergoes hyperemia and hypertrophy and there may be varying degree of synovial effusion. Generally, there are no systemic or laboratory signs of inflammation because osteoarthrosis is not a systemic disease. In advanced cases, there may be gross restriction of movements, however, the joint seldom undergoes spontaneous ankylosis.

Pathological changes are almost same in secondary osteoarthrosis, however, the wear and tear are preceded by an intra-articular fracture or juxta-articular fracture healed with some deformity **(Fig. 4.1)**. Altered

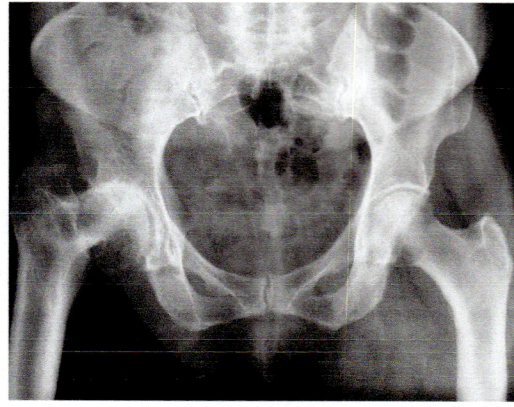

Fig. 4.1: Secondary osteoarthrosis: Comparison with normal (left) hip joint shows on the right side diminished joint (cartilage) space, sclerosis of joint margins and subchondral cysts. Disturbed kinematics due to coxa vara resulted in early degeneration.

biomechanics in the hip joint can also result in the degenerative changes many years after the healing of the primary defect such as Perthe's disease, slipped capital femoral epiphysis, avascular necrosis of femoral head, coxa vara, or healed infective lesion of long standing.

Main causes of secondary osteoarthrosis in the knee joint are osteochondral fractures, juxta-articular fractures healed with some malunion (genu varum, genu valgum), healed infection of long standing, loose bodies, rheumatoid disease, hyperuricemia and hemophilic arthritis **(Figs. 4.2 and 4.3)**. Similar pathologies can lead to osteoarthrosis in other weight-bearing or nonweight-bearing joints.

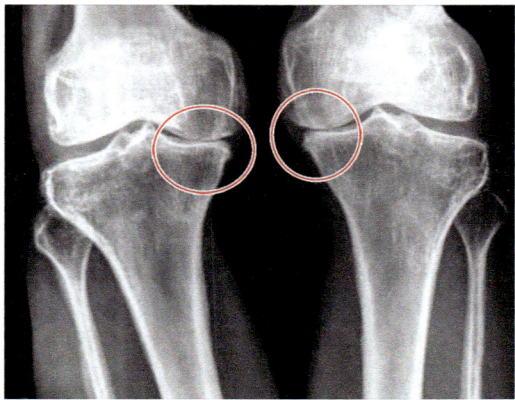

Fig. 4.2: Early osteoarthrosis: Reduction of joint space is due to loss of thickness of articular cartilage and semilunar cartilage. Early cases are suitable for joint repair (high tibial osteotomy).

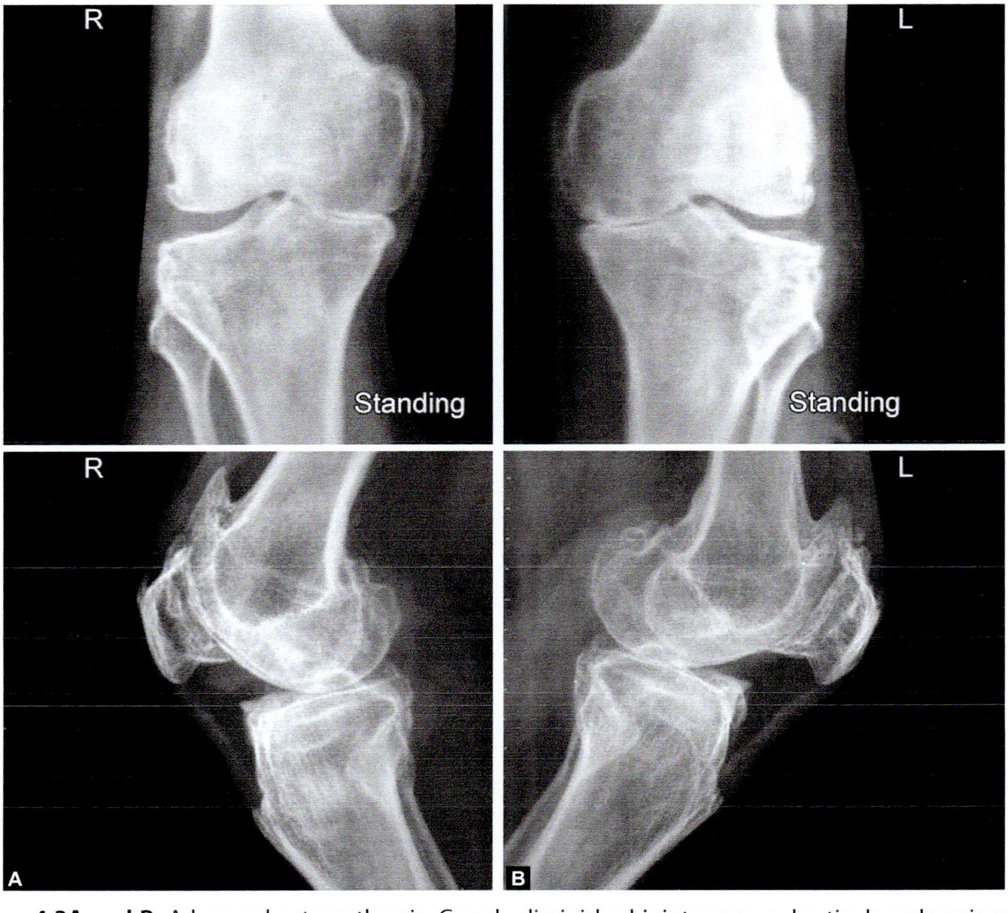

Figs. 4.3A and B: Advanced osteoarthrosis: Grossly diminished joint space, subarticular sclerosis and generalized osteophyte formation. Such cases are suitable for joint replacement procedures.

Symptoms

Generally, a middle-aged person presents with insidious symptoms of mild pain in the joints and moderate degree of restriction of terminal range of motion. Like many arthritides, the discomfort and restriction of movements is maximum when one starts activities after a long period of rest, typically the "joints loosen" after a few minutes of range of motion exercises and activities.

Examination of the involved knee and other superficial joints may show moderate degrees of swelling due to synovial effusion and thickening of the synovium and there may be restriction of terminal range of motion. One can elicit crepitations on joint movements and local tenderness along the joint margins. Wasting of the muscles can be appreciated by comparison with contralateral normal parts.

X-rays: Earliest changes seen are diminution of the joint space (cartilage space), sclerosis (eburnation) of the bony articular surfaces, subchondral cyst formation and periarticular osteophytosis. The clinical symptoms and signs are not proportional to the degree of radiological symptoms **(Figs. 4.1 to 4.3)**.

TREATMENT

Early Stage

The mainstay in early cases is to maintain the joint mobility and the strength of the muscles by repetitive active exercises. Exercises involving impact loading (jogging) should be avoided. Common sense measures like weight reduction for obese people and avoiding carrying weights >5–10 kg especially while negotiating stairs, use of a walking stick for outdoor activities are helpful. For painful hip disease, a stitch in the opposite hand is advised, however for the knee, the patient would choose the side according to his comfort. If pain is severe, the patient should be made comfortable by occasional use of nonsteroidal anti-inflammatory drugs (NSAIDs). Long-term use of NSAIDs have the potential of side effects in the older population, periodic appropriate laboratory investigations, e.g., hemogram and renal functions are mandatory.

Intermediate Stage

If clinical examination and imaging modalities suggest intra-articular debris or loose bodies, a joint debridement by arthroscopy or by open operation is justified and may give relief for some time. If there is malalignment of the articular surfaces, e.g., coxa vara, genu varum, genu valgum, deformity around the ankle, a suitable corrective osteotomy would slow down the degenerative process and give relief from pain with retention of movements for many years. Juxta-articular corrective osteotomy may help in repair and regeneration of articular cartilage.

Late Stage

Gross destruction of joint, increasing pain, marked limitations of movements, bone loss, deformity and previous surgery, especially in patients above the age of 60 years, are suitable candidates for joint replacement surgery. Total joint replacement of hip and knee should be considered after having tried adequate conservative treatment and lifestyle modifications. Generally one should aim at replacement at a mature age (60–65 years) so that need for repeat arthroplasty is minimal. Radiological appearance alone should not be the criteria for joint replacement. Hip arthroplasty is recommended for disabling joint pain, limitation of movements and gross deformity. Total knee replacement should be considered for end-stage tricompartmental osteoarthrosis having deformity of knee, gross reduction in range of motion and significant pain. Most suitable joints for replacement surgery are hip and knee, on an average, improvement obtained may last for 12–15 years. The contact between the articulating (weight-bearing) surfaces leads to the generation of wear debris, which compromises the long-term clinical results. Good results of joint replacement procedures are highly dependent upon the infrastructure facilities available and the surgical skills. Postoperative infection is the most serious complication and would be disastrous to the patient. Arthrodesis is a reasonable option for ankle and wrist, however at present it should be an extremely rare indication for hip and knee.

Surgery is usually confined to end-stage disease when pain has become refractory to other treatment options. Many seniors above the age of 60 years have multiple comorbidities which may make operative treatment more hazardous.

***Note*: Aritcular cartilage** → edema → degeneration → thinning → erosion → fragmentation → subchondral bone exposure → diminished joint space → subchondral sclerosis and osteophytes formation.

SUGGESTED READINGS

1. National Institute for Health and Care Excellence (NICE). Clinical guideline [CG177]: Osteoarthritis: Care and management, 2014.
2. Glyn-Jones S, Palmer AJR, Agricola R, Price AJ, Vincent TL, Weinans H, et al. Osteoarthritis. Lancet. 2015;386:376-87.

CHAPTER 5

Avascular Necrosis of Bone or Osteonecrosis

INTRODUCTION

Avascular necrosis (AVN) is a poorly understood derangement of the osseous circulation. The risk factors suspected to be responsible for the derangement are listed in **Box 5.1**; however, only about <5% of the people with risk factors may get the clinically manifest disorder. Most authors feel that development of osteonecrosis has involvement of multifactorial etiology/causes. Osteonecrosis is not life-threatening, however, it is very disabling because the onset of defect occurs mostly in young people between the age of 30 and 40 years, and in about 50% the disorder is bilateral (in hip disease). Most of the patients in early stage of disease exhibit selective restriction of range of motion.

> **BOX 5.1** **Common suspected risk factors of osteonecrosis.**
>
> - Prolonged use of corticosteroids
> - Abuse of ethanol
> - Abuse of nicotine
> - Dislocation of joint
> - Juxta-articular fractures
> - Hemoglobinopathies (Sickle-cell disease)
> - Myeloproliferative disorders (Goucher's)
> - Radiation exposure*
> - Pregnancies
> - Renal osteodystrophy
> - Systemic lupus erythematosus (SLE)
> - Idiopathic (10%)
> - Onco-chemotherapy
> - Cushing syndrome
>
> *Osteonecrosis occurs in the radiated region.
> Note: Risk higher with comorbidities.

Asymptomatic Contralateral Hip

It is likely to get involved with symptomatic affection as follows:
1. No evidence of X-rays and MRI abnormality—8% will get involved.
2. No evidence of X-rays abnormality, but MRI abnormality present—28% will get involved.
3. Contralateral hip has abnormal X-ray—82% will deteriorate and become symptomatic.

Theoretically, osteonecrosis can occur in any bone, however, most patients present with following symptomatic locations: femoral head, humeral head, lower end of femur, scaphoid, talus, lunate, distal humerus, and proximal tibia. Osteonecrosis has not been observed in the bone-ends with concave articular surfaces.

PATHOLOGY

Exact mechanism of pathological changes is not well-understood, however, thromboembolic causes and even increased intraosseous tension have been blamed to cause disruption of blood supply (nutrient end arterioles) leading to death of osteocytes and other marrow cells. Gross ischemia of bone leads to bone necrosis and collapse of the articular margins. Concomitant with the necrosis of bone, the adjacent living bone makes attempt to repair and invade the dead bone, and that is what makes the appearance in images at the dead and living bone 'interface' within a few weeks of ischemic episode. The penetration by reparative granulations is generally not >8–10 mm. The attempted repair ultimately shows as sclerotic lines in the X-rays.

DIAGNOSIS

Prompt diagnosis is important in the management because treatment at early stages of disease results in better outcome **(Figs. 5.1A and B)**. High suspicion index and history of risk factors should prompt the clinician for further investigations. The patient would generally present with deep vague pain in the joint, pain on weight-bearing (antalgic gait) and on use of the limb. In early stages, only terminal range of movements may show limitations. There is progressive loss of movements with advancing disease. The first investigation should be X-rays of the suspected joint with a concomitant X-ray of the contralateral normal (or abnormal) area in identical position. Osteonecrosis is the end result of severe and prolonged ischemia. X-rays at predestructive stage (preradiological stage, stage "O") show no difference between the living and necrosed bone. Any radiological changes that we see in clinical practice are due to the reaction of the living bone (living tissues) to the ischemic (necrotic) bone. The X-rays in earliest stages look normal (stage 0), however, if the history of disease is of a few months (about 3 months or more) duration, the plain X-rays may show a mottled appearance, cystic changes, sclerotic margin at the 'interface', crescent-like fragment of subchondral bone, and varying degree and extent of collapse of the articular margin. The joint space or cartilage space remains normal for a long time. Isotope bone scans may show a cold area (the dead bone) surrounded by a hot area (the hyperemic reparative response). MRI is the best diagnostic method in early stages in T1-weighted images. A low density single line demarcates the normal and ischemic bone interface. On T2-weighted image a double line (parallel lines) represents the demarcation interface and the adjacent repair response by granulations **(Tables 5.1 and 5.2, Fig. 5.2)**.

MRI scanning is at present the best modality to diagnose AVN at an early stage. T1 weighted images would show a geographical area (the necrosed bone) in the subchondral region limited by a wavy line. T2-weighted image would show a parallel double line, the proximal one (nearer to the articular margin), the boundary of the necrosed area and the caudal one (farther from joint margin) reparative hyperemic granulation tissue. In advanced stage of AVN, the MRI would show step-off sign, incongruity of the femoral head and degenerative changes in the

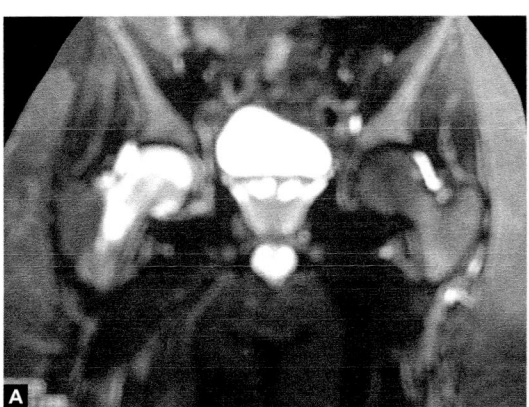 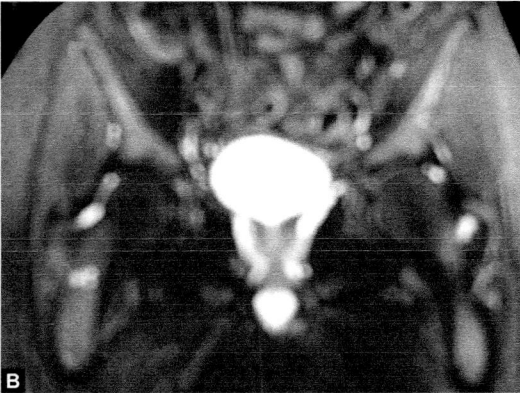

Figs. 5.1A and B: MRI of both hip joints. (A) Generalized bone edema in right femoral head and neck (Stage I), Complete resolution; (B) After 9 months of non-weight-bearing ambulation and use of bisphosphonates.

TABLE 5.1: Classification (Ficat 1985 is most practical).

Ficat and Arlet (based upon X-ray findings)

Stage I	Normal (MRI may show early signs)
Stage II	Sclerotic or cystic lesions without subchondral fracture
Stage III	Crescent sign (subchondral fracture) or step-off subchondral bone (depression of articular surface)
Stage IV	Diminished cartilage space, osteoarthrosis

Note: Minor modifications have been done by other workers incorporating the location of ischemic changes in the weight-bearing surface. This classification can be applied for AVN located in any bone.

TABLE 5.2: Japanese committee and Shimizu et al. (1994) proposed a classification based upon MRI observations for osteonecrosis of femoral head.

Grade I	Lesions occupying less than one-quarter of the femoral head in coronal diameter
Grade II	Lesions occupying one-half of the femoral head diameter (one-third to two-thirds) of weight-bearing surface
Grade III	Lesions involving more than two-thirds of the weight-bearing surface

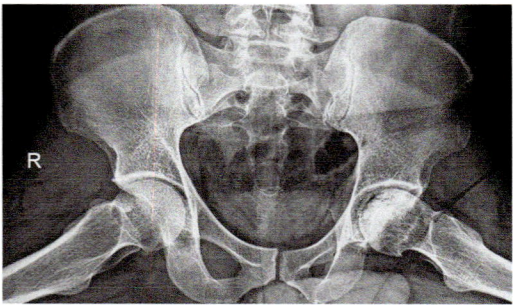

Fig. 5.2: Crescent shaped (sign) subchondral fracture seen in left hip joint in a patient with avascular necrosis.

joint (Ficat stage IV). Understanding of the pathomechanics of the vascular insult and observations in the MRI have suggested that the area of ischemic necrosis is determined at the time of insult. Its extent is unlikely to increase if the ischemic insult is not repeated. It is, therefore, important during treatment to stop or avoid the incriminating agents. Small ischemic areas in the non-loading parts are unlikely to collapse, whereas the large areas in the weight-bearing segment of the femoral head (or any other affected bone) may breakdown and collapse in nearly 60% of cases. Articular cartilage (joint space) retains its thickness for a long time.

TREATMENT

The goal of treatment is to relieve pain, retain a useful range of motion and maintain congruity of hip joint. Because of the young age of patients, the general advice is to stall total hip replacement and opt for procedures so that joint replacement is delayed or postponed to a more mature age, if possible above the age of 60 years. Radiographic features help predict the prognosis of treatment and also to formulate the treatment plans. Femoral head preservation procedures are justified if there is a functional range of motion, fairly preserved joint space and negligible involvement of acetabulum **(Figs. 5.1 and 5.3)**.

Femoral Head Preservation Techniques

Femoral heard preservation techniques are core decompression and autogenous bone grafting. One may insert a fibular graft to provide a support to a collapsing anterolateral segment of femoral head. Varus or valgus upper femoral osteotomy is another alternative to transfer the less affected femoral head segment to the weight-bearing area. Surface replacement is another bone preserving option, however in young

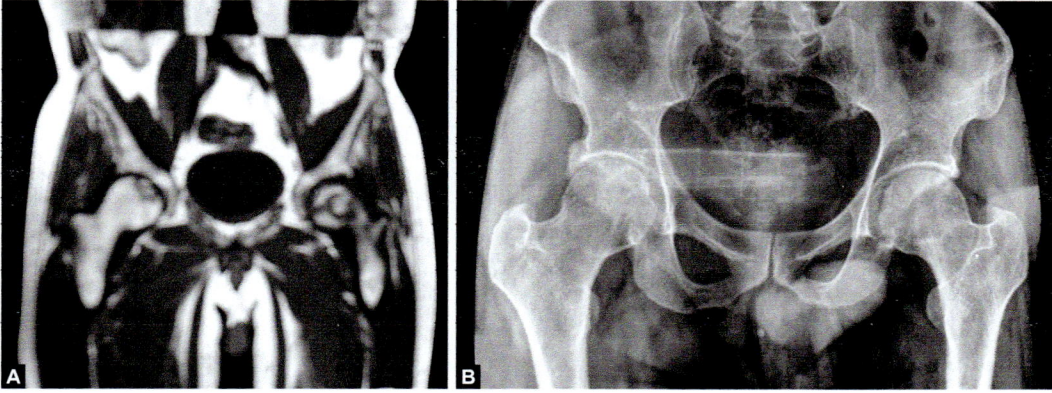

Figs. 5.3A and B: Avascular necrosis of both femoral heads: (A) MRI shows an early stage; (B) X-ray shows healing on conservative treatment.

persons (high demand patients) polyethylene wear and metal particles remain a concern **(Figs. 5.4 and 5.5)**.

Nonoperative Treatment

It is justified in lesions in Ficat stage I or Shimizu grade I or lesions less than one-third of the femoral head, and those in nonweight-bearing segment of femoral head in the precollapse stage. It comprises nonweight bearing walking for 2–3 months and protected weight-bearing for another 2–3 months. Full range of motion and active exercises are done for 10 minutes 6 times a day. Low dose anticoagulants or small dose aspirin may be tried for 3–6 months. Bisphosphonates have been found to be useful and may be tried for 6–12 months **(Figs. 5.1 and 5.3)**. Benefits of prolonged use of bisphosphonates are debatable because biologically it retards the process of bone turnover. Some of the smaller lesions may undergo resolution. More laterally placed lesions have the worst prognosis. Many pharmacological agents have been tried by various workers depending upon the philosophy or possibility of the causative factors. The trials have been made with lipid-lowering drugs, anticoagulants, vasodilators, and bisphosphonates. Biophysical modalities like pulsed electromagnetic field, extracorporeal shock therapy, ultrasonotherapy and hyperbaric oxygen (HBO), have also been tried. Hyperbaric oxygen therapy has limitations of intriguing facilities needed and the time needed.

Operative Treatment for Early Cases

Core decompression alone is based upon the reduction in intraosseous pressure to prevent further ischemia and infarction. It is most suitable for small lesions (<25% of weight-bearing area) in the precollapse stage. If the lesion is larger than 30% of weight-bearing area and it is precollapse or collapse with <5 mm of step-off, it is wise to do core decompression combined with fresh autologous cancellous bone grafting. The goal of femoral head preservation is to remove the necrotic bone and replace it with bone graft. A structural bone graft obtained from fibula or cancellous bone graft from the ipsilateral iliac bone can be inserted through the core decompression track or separately through an elliptical trapdoor made in front of the femoral neck near the articular margin. Core decompression is best done by making multiple tracks up to the lesion by using drill bit of the size of 3–5 mm. Best results are obtained with smaller lesions, more medially placed with no gross depression of the articular margins. This is a simple procedure best performed under C-arm, it fulfills four major objectives: Removes the necrotic bone, decompresses the intraosseous tension,

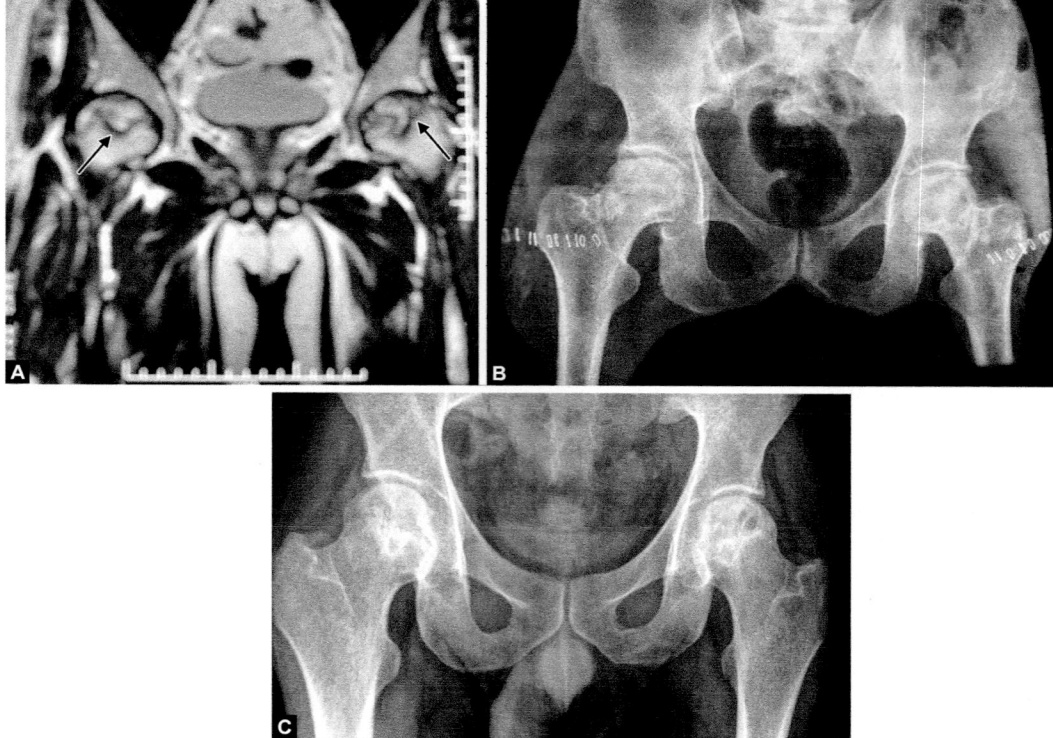

Figs. 5.4A to C: Avascular necrosis of bilateral femoral heads. (A) MRI-T1 image would show the earliest changes, hypodense bands are the hyperemic borders separating the proximal ischemic bone from the normal bone. Ischemic bone generally gives a "geographical" appearance, arrows show reparative granulation tissue; (B) X-ray soon after core decompression (forage) and bone grafting; (C) Femoral heads show increased density (new bone formation), spherical appearance and good cartilage space and function 9 years after core decompression operation.

bone grafts provide mechanical support for possible prevention of collapse of the weight-bearing articular surface, fresh grafts provide a source of pluripotent bone marrow stem cells (contained in autogenous cancellous bone) to produce neo-angiogenesis accompanied/followed by neo-osteogenesis. This procedure would possibly preserve and restore sphericity of femoral head and preserve the articular cartilage. If performed for Ficat II and early stages of Ficat III, 70% of patients were happy with the outcome at 10 years after the operation. Core decompression with or without bone grafts can be successfully done at hospitals with moderate infrastructure available. All such patients must be kept under observation, because 80% of them may need arthroplasty procedures after about 10–15 years **(Figs. 5.4 and 5.5)**.

Core decompression with or without bone grafting can be performed either (i) through the cores created from the lateral cortex of femur starting about one cm distal to the greater trochanter reaching up to the femor head, or (ii) through an hexagonal diamond-shaped window made through the anterior cortex of femoral neck almost reaching up to the articular cartilage. Using multiple drill holes and curets the avascular necrotic part of femoral head is enucleated. The void created is compactly packed with

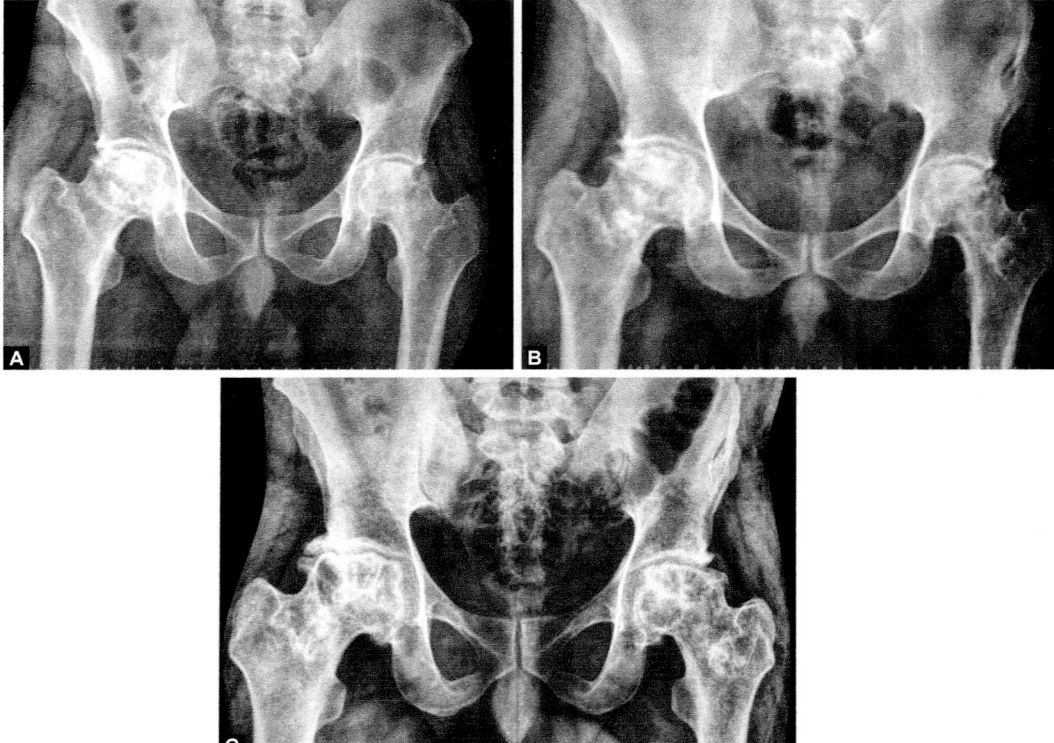

Figs. 5.5A to C: X-rays of osteonecrosis in a young patient of 22 years. (A) Advanced changes at presentation; (B) 3 years after core decompression and bone grafting; (C) At 12 years postoperation follow-up, heads show irregular texture and articular margins. The joint (cartilage) space is maintained. Patient is able to continue activities of daily living, thus, postponing the necessity of joint replacement.

fresh autogenous cancellous bone harvested from the neighboring iliac crest. The curetted material is sent for histological examination. Partial weight-bearing is permitted after 3–4 weeks for hips with core decompression alone, and after 6–8 weeks for hips who had core decompression with bone grafting.

The author tried **muscle-pedicled bone graft** by anterior route based upon sartorius (**Figs. 5.6 and 5.7**) or tensor fascia lata, and by posterior approach based upon quadratus femoris. These are, however, complicated operations with postoperative wound healing problems. Vascularized free fibular grafting has been tried by some workers, however, this is technically demanding and a time-consuming operation and it requires a highly specialized team. Other more "drastic procedures" are indicated for advanced cases of osteonecrosis and those who have failed the head preservation procedure; these are **osteotomies of proximal femur** to move the necrotic segment of femoral head away from the weight-bearing area and to bring the less involved segment of femoral head to the weight-bearing area. Femoral head resurfacing, or bipolar hip replacement or total hip replacement are indicated as changes in femoral head deteriorate. Arthrodesis is not considered a good option because the changes of AVN are present in both hips in 40–80% of patients.

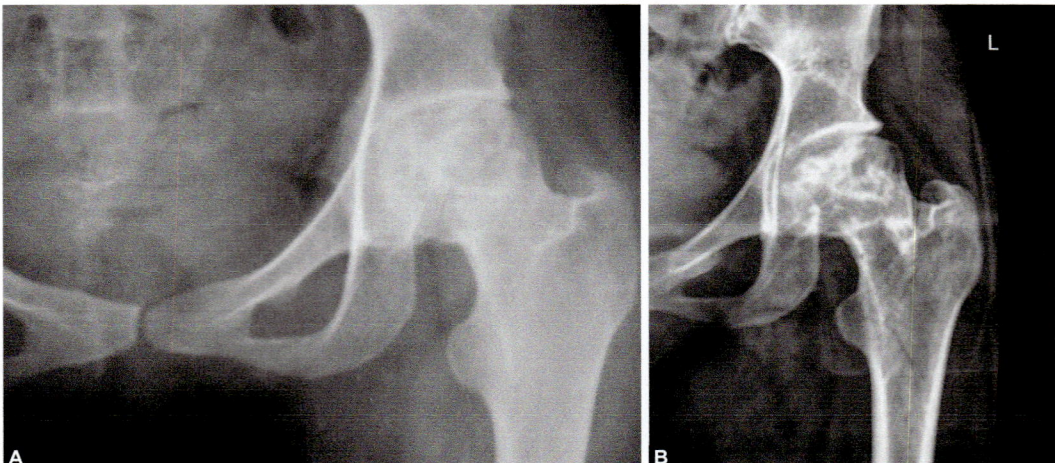

Figs. 5.6A and B: Post-pregnancy avascular necrosis of the femoral head in a young lady of 28 years. (A) A large necrotic segment of the femoral head is obvious, (B) Sartorius-based pedicled bone grafting was performed through anterior approach, 10 years after one can appreciate the incorporated bone graft, reasonable retention of the shape of femoral head and the joint cartilage space.

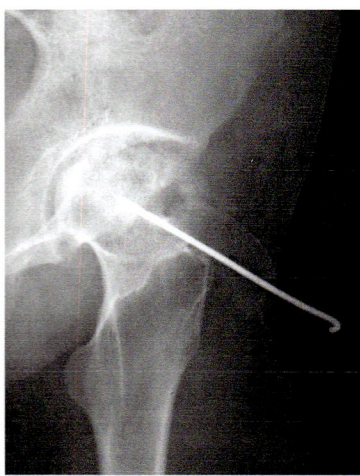

Fig. 5.7: Pedicle bone graft for avascular necrosis of left femoral head: This is an example of sartorius based iliac crest (4–6 cm) pedicled bone graft used for a large necrotic segment of femoral head. Soon after operation.

"Open" Operative Technique for Hip

Make a transverse incision almost parallel to the inguinal ligament from just lateral to the palpable femoral artery going laterally to about 1 cm medial to the prominence of the greater trochanter. Cut the skin and superficial fascia and expose the deep fascia. Split the deep fascia longitudinally for 8–10 cm. Now use deep retractors and retract the lateral lip of deep fascia and tensor fascia laterally, and retract the medial lip of deep fascia, sartorius, rectus femoris and iliopsoas medially. You are now in front of the femoral neck, still covered by the capsule. Slit the capsule from the articular margin to the base of femoral neck, expose the bone and make the window as needed in the anterior cortex of the femoral neck.

Any procedure where bone grafts are used, the repair takes place through neovascularization and neo-osteogenesis. The newly formed bone is very vascular and spongy. Under optimum environments adequate mineralization takes place in 2–3 months after the operation. Postoperatively encourage the patient to do active nonweight-bearing exercises (in bed or sitting on chair) from 3rd day onwards. Permit ambulation with walker on two crutches: no foot touch for 3 weeks, only toe touch for 3 weeks, forefoot touch for 3 weeks, full-foot touch for 3 weeks. Most of the patients are able to manage normal activities for 15–20 years after the femoral head preservation operations.

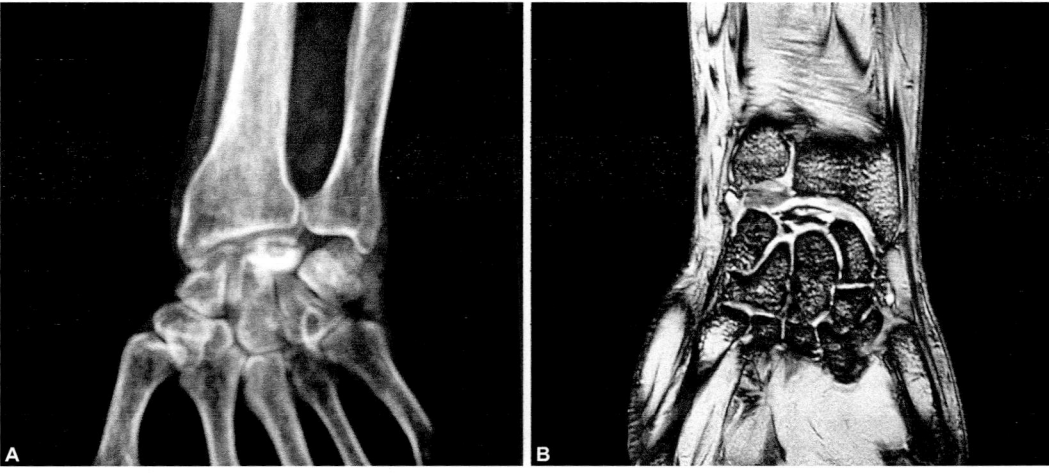

Figs. 5.8A and B: (A) Classical avascular necrosis of the lunate bone (Kienböck's disease) showing increased density and fragmentation; (B) MRI of another patient showing complete collapse of the lunate.

OSTEONECROSIS OTHER THAN FEMORAL HEAD

Avascular necrosis of humeral head and other nonweight-bearing bones are best treated by range of motion exercises, symptomatic treatment and bisphosphonates **(Figs. 5.8A and B)**. In general, symptoms are mild and intermittent; rarely you may need core-decompression with or without bone grafting. AVN in other weight-bearing bones like lower end of femur, talus, or upper end of tibia occurs rarely. In general, treatment is nonoperative; however, for disabling pain core decompression with bone grafting is suggested. In advanced stage of disease with disabling pain, gross reduction in the cartilage space, significant incongruity of the articular surfaces and absence of useful motion, "drastic options" may be justified. Arthroplasty becomes an inevitable option in such cases.

No single procedure has emerged as the gold standard for all patients largely because of many variables in each case such as the age, possible causative agent, stage and extent of disease, concomitant medical comorbidities, and patient's expectations. By no means one can give a normal hip joint, therefore, expectations of patient and family must be tempered.

SUGGESTED READINGS

1. Ficat RP. Idiopathic bone necrosis of the femoral head; Early diagnosis and treatment. J Bone Joint Surg. 1985;67B:3-9.
2. Shimizu K, Moriya H, Akita T, Sakamoto M, Suguro T. Prediction of collapse with magnetic resonance imaging of avascular necrosis of the femoral head. J Bone Joint Surg Am. 1994;76A:215-23.
3. Agarwala S, Shah SB. Ten-year follow-up of avascular necrosis of femoral head treated with alendronate for 3 years. J Arthroplasty. 2011;26:1128-34.
4. Chughtai M, Piuzzi NS, Khlopas A, Jones LC, Goodman SB, Mont MA. An evidence-based guide to the treatment of osteonecrosis of the femoral head. Bone Joint J. 2017;99-B:1267-79.
5. Ververidis AN, Paraskevopoulos K, Keskinis A, Ververidis NA, Moustafa RM, Tilkeridis K. Bone marrow edema syndrome/transient osteoporosis of the hip joint and management with the utilization of hyperbaric oxygen therapy. J Orthop. 2020;22: 29-32.

CHAPTER 6

Common Metabolic Bone Disorders

Calcium is an important regulator of many cellular functions including muscle contraction, intracellular signal transmission and control of cell membrane potentials. Calcium homeostasis is maintained through interactive influence between skin, intestines, liver, kidneys and bones. Though skeleton is used as a reservoir of calcium, however, calcium metabolism is influenced almost by all major hormones in the body such as vitamin D, parathormones, estrogens, androgens, corticosteroids, thyroid hormones and calcitonin. Metabolic bone diseases result from a disruption in the balance between the normal process of bone formation, mineralization, and bone remodeling. Calcium and phosphorus have an essential role in many physiological processes in the body. Over 98% of body's calcium and 85% of phosphorus are tightly packed as hydroxyapatite crystals in the bone. A small amount exists in a rapidly exchangeable form in blood and extra-cellular fluids in the body.

NORMAL AGE-RELATED CHANGES IN BONES

During **childhood or growing age**, each bone increases in size; bones get longer and wider, though the bone tissue remains quite (somewhat) porous till the age of puberty. Diaphyseal areas of bone increase in diameter by subperiosteal appositional bone deposition, medullary canal widens by endosteal resorption and the bulbous bone ends are sculpted and grow in height and width by endochondral bone formation by the growth plate, the physis.

Between **puberty and 30 years** of age, the bone texture becomes filled up, the cortices become thicker and in general bones become heavier and stronger. Bone mass increases at the rate of about 3% per year and during the third decade, each individual attains a state of "peak bone mass". In general, peak bone mass is 5–10% greater in men than in young women. The peak bone mass depends upon nutritional status, exercises, genetics, environments and hormonal factors. The greater is the peak bone mass, the less marked will be the effects of the inevitable depletion of bone mass, which starts in later life.

Between **30 and 40 years** of life, there is very small bone loss—about 0.3% per year in men and 0.5% is women. However, from the onset of menopause (40–50 years) in women and climacteric (60–70 years) in men, the rate of loss of bone mass accelerates to about 3% per year. With **advancing years of age**, the loss of peak bone mass is accompanied by loss of bone strength. During each remodeling cycle, bone resorption exceeds the bone formation. The maximum changes are seen in the trabecular bones; perforations and gaps appear in the plates and cross-spars. Radiologically, the first trabeculae to disappear are the secondary tensile trabeculae followed by secondary compression trabeculae, primary tensile trabeculae and finally the primary compression trabeculae. These changes lead to increased bone fragility (clinically addressed as osteoporosis) resulting in fractures due to trivial trauma or insufficiency fractures without trauma. Stress fractures have been observed even in apparently healthy persons (not used to physical activities), newly recruited soldiers, ballet dancers and newly appointed nurses. Osteoporosis is defined as reduction in the amount of bone per given volume of bone, without a change in its composition. Aging individuals may also have some degree of concomitant osteomalacia due to lack of dietary vitamin D and poor exposure to sunlight. During the repair cycle of bone remodeling, the osteoid does not get mineralized and one can observe Looser's zones (or lines) on the concave sides of femoral neck, superior and inferior pubic rami and proximal tibia, fibula, humerus, axillary border of scapula and any other bone **(Figs. 6.1A to C)**. Mass of skeleton, architecture, thickness and direction of trabeculae are adjusted according to functional load bearing (function determines form—Wolff's law).

RICKETS IN CHILDREN AND OSTEOMALACIA IN ADULTS

In these conditions, osteoid formation is normal but there is deficiency in the mineralization of the osteoid **(Figs. 6.2 and 6.3)**.

Rickets in growing children and osteomalacia in adults are (with rare exceptions) caused by deficiency of vitamin D or a disturbance in its absorption and metabolism. In children, at the calcification front, bone matrix is formed, however, it does

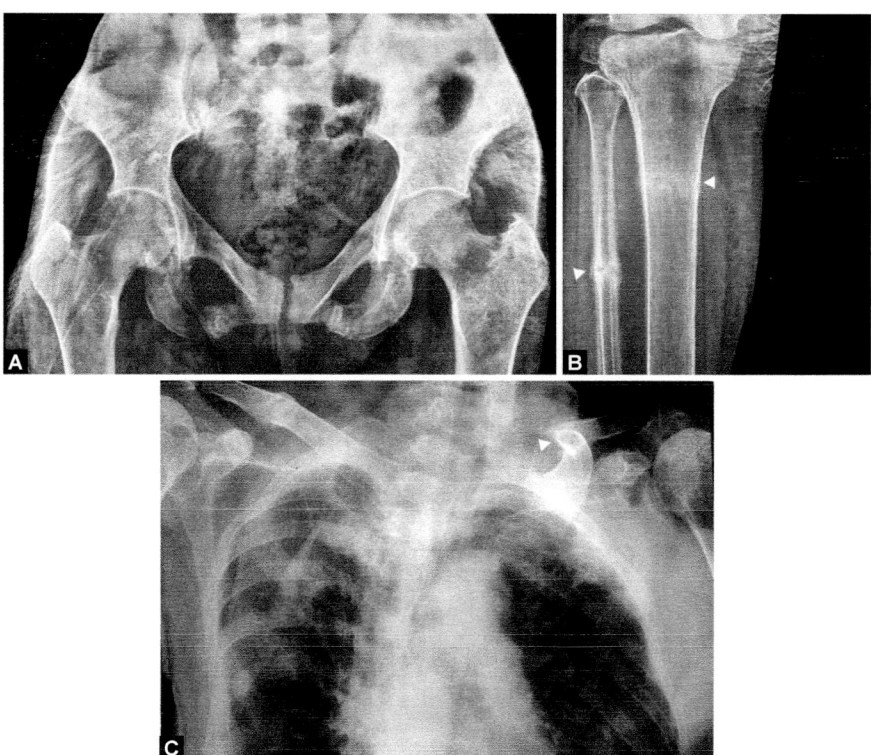

Figs. 6.1A to C: Characteristic radiological features of osteomalacia showing Looser's zones: (A) In pubic rami; (B) Fibula, and tibia; (C) Clavicles and ribs. It takes a few weeks for such fracture lines to be appreciated in conventional X-rays, however earliest evidence is possible by the use of MRIs and ultrasonography.

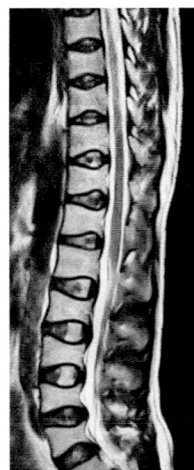

Fig. 6.2: Osteomalacia in young person: Showing generalized biconcave vertebral bodies and biconvex discs.

not get mineralized. In adults, at the site of (rapid) bone turn-over, the bone matrix is formed, however, (like children) it does not get mineralized. These conditions occur in underprivileged populations throughout the world due to lack of exposure to sunrays, social customs of using veils, due to compromised living conditions and diet poor in dairy products (milk and curd) and vitamin D. Compromised liver and renal function and prolonged use of anticonvulsants can also lead to changes like rickets and osteomalacia.

Children with nutritional rickets present with delayed growth, bony deformities around the wrists, ankles and the epiphyseal region of long bones, costochondral junctions

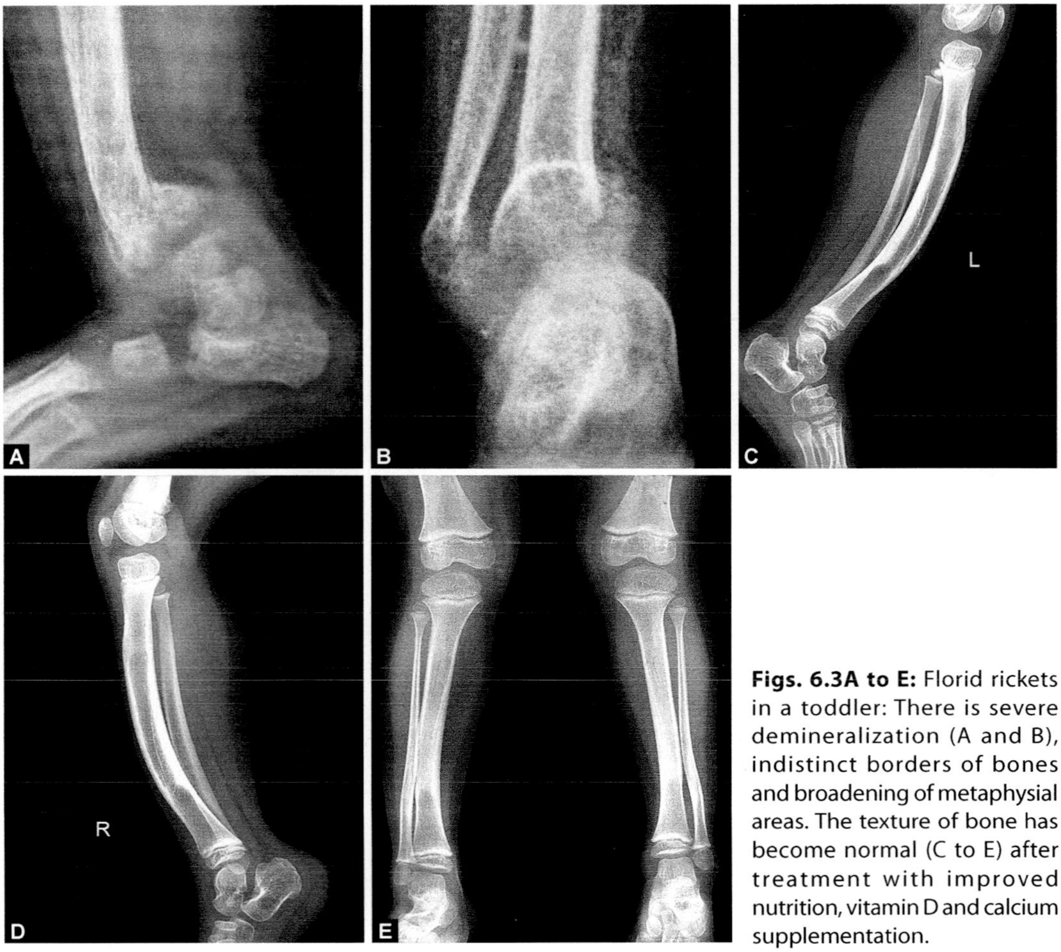

Figs. 6.3A to E: Florid rickets in a toddler: There is severe demineralization (A and B), indistinct borders of bones and broadening of metaphysial areas. The texture of bone has become normal (C to E) after treatment with improved nutrition, vitamin D and calcium supplementation.

(producing rickety rosary) and bossing of forehead. In general, normal lower limb alignment in children varies up to the age of 12 years: from birth to 2 years varus angulation of 10–15 degrees, from 2 to 3 years neutral alignment, from 3 years onwards valgus angulation of 10–15 degrees, around 10–12 years almost an adult pattern of about 6–8 degrees of valgus is achieved. Deformities created by endocrine defects like genu varum or genu valgum are an accentuation of the pre-existing physiological alignment in the growing age: generally below the age of 3 years genu varum and above the age of 3 years genu valgum is observed **(Figs. 6.4A and B)**. Deformities in the weight-bearing bones may also occur leading to genu valgum (knock knees), bowed legs (genu varum and tibia varum). In severe cases, weakness of muscles around the hips (proximal myopathy) may produce difficulty in getting up from the floor or low chair, and difficulty in walking. In more severe cases, hypocalcemia may produce tetany, carpopedal spasm and rarely stridor.

In rickets, radiographs show a widening of the growth plate and increase in the vertical height of the growth plate (due to lack of mineralization of proliferated cartilage zone), the metaphyses appear cup shaped, widened and ragged. Generalized demineralization of the skeleton (thinning of bone cortices) is present. In adolescents and adults, Looser's lines (unmineralized osteoid) can be detected on the medial borders of femoral neck, long bones, pubic rami, axillary borders of scapulae and other bones **(Figs. 6.5 to 6.9)**.

Renal Rickets

The commonest variety is nutritional rickets or malabsorption rickets, however, rickets are also caused by various defects in the renal functions. Renal rickets may be caused by defective glomeruli and tubules (chronic nephritis, polycystic kidneys). Dysfunction of tubules to re-absorb phosphates from the glomerular filtrate leads to "vitamin D resistant rickets", and such patients respond to massive doses of vitamins. Inability of proximal renal tubules to re-absorb phosphates, glucose and amino acids also cause rickets known as Fanconi syndrome **(Table 6.1)**.

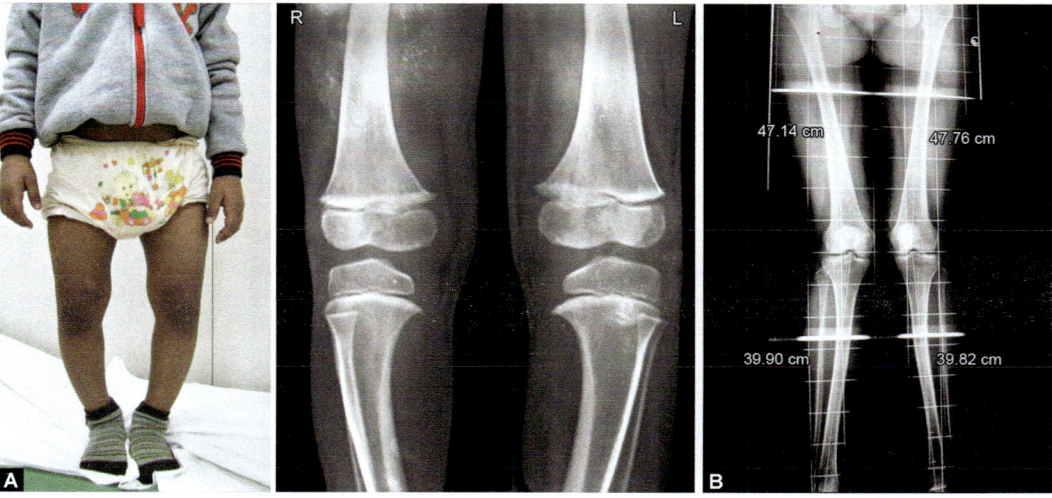

Figs. 6.4A and B: (A) Clinical picture and X-rays of genu varum usually initiated below the age of 3 years; (B) A scanogram of both lower limbs showing genu valgum deformity usually initiated after 3 years of age.

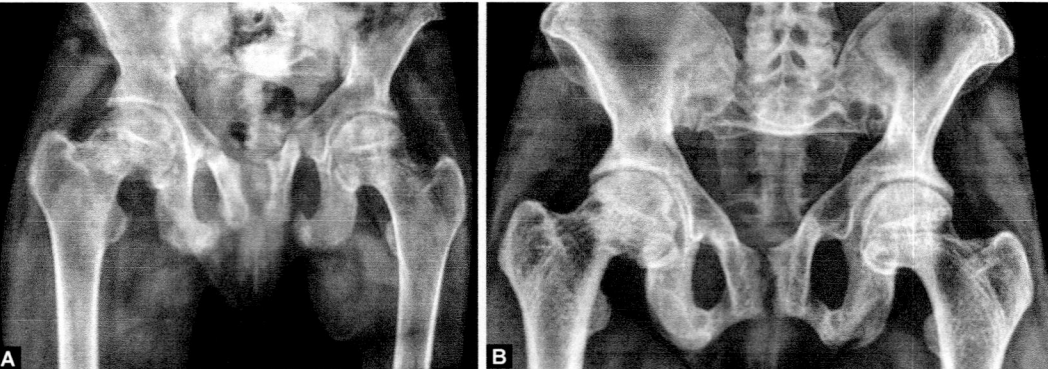

Figs. 6.5A and B: (A) X-ray of a young lady (20 years) showing Looser's zones in pubic rami and femoral neck, and generalized demineralization of visible bones in a case of severe osteomalacia; (B) X-ray of the same patient 1 year after the treatment. Note healed Looser's zones and remineralization of the visible bones, however the triradiate shape of the pelvis persists.

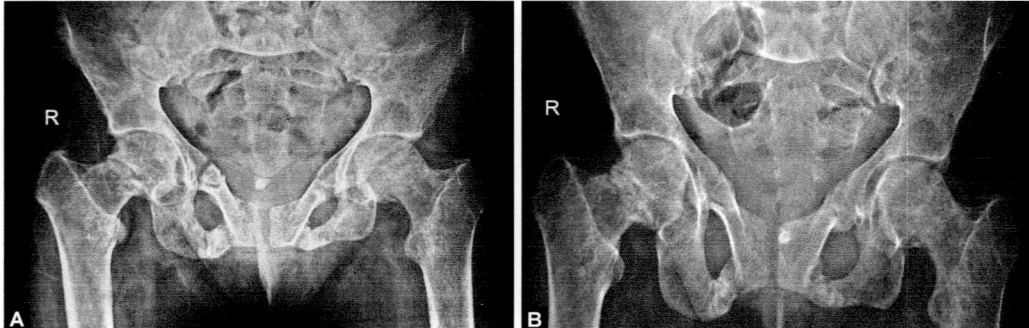

Figs. 6.6A and B: Osteomalacia: Inadequate mineralization of skeleton in adults is addressed as osteomalacia. The osteoid throughout the bones is poorly mineralized showing as Looser's zones (A) in this patient in pelvic bones and femora. After treatment (B) the Looser's zones have healed, however the trefoil (triradiate pelvis)shape of pelvis has not changed.

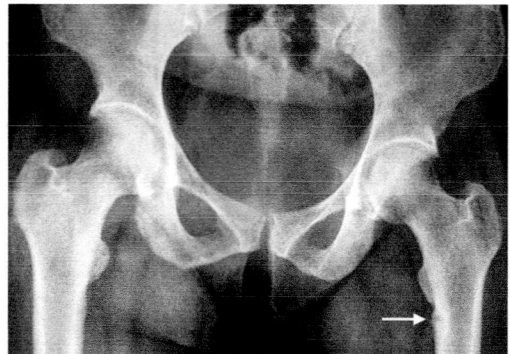

Fig. 6.7: Insufficiency fracture or Looser's zone in left femur.

CORRECTION OF DEFORMITIES

Regardless of the causes of abnormal metabolism, children with rickets have similar long bones and trunk deformities. In very young children (younger than 5 years), medical treatment of metabolic defects supplemented by corrective splinting or bracing for 6–12 months may correct the deformity. Between the age of 6 and 12 years most of the patients would require corrective osteotomy for unacceptable deformities of the lower extremities. Deformities near the joints are best corrected by osteotomies at

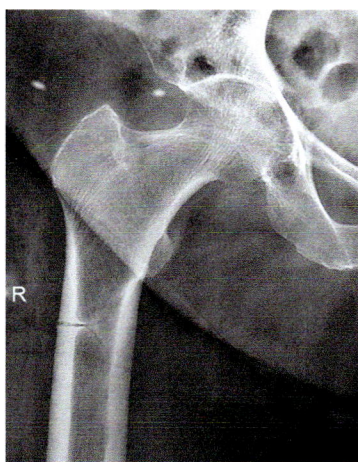

Fig. 6.8: Stress fracture (also called Fatigue, Insufficiency, March fracture): A break in continuity of an apparently healthy bone, caused by recurring and repetitive unaccustomed trauma.

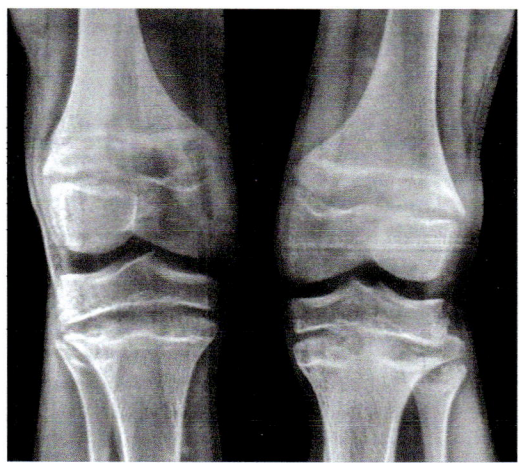

Fig. 6.9: X-rays of active rickets in a child. Note widening (flared) and cupping of growth plates, widening of metaphyseal area and generalized demineralization.

Table 6.1: Biochemical changes in different types of rickets.			
	Nutritional rickets	Renal tubular (Vitamin D resistant)	Renal (failure) glomerular
Plasma			
Ca	↓	N	↓
P	↓	↓	↑
Alkaline phosphatase	↑	↑	↑
Urine			
Ca	↓	↓	↓
P	↓	↑	↓
(N: normal; Ca: calcium; P: phosphorus)			

metaphyseal–diaphyseal junction. Those involving the generalized diaphyseal bowing can be corrected by one or two osteotomies stabilized with intramedullary elastic nails. Attempts should be made to achieve correction before the age of puberty to minimize development of osteochondritis lesions (shedding of articular cartilage) in the neighboring joints.

Preoperative Planning

Before surgery medical management of the basic metabolic defects with vitamin D, phosphorus, calcium, supportive therapy should be carried out for a few months. Corrective osteotomies are best performed when the patient is metabolically stabilized before surgery, however massive doses of vitamin D should be discontinued for 7–10 days to avoid hypercalcemia during paraoperative immobilization. Mobilization of the patient as early as possible after operation should allow resumption of medical treatment.

The deformities that require surgical correction most often are genu varum and genu valgum. In genu valgum, most of the deformity is in femur and is corrected by supracondylar femoral osteotomy. In genu varum, there is usually a concomitant internal torsion of tibia, both are corrected by upper tibial osteotomy. Any correction of these deformities should also ensure that upper tibial joint line is horizontal (parallel to the ground) as seen in standing X-rays of knee joints.

GROWTH PLATE (PHYSIS) MODULATIONS (FIGS. 6.10A AND B)

An alternative to corrective osteotomies is growth modulations by physeal surgery. These procedures require close observations of the growth pattern of the involved bones. The best age to perform such procedures is between 7 to 11 years. The behavior of deformities is best judged by measuring the intercondylar distance in genu varum, and intermalleolar distance in genu valgum at each visit, rather than doing frequent X-rays. All procedures of "accelerating" the growth potential of the physis or it's selective "arrest" to correct deformity during growing age need more precision. Chondrodiastasis (physis stimulation) may lead to premature apoptosis of the physeal cells.

Risser's sign (Fig. 6.11) is a radiological ossification of the iliac crest apophysis. It become visible during late adolescence starting from anterior superior iliac spine proceeding up to posterior iliac spine. From start to the complete formation takes about 2 years. Once fused (stage 5), no appreciable growth of the skeleton takes place. Spinal deformity deteriorates most during the spikes of growth. Mild vertebral growth may take place even after complete fusion of iliac apophysis (stage 5). Risser's sign may help while planning growth modulation techniques for lower limb deformities

A physeal bar occupying the physis may be excised and replaced with autogenous

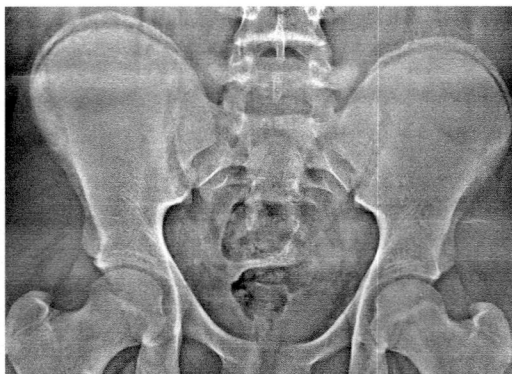

Fig. 6.11: Risser's sign: Iliac crest apophysis proceeds from anterolateral part to posteromedial area, Generally it takes 2 years for complete formation fron anterior to posterior end. Once the apophysis is fused no significant growth of vertebral column occurs thereafter.

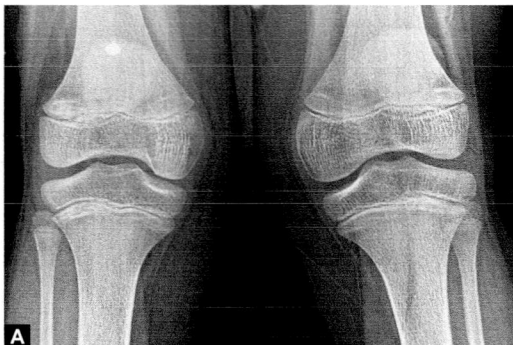
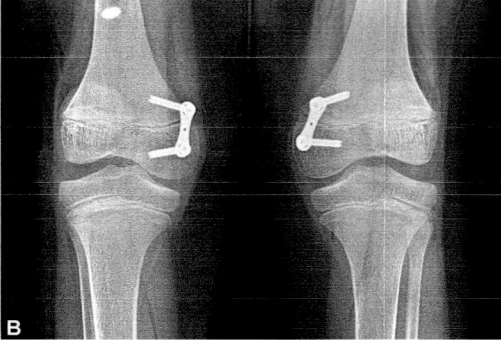

Figs. 6.10A and B: Significant genu valgum deformity: During growing age can be rectified by growth modulation techniques. Medial part of femoral physis has been arrested using plate and screws. One can appreciate the correction achieved.

fat, this may permit natural growth of the physis. Temporary arrest of the growth plate (physis) may be achieved by inserting staples or a small plate inserted astride the physis. The implants are retained till the deformity has been corrected, removal of the implants permits the resumption of growth. Epiphysiodesis may be used to arrest the growth of bones and chondrodiastasis may be used for lengthening of bone, close to the end of growth of the bone. Chondrodiastasis or physeal growth stimulation may gain some length, however the stimulated cells may undergo early apoptosis.

OSTEOPOROSIS

With changing demographics of the global population osteoporosis is probably the most important of the metabolic disorders of the bones.

It is a clinical disorder characterized by marked reduction of bone mass per unit volume of bone. Though histologically the remaining bone may not be very abnormal, however, in addition to reduction of bone mass there may be structural bone defects such as break in trabeculae and connecting bars. This combination of reduction of bone mass and mechanical breaks in structural connectivity results in (porous bones) reduction in the strength of bone. As a consequence the bones particularly around metaphyseal–diaphyseal junctions and cancellous bones especially in the vertebral column can get fractured even with modest trauma or without history of significant trauma. This description is applicable to generalized osteoporosis. However, in orthopedic practice one must be cognizant of the localized osteoporosis associated with immobilization and any inflammatory condition **(Table 6.2)**.

Commonly generalized osteoporosis is associated with exaggerated bone loss/depletion associated with postmenopausal or postclimacteric state, however, prolonged nutritional deficiency, oophorectomy, early hysterectomy, tobacco consumption

Table 6.2: Common causes of secondary osteoporosis unrelated to age.

Nutritional	Endocrine disorders
Malabsorption	Gonadal insufficiency
Malnutrition	Early menopause
Lack of vitamin D and calcium	Hyperparathyroidism
Scurvy	Thyrotoxicosis
	Cushing's disease
Inflammatory disorders	**Malignant diseases**
Rheumatoid disease	Carcinomatosis
Ankylosing spondylitis	Multiple myeloma
Tuberculosis	Leukemia
Drug induced	**Miscellaneous**
Corticosteroids	Smoking
Excessive alcohol consumption	Chronic obstructive pulmonary disease
Anticonvulsants	Osteogenesis imperfecta
Heparin	Chronic renal disease
Immunosuppressives	Poor exposure to sun-rays

(smoking or chewing), alcohol and substance abuse, sedentary lifestyle and chronic lack of exercise, and prolonged use of steroids and anticonvulsive drugs are also responsible for generalized osteoporosis. Genetic influences and family history of osteoporosis also play a role. Chronic diseases of kidney, lungs, and intestines may also contribute to the development of osteoporosis. Healthy lifestyle including exercises and diet are important to minimize the severity of osteoporosis. Common sources of calcium are milk and milk products, green leafy vegetables, beans and animal products.

Diagnosis

Generally, a woman near the menopausal age develops backache, increase in dorsal (round) kyphosis and slight diminution of her height. There may be history of fracture of distal radius or hip or ankle caused by low impact (fragility fractures) trauma. X-rays of spine may show wedging of one or more vertebral bodies, and generalized osteoporosis. The earliest radiological feature may be depression of proximal (upper) end plates of vertebral bodies. The common site for earliest changes is at dorsolumbar junction. Many of these patients may show calcification of the aorta, especially observed in patients having concomitant diabetes **(Fig. 6.12)**. Once osteoporosis is suspected in early cases, bone mineral density (BMD) measurements may help reach the diagnosis. Dexa scan may be helpful in suspected cases of premature osteoporosis, premature menopause, or patients on long-term steroids or for assessing the response to treatment in such patients. In an established case with clear radiological findings, BMD measurements are of no significance. Further investigations may be needed to exclude other pathologies like hyperparathyroidism, malignant disease (oncogenic osteoporosis), and hypercortisonism. Serum alkaline phosphatase is a reliable index of osteoblastic activity, the level is increased in osteomalacia, osteoporosis, bone metastasis, hyperparathyroidism, and Paget's disease.

Treatment

Women approaching menopausal age should be advised to maintain adequate intake of dietary calcium, vitamin D, and proteins. Active exercises of spine and whole body must be encouraged. Most of the patients would need nutritional supplements of calcium, vitamin D, and proteins. About 20 minutes of sun-rays exposure daily may also be helpful.

Hormone replacement therapy which was popular in twentieth century is rarely advised now because of growing concerns about apparent increased risk of thromboembolism, stroke, breast and uterine cancer. Bisphosphonates are now regarded as preferred antiresorptive drugs. These act by reducing osteoclastic activity and by reduction of overall bone turnover. The bone trabeculae laid over under the influence of bisphosphonates are, however, not exactly in the direction of functional stress (adynamic). Prolonged uninterrupted use has been reported to cause subtrochanteric fractures in active patients. Safe dose schedule suggested is continuous use for 9–12 months followed by a gap of 3–4 months. Parathyroid hormone, calcitonin and raloxifene (selective estrogen receptor modulator) have also been recommended in patients who do not respond to dietary supplements and bisphosphonates.

Bisphosphonates in Clinical Settings

Bisphosphonates are used in clinical practice in the treatment of osteoporosis, osteogenesis imperfecta, Paget's disease, osteonecrosis, Sudeck's complex regional pain syndrome (CRPS), and during the postoperative phase in incorporation of grafted bones (postoperative phase).

The normal bone turnover is a balance between the activities of osteoclastogenesis and osteoblastogenesis, use of bisphosphonates suppresses the osteoclastic activity

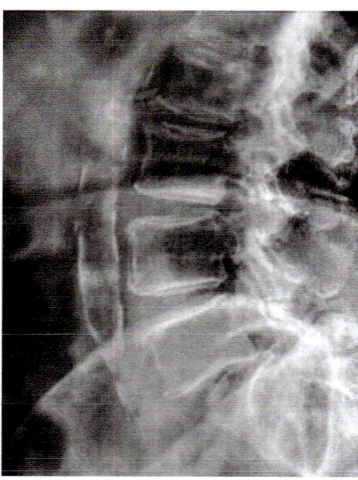

Fig. 6.12: Classical appearance of osteoporosis of spine. X-rays may show wedging of vertebral bodies and biconcave vertebral bodies. Many patients suffering from osteoporosis may show aortic calcification as in this X-ray. Most of these patients have concomitant diabetes. Mild listhesis is also present at L5-S1 level.

of bone resorption without any effect on mineralization. This temporarily increases the bone density. The new bone laid down during the period of influence of bisphosphonates is not laid down according to the pattern of functional needs of the bone. The pattern of bone trabeculae is in a "mosaic fashion" almost like Paget's disease. Continuous prolonged use (about 2 years or more) of bisphosphonates has been observed with atypical pathological or stress fracture in the subtrochanteric region of femur. About 1–2 years of treatment by bisphosphonates probably reduces the risk of fractures (vertebral and hip fractures) for the next 2–3 years. Despite the introduction of bisphosphonates for clinical use in 1995, the analysis of clinical observations have not been able to reach at consensus regarding the duration of use, possible effect of duration on fracture prevention, and prevention of complications (atypical subtrochanteric fracture) of long-term medication **(Fig. 6.13)**.

At present, there are many salts of bisphosphonates however in general clinical settings alendronate 35–70 mg is given every week with a full glass of water on empty stomach (about 30 minutes before breakfast), the patient is advised to walk for about 30 minutes or remain upright after taking the medication, to avoid esophageal irritation. After 9–12 months of use one should give a gap of 4–6 months before one starts the next course of bisphosphonates. There is at present probably no optimal bisphosphonate treatment regime, however it may depend upon bone turnover, age, fracture risk, renal function and the clinical conditions. In addition to bisphosphonates a variety of anti-resorptives are being tried and analyzed in clinical cases. In case of renal compromise calcitonin can be used safely.

Operative Intervention

Femoral neck fractures and fractures of other bones may need operative treatment or closed treatment. One should choose the methods which do not restrict the mobility of patients. Diaphyseal fractures are preferred to be treated by intramedullary nails. Most of the osteoporotic vertebral compression fractures can be treated successfully by nonoperative measures. Vertebral fractures are painful and these patients require rest in recumbent position for 3–6 weeks. As soon as pain subsides, the patient may be permitted partial activities for personal care with suitable spinal braces, spinal exercises must be continued on long-term bases. Operative intervention may be called for if there are neural complications.

In the presence of neural complications, anterior decompression of the dural tube is mandatory, with concomitant stabilization of the vertebral column. Less invasive techniques of vertebroplasty and balloon kyphoplasty are being tried to augment the height and strength of collapsed osteoporotic vertebrae under image intensifying facilities. These procedures need specialized training and sophisticated infrastructure facilities. Potential risks include cement leakage, infection, pulmonary embolus, pneumonia and adjacent level compression fractures. The author has seen (since 2005) two cases of cauda equina syndrome and one case of paraplegia with perpetuation of dorsal spine tuberculosis related to cementation.

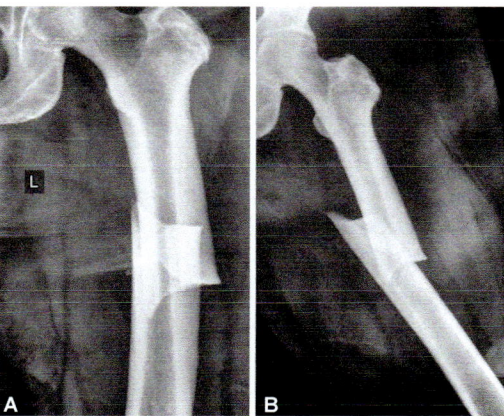

Figs. 6.13A and B: X-rays of femur showing prolonged use of bisphosphonates which may lead to an atypical (beak shaped) subtrochanteric fracture preceded by negligible trauma.

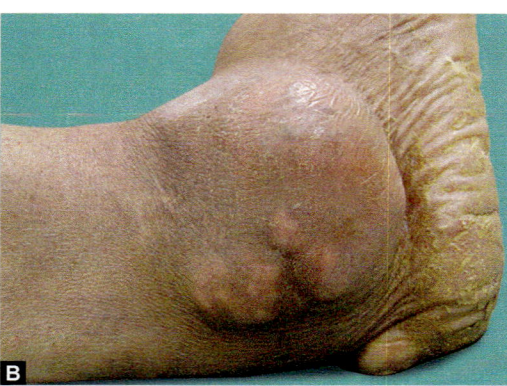
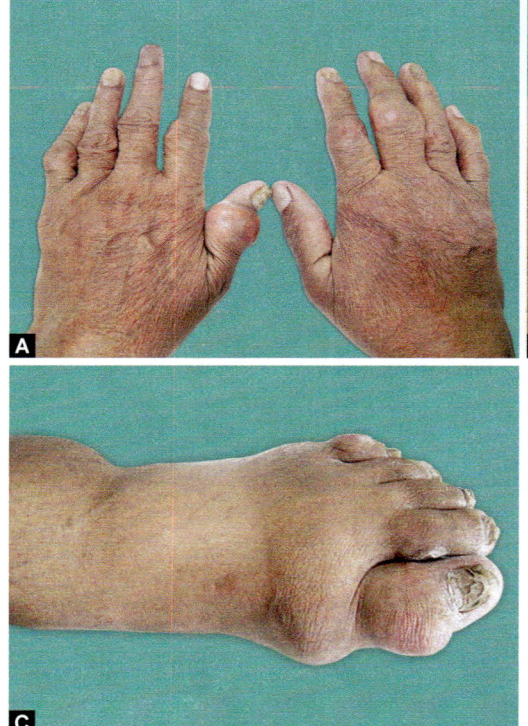

Figs. 6.14A to C: Gouty arthropathy: One can see large tophaceous gouty swelling of (A) hand, (B) ankle and (C) foot. The swelling around the great toe is the most typical. These swellings are the result of deposits of monosodium urate crystals in and around joints.

Gout (See also Chapter 18)

Gout is a metabolic disorder of the skeletal system caused by deposition of monosodium urate (MSU) crystals in and around the joints. Most commonly involved joints are first metatarsophalangeal joint, foot, ankle and knees. Generally affecting men above 40 years of age **(Figs. 6.14)**.

SUGGESTED READINGS

1. Mirsky EC, Einhorn TA. Bone densitometry in orthopaedic-practice. J Bone Joint Surg. 1998; 80A:1687-98.
2. Morris CD, Einhorn TA. Bisphosphonates in Orthopaedic surgery. J Bone Joint Surg. 2005; 87A:1609-18.
3. Pettifor JM. Vitamin D and/or calcium deficiency rickets in infants and children: a global perspective. Indian J Med Res. 2008;127:245-49.
4. Capeci CM, Tejwani NC. Bilateral low-energy simultaneous or sequential femoral fractures in patients on long-term alendronate therapy. J Bone Joint Surg Am. 2009;91A:2556-61.
5. Rosen CJ, Bouillon R, Compston JE, Rosen V, (Eds). Primer on the Metabolic Bone Diseases and Disorders of Mineral Metabolism. Oxford: Wiley-Blackwell, 2013.
6. Al-Rashid M, Ramkumar DB, Raskin K, Schwab J, Hornicek FJ, Lozano-Calderón SA. Paget disease of Bone. Orthop Clin North Am. 2015;46:577-85.

CHAPTER 7
Common Generalized Congenital Deformities and Dysplasias in Orthopedics

INTRODUCTION

The exact cause of congenital malformations and defects is not always clear. However, at present, intrinsic genetic factors, or mutations due to teratogenic agents working on the developing fetus, especially in the first trimester of pregnancy have been incriminated. Some few examples of teratogenic agents suspected in many congenital malformations and generalized dysplasias are German measles, cytomegalovirus, thalidomide, excessive maternal smoking and use of alcohol, prepregnancy folic acid deficiency, use of valproate, X-rays, ionizing radiation (e.g., post-atomic bomb radiation of Hiroshima and Nagasaki 1945), cyclophosphamides, anti-metabolic agents (methotrexate, leflunomide and antimitotic agents). Suspected teratogenic agents affect the embryo most, during the phase of tissue differentiation and organ formation (first trimester). Certain conditions such as congenital club feet, arthrogryposis tend to exhibit occurrence in many siblings and suggest the possibility of genetic transmission. All types of genetic disorders are more likely to occur in children of consanguineous marriages. Many rarer recessive defects and malformations have also been observed in these circumstances.

Single alleles of chromosome is addressed as carrier of a faulty trait, this however does not produce a clinically manifest disease/disorder. Contribution of two faulty genes (one from father and one from mother) in the making of the offspring would develop the disease; osteogenesis imperfecta is an example.

A large number of congenital musculoskeletal defects have been recognized, those with generalized manifestations have been "classified", however, there are others which still remain "unclassified". Outline of the least uncommon congenital defects is given in the following write up. Every time a patient presents with a congenital defect, we must determine whether the deformity is primary (due to local defects) or secondary (due to a defect in other parts of body) or compensatory (e.g., an equinus deformity acquired by the patient to compensate for the shortening of limb). Clinical examination must also determine whether the deformity is mobile (supple) and correctable, or fixed, uncorrectable by passive manipulations, is there any loss of sensations or circulation.

The complexities and subtleties of congenital abnormalities must be kept in mind while counseling the parents and families. With more awareness and available investigative facilities there is a constant subtle change in classifications.

CLINICAL DIAGNOSIS

All the skeletal dysplasias may not be obvious at birth. Whenever there is suspicion, such children must be kept under observation till maturity or puberty. Normal body proportions are achieved at the maturity of skeleton. From puberty onwards, length of upper segment (top of pubic symphysis to top of cranium) is equal to the length of lower segment (top

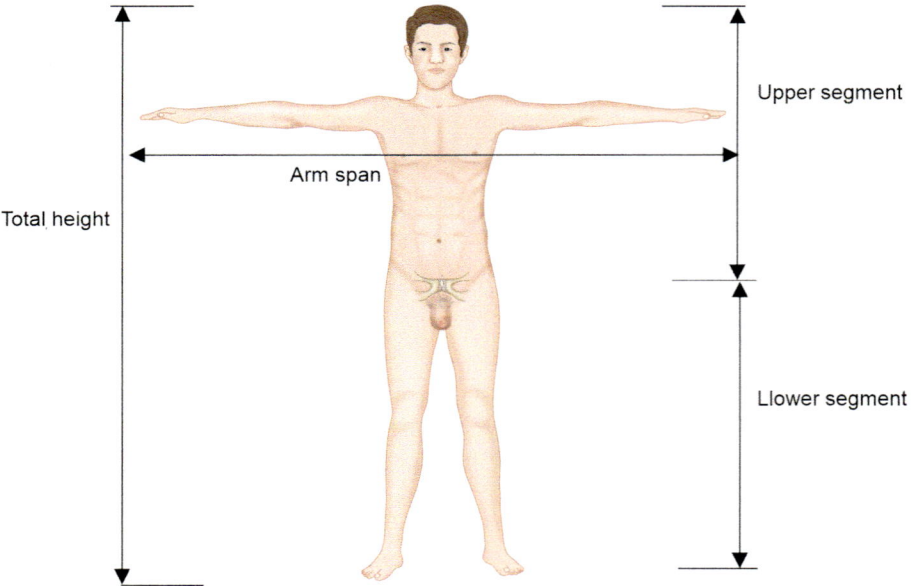

Fig. 7.1: Normal proportions. Upper segment = Lower segment; total height = Arm span.

of symphysis pubis to heel). Arm span (tip of left middle finger to tip of right middle finger in 90 degrees abduction of shoulders) is equal to the body height (top of the cranium to heels) **(Fig. 7.1)**. Retarted generalized growth, disproportionate length of trunk and limbs, localized deformities and soft tissue contractures and hyperlaxity suggest the possibilities of congenital dysplasias and deformities. Suspicion of a congenital defect warrants appropriate local X-rays; and in generalized dysplasia, limited skeletal survey which must include anteroposterior view of the pelvis including both hip joints. Attempt should be made to exclude metabolic skeletal disorders by blood examination for diabetes, thyroid, renal and hepatic functions.

Clinicoradiologically, **osteochondral skeletal deformities (Figs. 7.2 and 7.3) (dyplasias)** may be caused by:
- Predominantly epiphyseal changes—least uncommon = multiple epiphyseal dysplasia.
- Predominantly physeal and metaphyseal changes—least uncommon = hereditary multiple exostosis, achondroplasia, enchondromatosis.
- Predominantly diaphyseal changes least uncommon = osteopetrosis.
- Mixture of abnormalities least uncommon = spondylometaphyseal dysplasia.

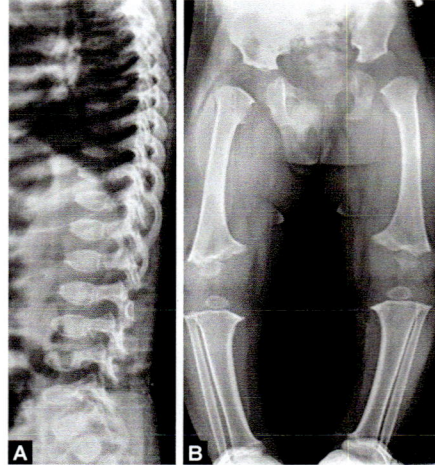

Figs. 7.2A and B: Osteochondral dysplasia: X-rays of a child showing abnormal development of all vertebrae and limb bones.

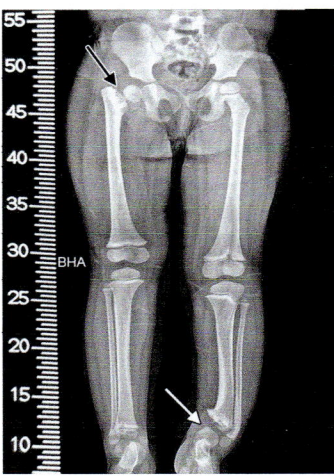

Fig. 7.3: Epiphyseal dysplasia: Note localized epiphyseal defect, right femoral neck showing congenital coxa vara, distal end left tibia showing dysplasia.

- Different segments of limbs may develop disproportionately, for general communication usual terminologies used are "Rhizomelia" = short proximal segments (femora, humeri), "Mesomelia" = short middle segments (forearm and legs), "Acromelia" = shortening of hands and feet, "Phocomelia" = attachment of hand or foot almost to trunk. In clinical practice however, one will find many overlapping combinations.

CONGENITAL CONNECTIVE TISSUE DISORDERS

Collagen is the commonest form of protein making 90 percent of matrix for mineralized tissues (bone), and 70 percent of the structure of ligaments and tendons. Heritable disorders of collagen synthesis result in a number of defects.
- Predominant defect in soft tissues: Least uncommon = generalized familial joint laxity, Marfan's syndrome.
- Predominant defect in bones: Least uncommon = osteogenesis imperfecta.
- Combined soft tissue and bones: Least uncommon = neurofibromatosis **(Fig. 7.4)**.

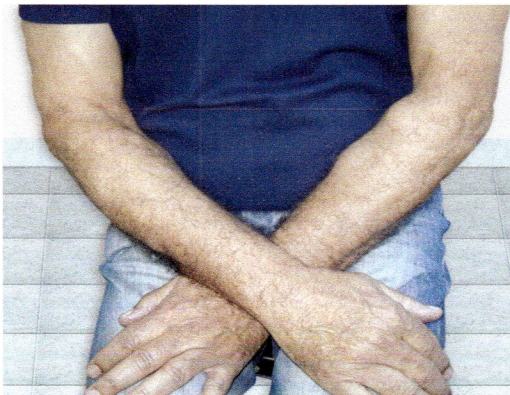

Fig. 7.4: Generalized neurofibromatosis. Note multiple subcutaneous "nodules" shown here on forearms.

GENERALIZED SKELETAL DYSPLASIAS

Neurofibromatosis

It is a genetic condition, which runs in families. The patients present with multiple neurofibromata in the skin. There may be associated deformities of the skeletal system like scoliosis, bone deformities, pseudarthrosis of tibia, and local gigantism of fingers or toes (macrodactyly). The nerve swellings in the spine may rarely lead to neural signs. Operative removal of the tumor must be confined to the neurofibromatas causing pressure symptoms. Many patients may have café-au-lait patches **(Figs. 7.5A to D)**. Café-au-lait spots may be present in normal population, however multiple spots may be associated with neurofibromatosis, polyostotic fibrous dysplasia, or Caffey's disease (infantile cortical hyperostosis).

Fibrous Dysplasia

In the normal skeleton, there is a balance between the process of bone resorption (osteoclastic activity) and the process of bone deposition (osteoblastic activity). In fibrous dysplasia, this balance is disturbed; the resorbed bone is replaced by fibro-osseous

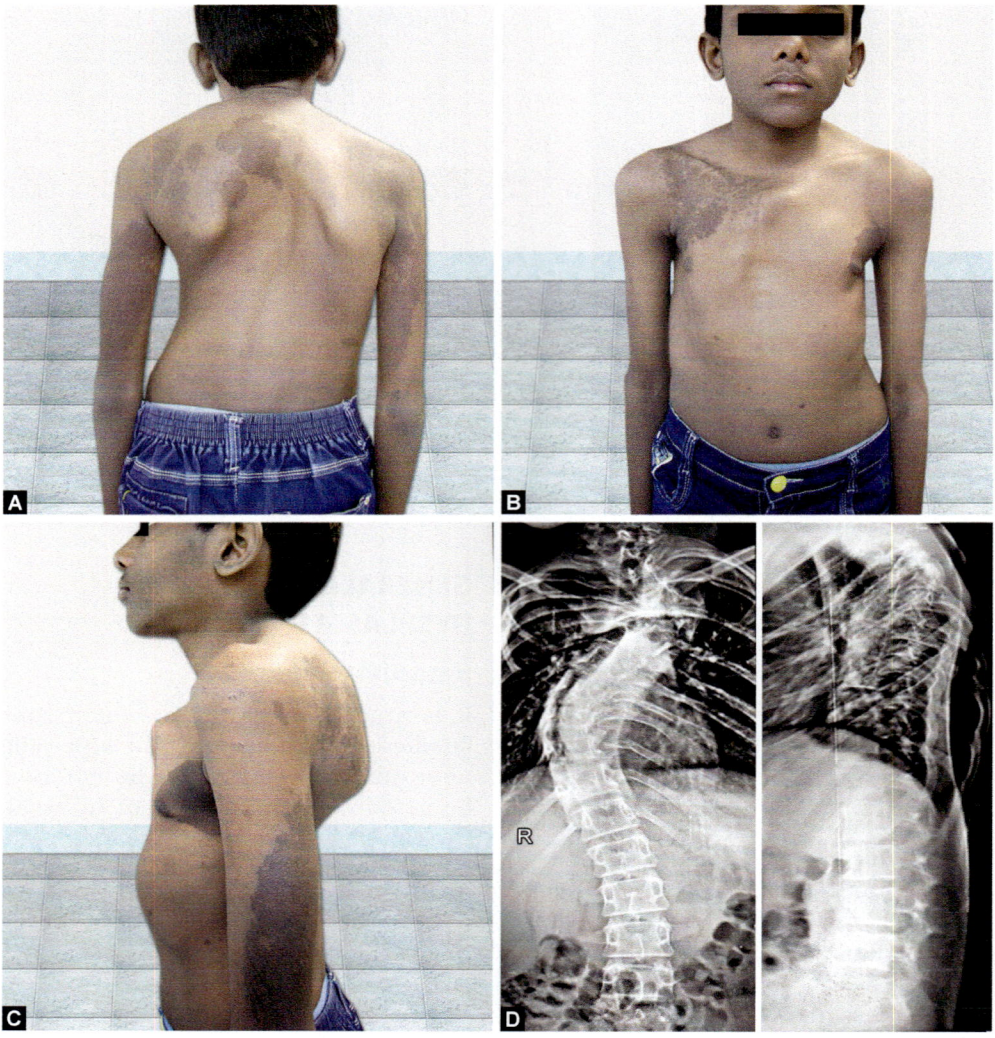

Figs. 7.5A to D: Generalized neurofibromatosis (a genetic disorder). Note large café-au-lait patches and kyphoscoliosis.

tissues rather than the normal osseous tissue. This leads to "cavitations" in bones, thinning of cortices, deformation or pathological fractures. The lesion may be monostotic or polyostotic. In a symptomatic patient, the bones commonly affected are femur, tibia, pelvis, humerus and facial bones. The lesions threatening the integrity of bone and ambulation must be treated by bone grafting after curettage. In the weight-bearing bones if the involvement is more than one third of the diameter, bone grafting is desirable. In a polyostotic condition, allogenic bank bone, repeated operations and use of bisphosphonates may keep such patients ambulatory. Autogenous bone grafts as a rule undergo resorption **(Figs. 7.6 and 7.7)**, because these may be "inherently defective".

Osteogenesis Imperfecta

This condition is an inherited disorder, a vast majority are the result of a defective autosomal dominant trait. The osteoblast is not able to produce adequate intercellular substances like osteoid, collagen and dentine. Prominent clinical features are multiple fractures with minimal trauma, blue sclera, early deafness, poor dentition, and joint laxity. "Osteogenesis imperfecta congenita" manifests in utero or at birth. "Osteogenesis imperfecta tarda" manifests later in childhood with delayed onset of fractures and milder manifestations. Fractures heal normally. The tendency to fractures decreases as the child reaches adulthood. Established deformities of femur or tibia may be corrected by multiple corrective osteotomies and intramedullary nailing using elastic nails. Bisphosphonates in a cyclical fashion are being tried to minimize the tendency to fracturing **(Figs. 7.8 and 7.9)**.

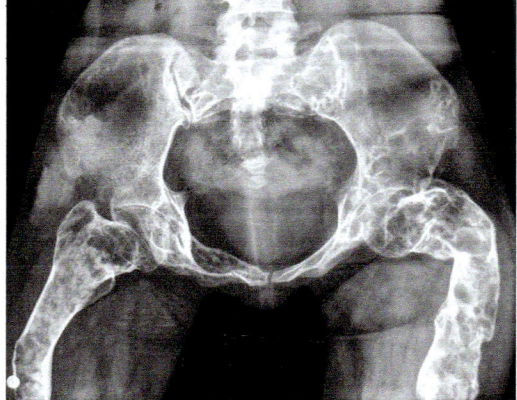

Fig. 7.6: Polyostotic fibrous dysplasia. Note involvement of all the bones visible in this X-ray. Because of softening of bones and multiple fractures, most of the weight-bearing bones would show deformations. Left hip in this X-ray shows the typical "Shepherd's crook" deformity.

Chondro-osteodystrophies

Chondro-osteodystrophies or generalized skeletal dysplasias are a heterogenous group of disorders characterized by abnormal cartilage and bone growth. In clinical practice, the predominant abnormalities may be in epiphyseal region, physeal and metaphyseal region, diaphyseal areas or a mixture of all these. When a patient

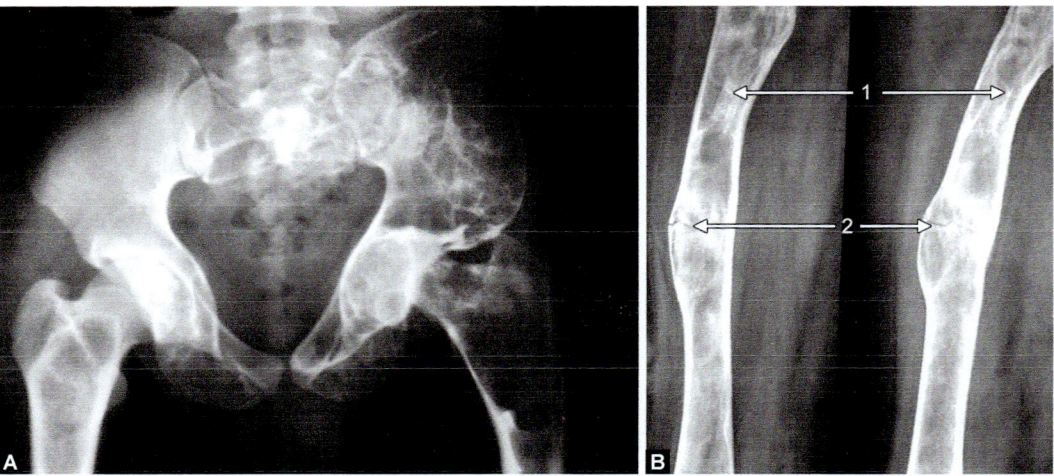

Figs. 7.7A and B: Polyostotic fibrous dysplasia showing involvement of all visible bones and a pathological fracture in the femur. Autogenous fibular graft inserted in the femur is showing resorption. (1) Resorbed fibula; (2) Stress fracture.

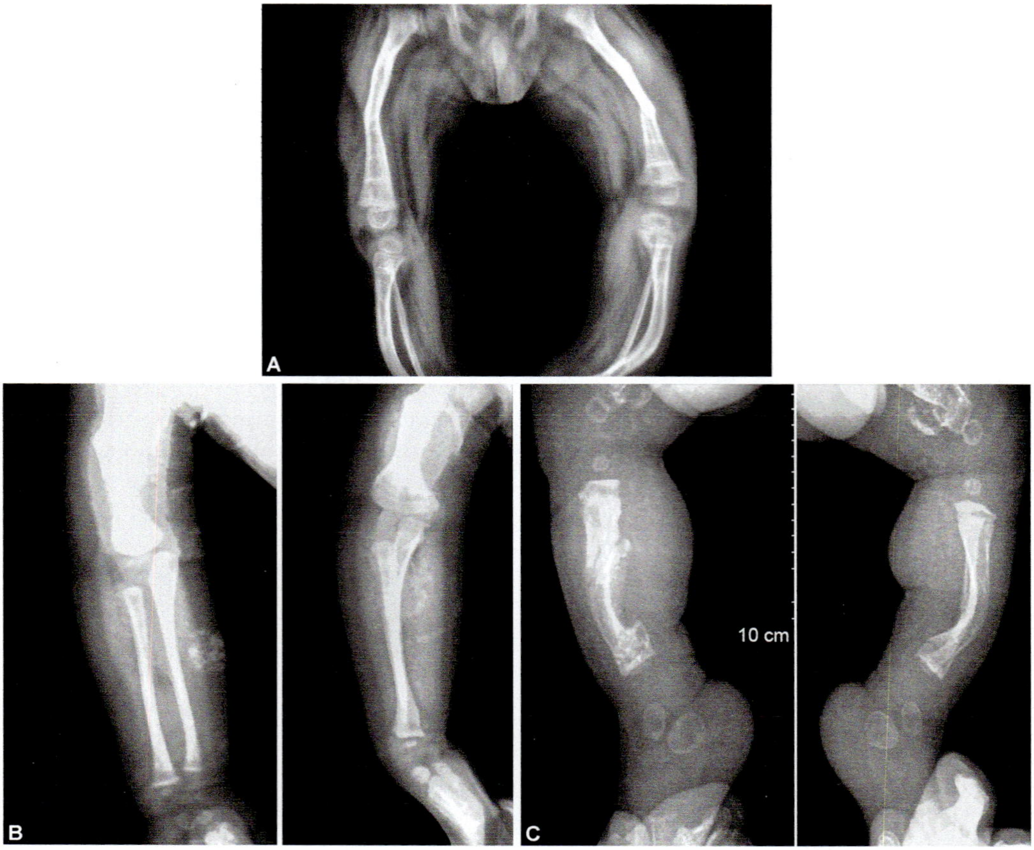

Figs. 7.8A to C: Osteogenesis imperfecta congenita: All bones of the limbs are showing fractures and deformities.

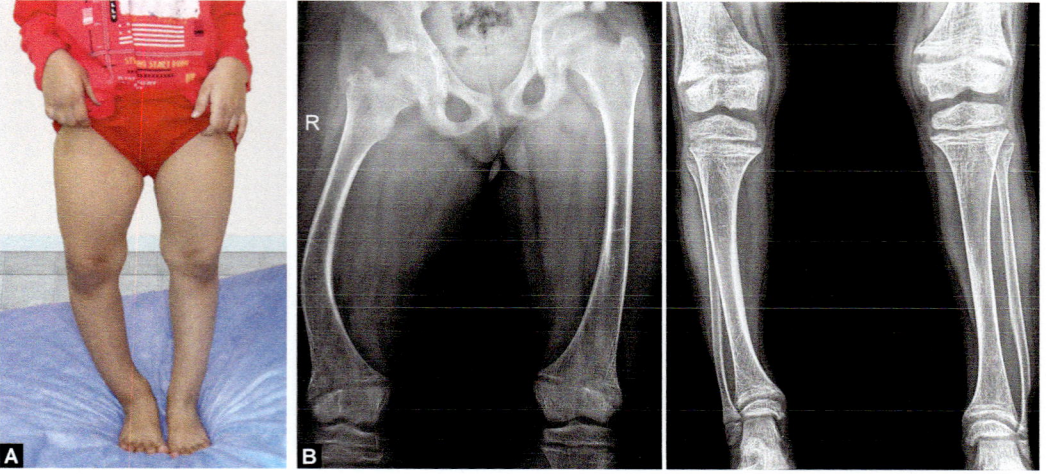

Figs. 7.9A to C: Osteogenesis imperfect tarda: The standing clinical picture (A) shows multilevel diaphyseal deformities of both lower limbs. X-rays (B) show the deformities of bones of low limbs.

presents with bilateral Perthes' disease, one must exclude generalized skeletal dysplasia, spondyloepiphyseal dysplasia, epiphyseal dysplasia, and hypothyroidism (in childhood). Symptomatic treatment is required to keep these children comfortable. After adulthood joint replacement for painful osteoarthrosis of hip or knee may be needed **(Figs. 7.10 and 7.11)**.

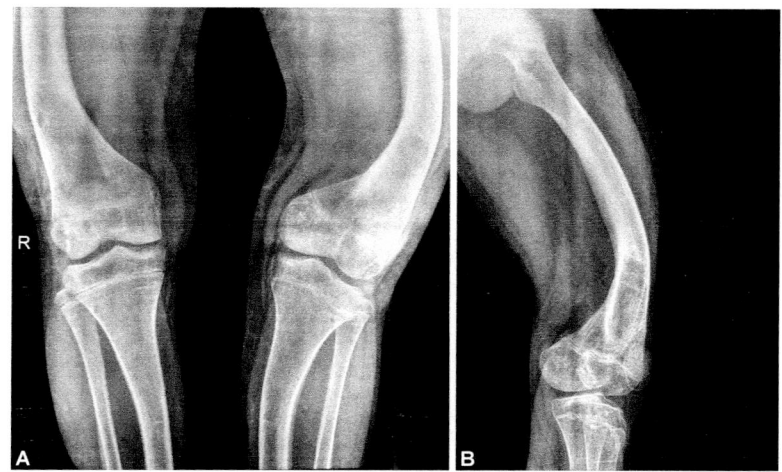

Figs. 7.10A and B: X-rays of a young child showing bowing (almost like kyphoscoliosis) of all bones of lower limbs. The condition may be addressed as a mild type of osteogenesis imperfecta tarda or unclassified generalized skeletal dysplasia. To keep the patient ambulatory, repeated corrective osteotomies were performed till the age of skeletal maturity.

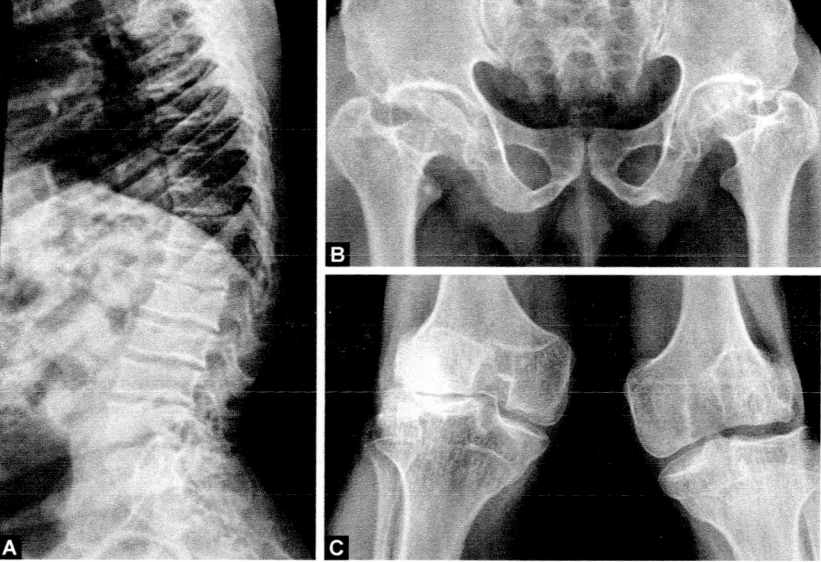

Figs. 7.11A to C: Classical appearance of generalized spondyloepiphyseal dysplasia. Note flattening of vertebral bodies, poorly formed hip joints and deformed knees.

BASIC PRINCIPLES OF DEFORMITY CORRECTION

Corrective Manipulations

Attempt for correction must be initiated soon after birth or as soon as the patient is attended by an orthopedician. Gently correct the deformity and hold in corrected position for about 10 seconds, about 15 excursions 4–5 times a day, in a child less than 4-weeks-old. When the child is about one-month-old, correct the deformities by gentle manipulations and hold in corrected position by strapping or by corrective plasters. The corrective plaster cast is changed every 3–4 weeks with addition to further correction. Generally, maximum correction can be achieved by the end of 4–6 manipulations. "Inevitability of gradual correction" (as emphasised by Paul Brand) is a universal rule for correction of any deformity by any technique.

Correction by "Wedging"

Flexion deformities of knee can be corrected by applying a padded plaster cast in maximum correction. A transverse cut is made on the concave side (popliteal aspect) running half-way around the girth of plaster. The cut plaster is opened to further correction (10–15 degrees at a time) and held in the corrected position by insertion of wooden wedge driven in the plaster gap. This "correction by wedging" can be repeated at 7–10 days interval. One can obtain a correction of up to 60–80 degrees by doing careful wedging over a period of 4–6 weeks. The transverse cut in the plaster cast is clinically made at the site of maximum deformity; however, error slightly toward proximal site is acceptable.

Wedge Correction by "Turn-buckle" Method

After making a cut in the plaster-cast (like wedging procedure), a turnbuckle is fixed onto the plaster in (along) the axis of the limb on the concave side of the deformity. The turnbuckle is slowly wound up to correct the deformity (not unlike Ilizarov's technique) over the next 3–4 weeks.

Botulinum toxin A (BTX-A) injections have been tried as intramuscular injection into the spastic muscle responsible for a deformity. The injection results in a temporary paralysis of the spastic muscle which facilitates stretch to correct the deformity by physiotherapy and/or by serial casting. There is however no clear evidence at present to suggest long-term benefits regarding time, expense and effort involved. BTX-A may help judge the efficacy of planned "Surgical Release" of the deforming muscles.

Correction Attempted Under Anesthesia

Sometimes, one may use manipulation under anesthesia. Correct the deformity by gentle sustained pressure and apply a well-padded plaster cast in the position of maximum correction. Taking advantage of anesthesia, one may be able to achieve more correction by careful selective percutaneous fasciotomy, limited capsulotomy, partial tenotomy and section of intra-articular fibrous adhesions (fibrolysis), resembling Ponseti technique.

Operative Correction

When conservative measures have failed or the patient presents to you with severe disabling or unacceptable deformity, operative intervention is justified. Soft tissues are always released first (especially in children) when permanent bone deformities have not yet occurred. The deformities persisting after the release of contracted soft tissues require operations on bones.

In growing children, major resection of bones is unjustified. One may, however do limited enucleation of small bones (of feet) or perform an extra-articular fusion to hold the foot in best corrected shape. In adults where permanent bone changes have occurred, further correction will require bone-resection with/without fusion of small joints. Bony procedures that can be safely performed with moderate infrastructure are wedge resection of small bones, arthrodesis of foot bones, distal femoral osteotomy for genu valgum, upper tibial osteotomy for genu varum, multiple diaphyseal osteotomies for severe deformities of long bones, centralization of ulna in radial club hand, proximal femoral osteotomies for coxa valga or coxa vara, distal humeral osteotomies for deformities around elbow. Currently fusion of major joints like hip, knees and elbow are not generally recommended because of excessive disturbance of kinematics of locomotion. For absolute indications, however, one can accept fusion (in best functional position) for small joints like wrist and hand, ankle and feet.

Having achieved the correction of deformities, the limb must be held in a plaster cast for 3-4 months to be followed by a removable corrective splint for a further 3-4 months. The plaster casts and splints may help improve the correction of deformity and prevent its recurrence.

More sophisticated and specialized techniques of correction like Ilizarov's technique, Jess technique, arthroscopic release are also available. However, these require especially trained orthopedic surgeons and superspecialty infrastructures. Such procedures are justified for highly complex deformities, and for limb lengthening. Rare developmental defects, spinal dysraphism and scoliosis are best treated in specialized centers.

The risks of any complex surgery should be carefully explained and the expected benefits should not be exaggerated to minimize future litigations. In generalized skeletal deformities, operative correction is justified for improvement of function rather than for cosmetics.

COMMON SOFT TISSUE PROCEDURES

A few examples of common and useful soft tissue procedures are: Medial soft tissue release for club foot deformities, plantar fasciotomy for pes cavus; tendo calcaneus lengthening and posterior capsulotomy for equinus foot, Soutter's operative release for flexion deformity of hip: (sartorius and tensor fascia lata release), adductor tenotomy for adduction deformity of hips (scissoring deformity in cerebral palsy), sternomastoid tenotomy for congenital torticollis, lengthening of flexor tendons (of hand) in established Volkmann's ischemic contracture. Currently, the preferred method for lengthening (e.g., tendo calcaneus) is by incising the musculotendinous junction in a Y-shaped fashion or as an inverted V-shape. Correct the deformity by gentle stretching. Suture the musculotendinous junction and apply a suitable plaster cast in the best corrected position.

Any gross deformity of foot when the foot is not plantigrade is defined as "club foot". During childhood ideally one should aim to achieve full correction by soft tissue release and corrective plaster-casts. Residual deformities and those in adults more often would need supplementation with bony procedures to achieve a satisfactory correction.

DYSCHONDROPLASIA, ENCHONDROMATOSIS (OLLIER'S DISEASE) AND ENCHONDROMA

It is a rare nonhereditary condition characterized by asymmetrical polyostotic distribution of radiolucent lesions in the skeleton. The lesion may be mono-ostotic, monomelic, hemimelic, or polymelic. Probably, the cartilage cells from the physeal cartilage plate get disrupted and keep on proliferating within the bone either as globular masses (chondroma-mostly in hands), as columns (mostly in tubular bones of extremities) or as cartilage sheats in iliac bones. Most of the patients present between 10 to 20 years for consultation for swelling of bones, deformities (most common genu varum), or shortening of extremities. Rarely multiple enchondromatosis may be associated with soft tissue angiomas (Maffucci's syndrome), or a chondroma may present as a solitary lesion. As adolescence approaches the cartilage may start showing flecks of calcification within the lucent zones.

Operative intervention is indicated for prevention or treatment of pathological fractures (thorough curettage and bone grafting), for cosmetic reduction of large swellings or for correction of deformity. For fractures of tubular bones (femur or tibia) insert intramedullary elastic nails along with bone grafting, for expandable sites (fibula) the tumor may be excised en bloc, correction of deformity is best advised a few years before skeletal maturity. Irrespective of the treatment, these patients must be regularly monitored for malignant transformation especially in lesions situated in rhizomelic locations.

SUGGESTED READINGS

1. Bergsma D. Skeletal dysplasias. Birth Defects Original Article Series. The National Foundation. March of Dimes. New York, NY: Intercontinental Medical Book Corp. 1974;10(12).
2. Kocher MS, Shapiro F. Osteogenesis imperfecta. J Am Acad Orthop Surg. 1998;6:225-36.
3. DiCaprio MR, Enneking WF. Fibrous dysplasia. Pathophysiology, evaluation and treatment. Current Concepts Review. J Bone Joint Surg. 2005: 87(8):1848-64.
4. Ippolito E, Farsetti P, Boyce AM, Corci A, Maio FD, Collins MT. Rdiographic classification of coronal plane femoral deformities in polyostotic fibrous dysplasia. Clin Orthop Relat Res. 2014;472: 1558-67.

CHAPTER 8

Localized Congenital Deformities (Anomalies) of Limbs

Localized deformities include extra bones, absent or hypoplastic bones, and incomplete formation of joints. Certain expressions are universally used; however, these many not be the ideal, nor can these express all deformities:

Complete absence of limb = amelia; subtotal absence of limb represented by a small stub = phocomelia; partial absence of limbs = ectromelia. The defect may be transverse or paraxial. In the hands and feet, brachydactyly (short bones), syndactyly (fused fingers), polydactyly (multiple extra fingers), symphalangism (fused phalanges) may be present. Some of the least rare local deformities are described below. Any congenital deformity of the skeletal system may be associated with anomalies of other systems like visceral, cardiac, renal and neurological system.

RADIAL DEFICIENCY

The radius may be absent or hypoplastic; in about 40%, the condition is bilateral. The hand is underdeveloped, wrist and hand are radially deviated, thumb is absent or hypoplastic and the radial side of hand may be hypoplastic, the forearm is smaller in size and there is a deformity or bowing of ulna with convexity toward ulnar (medial) side **(Fig. 8.1)**. Despite the deformity and hypoplasia, children often acquire good function. As soon as the deformity is detected, corrective stretching and splintage may help to minimize the deformity till the child grows and operative options are considered.

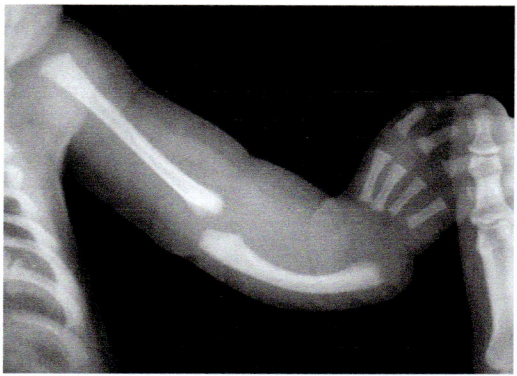

Fig. 8.1: Congenital absence of radius. Note curvature of ulna, radial deviation of hand, absence of first ray and a soft tag of thumb.

To improve the cosmetics during growing age, the distal end of ulna is centralized in the carpal bones. Generally, the space for distal ulna is created by the excision of lunate bone. Ulna is fixed in the wrist using one or two Kirschner wires (K-wires). The deformity must be observed up to the stage of skeletal maturity. Convex deformity of ulna may be corrected by multiple osteotomies, and the wrist may need fusion with centralized ulna in about 10 degrees of dorsiflexion after skeletal maturity.

Congenital Radioulnar Synostosis

There is fusion of superior radioulnar joint, the condition may be bilateral in about 30% of cases. The fusion may occur with the radial head placed posterolaterally. The condition is generally detected at the age of 3–4 years when the child starts using the hand for various activities. The delay in diagnosis is because the child manages most of the functions using compensatory movements at shoulder. On clinical examination, there is no movement palpable at the radial head and there in loss of pronation and supination. Attempted excision of the upper end of radius generally fails to restore pronation—supination because of absence of supinator and other muscles of the forearm. In cases where the forearm is fixed in extreme pronation, a corrective derotational osteotomy can provide a more suitable (generally mid-pone) angle for better function. Some patients may present with partial synostosis.

Syndactylism

There is fusion of two or more fingers (or toes). The fusion of two fingers is generally total. The fingers (or toes) can be separated by operation with careful planning of local skin flaps or use of skin-grafts, if required.

Polydactylism

There is presence of extra fingers (or toes) attached to the medial or lateral aspect of hand (or foot). If the main fingers have functioning tendons and nerves, the extra fingers (or toes) may be excised to improve the appearance of hand (or foot). If the extra fingers have functioning tendons, these may be transferred to the neighboring finger to augment the function.

Hallux Valgus

This is a deformity of the great toe, where the toe is deviated outwards at the metatarso-phalangeal joint (MTPJ). The acquired type of hallux valgus is common in middle-aged ladies in the European countries due to habitual wearing of high heel tight toes fitting shoes. Acquired deformity is not uncommon in the Indian subcontinent and other countries with warm climate. A congenital type of hallux valgus is also found in some families, where in addition to the valgus deformity at MTPJ, generally there is marked varus of the first metatarsal bone (metatarsus varus) with increased gap between the heads of first and second metatarsals. Minor hallux valgus (about 30 degrees) at the first MTPJ does not cause any symptoms. However, deformities of >40 degrees lead to crowding of other (lateral) toes with overriding of toes (e.g., second over the third). There is subluxation at the MTPJ, prominence of the first metatarsal head, formation of an adventitious bursa over the prominent metatarsal head (bunion formation), and periodic painful inflammation at the bunion. Gross deformity makes it difficult to wear the shoes; due to abnormal stress on the anterior metatarsal arc and inflammation of the bunion, there is pain and metatarsalgia on walking.

Due to damage to ligaments and joints a similar deformity may be induced in rheumatoid disorder.

In a patient with long-standing deformities, hallux valgus >30 degrees, and metatarsus adduction >15 degrees, in addition to soft tissue release and reefing, corrective osteotomy concomitantly at the base of first metatarsal and near it's neck is advised to correct the deformity. There are many methods to hold the corrected position, use of two or three K-wires provides us the simpler and effective method.

Treatment

Exercises help to keep the joints flexible; however, 'spacers' or strappings have no effective role. Operation for cosmetic purposes is rarely indicated; however, deformities with pain and difficulty in foot wear are appropriate indications for surgical correction. A number of corrective osteotomies are described in the literature. Simple and effective is an osteotomy around the neck of first metatarsal (with or without wedge resection), if there is severe metatarsus primus varus, it is wise to do corrective osteotomy near the base of first metatarsal bone (with or without wedge resection); and in the presence of gross osteoarthrosis of first MTPJ, resection of the joint may be needed concomitantly. In long-standing cases, soft tissues (capsule and adductor hallucis) on the concave side of deformity at MTPJ would require release near their bony attachments. Bony prominence under the bunion may be excised; however, soft tissue elements of "bunion" reduce in due course with correction of deformity. Postoperatively hold the correction achieved (aim at 10 degrees over correction) by two K-wires and corrective padded plaster, permit nonweight bearing ambulation soon after surgery, start weight-bearing after 3 weeks, and remove plaster and K-wires after 8–12 weeks.

DEVELOPMENTAL DYSPLASIA OF THE HIP (CONGENITAL DISLOCATION OF HIP JOINT)

Congenital dislocation of the hip is considered to be the result of defective development of acetabulum leading to loss of containment of the femoral head in the depth of acetabular cup. Probably there is simultaneous dysplasia of proximal femur as well, the term "developmental dysplasia of hip (DDH)" is, therefore, preferably used now. Partial displacement is called subluxation, and complete dislocation is addressed as dislocation. In long standing cases, secondary changes take place in the upper end of femur. It is not an uncommon defect in Latin and Anglo-Saxon races. The incidence is low in Indian-subcontinent and in the Eastern countries. Probably many cases of subluxation of hip get reduced and stabilized by the "frog position of hips"—legs widely abducted assumed by the child when carried astride the back or the side of the mother or attendant, as is prevalent in the Indian-subcontinent and in far Eastern countries. Carrying the babies in swaddled posture, legs together with hips and knees fully extended probably converted unstable hips to complete dislocation.

Clinical Features

All neonates must be subjected to clinical examination of their hips to suspect hips "at risk of instability". Three clinical tests that have been found useful are shown in the figures or diagrams here **(Figs. 8.2A to D)**. Ortolani and Barlow tests are best performed with the child in lying down position. The examiner places the palm over the infant's knee and the contralateral middle-finger-tip over the top of greater trochanter. **Ortolani's test** is like a subluxated hip relocation of femoral head into acetabulum (reducibility test). **Barlow's test** is like provocative test, subluxating the femoral head posteriorly and upwards out of the shallow acetabulum (dislocatability test). **Galeazzi test** would reveal shortening of limb and limitation of abduction of hip joint in an establised case of hip dislocation.

The condition often escapes notice till the child begins to walk, when a limp is noticed, in unilateral cases, the affected limb is short, looking at back of child may show extra creases on the affected side and a broad perineum as compared to the normal side. With child lying on its back, the hips and knees are flexed to 90 degrees, and both feet at the same level would show the knee at lower and proximal level on the dislocated side (Galeazzi test). In the same position on pushing and pulling vertically at the knee, the femoral head will be felt to travel up and down in the gluteal region (Ortolani maneuver). Observation of the walking child would show a Trendelenburg gait on the dislocated/subluxated side.

In bilateral hip dislocations/sub-luxations, the diagnosis may be delayed because there is no difference between the two limbs. Careful examination would, however, show widening of perineum, Trendelenburg telescopy would be present in both hips. On walking, such patients would be swaying from side-to-side with increased lumbar lordosis. Children do not have any pain walking on dislocated hips.

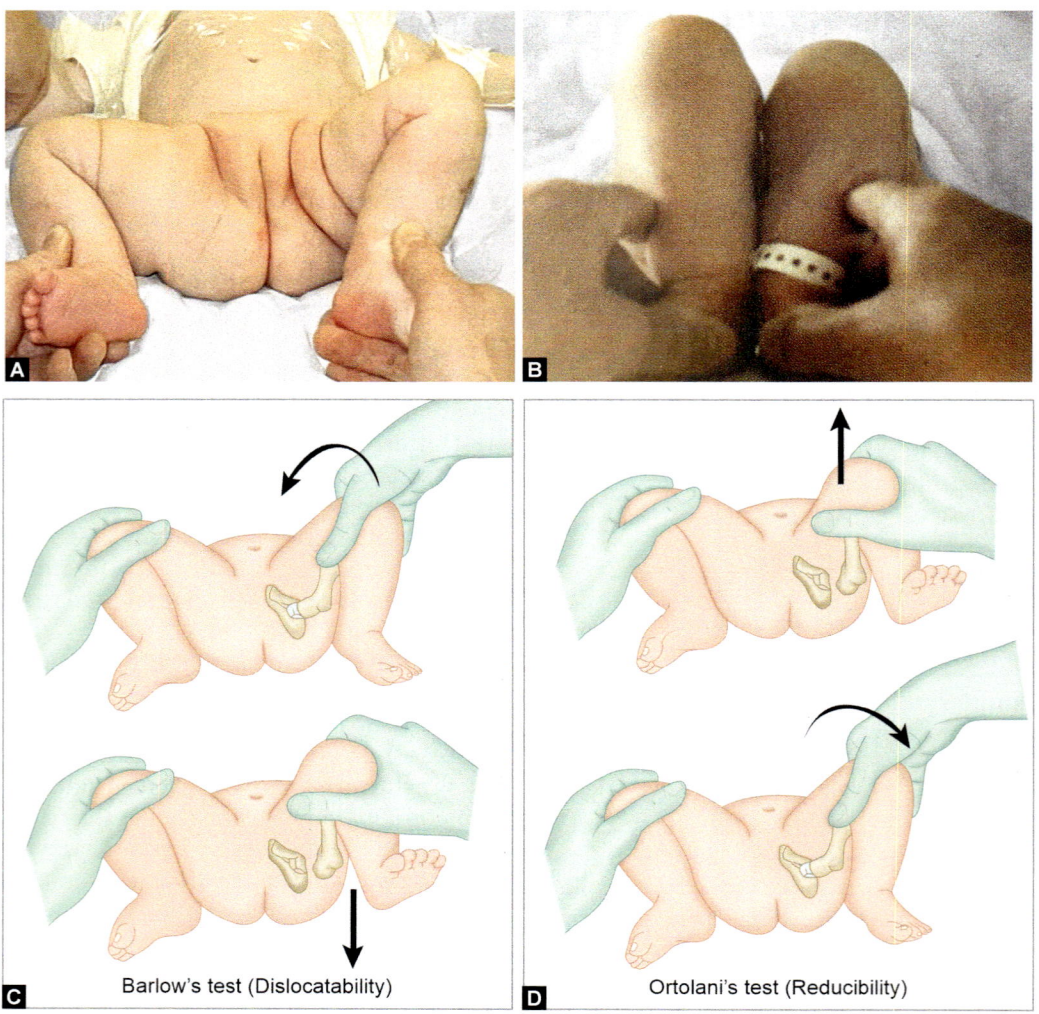

Figs. 8.2A to D: (A) Observe abnormal extra crease around left groin, suggesting congenital hip dysplasia. (B) Galeazzi test showing shorting of left lower limb. (C) Barlow's test and (D) Ortolani's test.

Radiological Features

X-ray of the pelvis including both hips helps suspect and diagnose the condition by comparing the "abnormal to normal". In a newborn between 6 months to 1 year of age, the femoral head epiphysis is not visible. Suspect the condition by observing excessive (broad) joint space, and the femoral neck staying far away from the acetabulum. In children above the age of 1 year (when femoral head epiphysis on the normal side becomes radiologically visible), the femoral head can be seen lying outside the acetabulum and at a higher level. The roof of the acetabulum is poorly developed and slopes vertically upwards.

Ultrasonography

Ultrasonography (US) has replaced X-rays for periodic assessment of the hip joint in newborn babies. Sequential assessment monitors the development of hip joint and quality of reduction. In addition to clinical examination, hip ultrasonography is accepted as a useful tool for screening DDH especially in the newborns up to 6 months. Ultrasonic morphology of hip has been expressed as "alpha angle" for osseous acetabular roof and "beta angle" for cartilaginous acetabular roof development. Once capital femoral epiphysis starts to ossify (around 4–6 months) radiological imaging is considered as the gold standard. There are however clinicians who would still use ultrasonic assessment to reduce the number of radiological exposures in these children.

Pathology-adaptive Changes

After weight-bearing (walking), the morbid anatomy or pathological changes in the hip joint get more exaggerated (intensified). Radiologically the femoral head is dislocated upward and backward in relation to the acetabulum, the superior lip of acetabulum is flat or hypoplastic and the ossific nucleus of femoral head is absent or appears late. The femoral head-neck and acetabulum remain anteverted, the misplaced femoral head may form a false socket above the acetabulum. The superior capsule is stretched, redundant and thickened, the ligamentum teres gets elongated and hypertrophied, the superior fibrocartilaginous limbus may get inverted, superior capsule between the misplaced femoral head and outer surface of iliac bone may become adherent to iliac bone, and the capsule may get squeezed between the acetabulum and the ilio-psoas muscle (proceeding to lesser trochanter for insertion) creating an "hour-glass appearance" of the capsule. It is mandatory to keep these adaptive changes in mind while attempting an operative reduction in patients who are walking and present late for treatment.

Treatment

Whenever there is suspicion of instability, the babies are nursed in broad napkins. In children younger than one year of age, the hip joints are maintained in wide abduction by nursing them in broad napkins or cushions placed between the thighs. One can use a splint to keep the thighs in abduction. When a newborn is suspected to have a dislocatable hip or a dysplastic hip even without subluxation use of Pavlik harness **(Fig. 8.3)** in strongly suggested. The harness holds the hips in the human position: about 100 degrees of flexion and about 45 degrees of abduction (the angle between the two thighs should not be >100 degrees), more wide abduction may jeopardise blood supply of the femoral head. The kicking motions allowed in the harness, promotes and maintains the spontaneous reduction of the dislocatable or dysplastic hip. Pavlik harness is most useful for children below the age of 10 months. The abduction maintained for 6–9 months would reduce the unstable hip joint and the acetabulum would develop normally.

In Children between 1 and 3 Years

One may apply skin traction for about 2 weeks. Role of traction is, however, debated probably because of the necessity of hospitalization or care at home. After traction of 10–20 days, under anesthesia gentle manipulation is done to reduce the femoral head into the acetabulum, presently under C-arm observations. If successful, limbs are held in the best stable position, frog position in younger children, or abduction 40 degrees, flexion 60 degrees and internal rotation 20 degrees in older children. Three

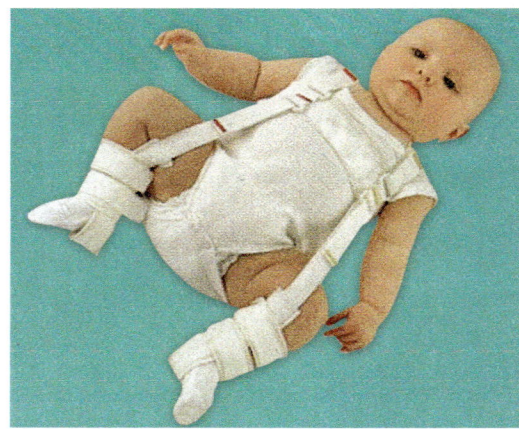

Fig. 8.3: Pavlik harness (Flexion-abduction orthosis).

months after the closed reduction, change the hip spica to "human position" about 45 degrees of flexion, 40 degrees of abduction and 15 degrees of external rotation. The plaster cast is changed every 3 months. About 6-9 months after the closed reduction, the limb should be held in abduction while sleeping (broom stick like splint or plaster) and the child is encouraged gradual weight-bearing. Golden rules of splintage must be followed (Apley, 9th edition):

1. Ensure concentric reduction before splintage
2. Extremes of position must be avoided
3. Some degree of mobility of hip joint should be possible.

Child Aged 3–6 Years

After 10–20 days of traction, closed reduction is given a trial; however, if it fails, operative reduction is done followed by plaster cast hip spica for about 3 months. If the reduction is unstable on the operation-table, a shelf operation is performed. The acetabular roof is augmented by doing a Salter's innominate osteotomy (redirectional) or by Chiari's osteotomy (displacement) or increase the acetabular roof by turning down a flap of bone from the outer table of iliac bone (Pemberton's or Dega's pelvic osteotomy, with impaction bone grafting). Dega's pelvic osteotomy is similar to Pemberton's except that the curvilinear osteotomy is about 2 cm above and paralle to the acetabular margin. Once complete the outer table of iliac bone above the acetabulum is levered down over the femoral head capsule, and held in position by impaction bone grafts. This is suitable for patients aged 3–11 years **(Figs. 8.4A to C, also see Chapter 16)**.

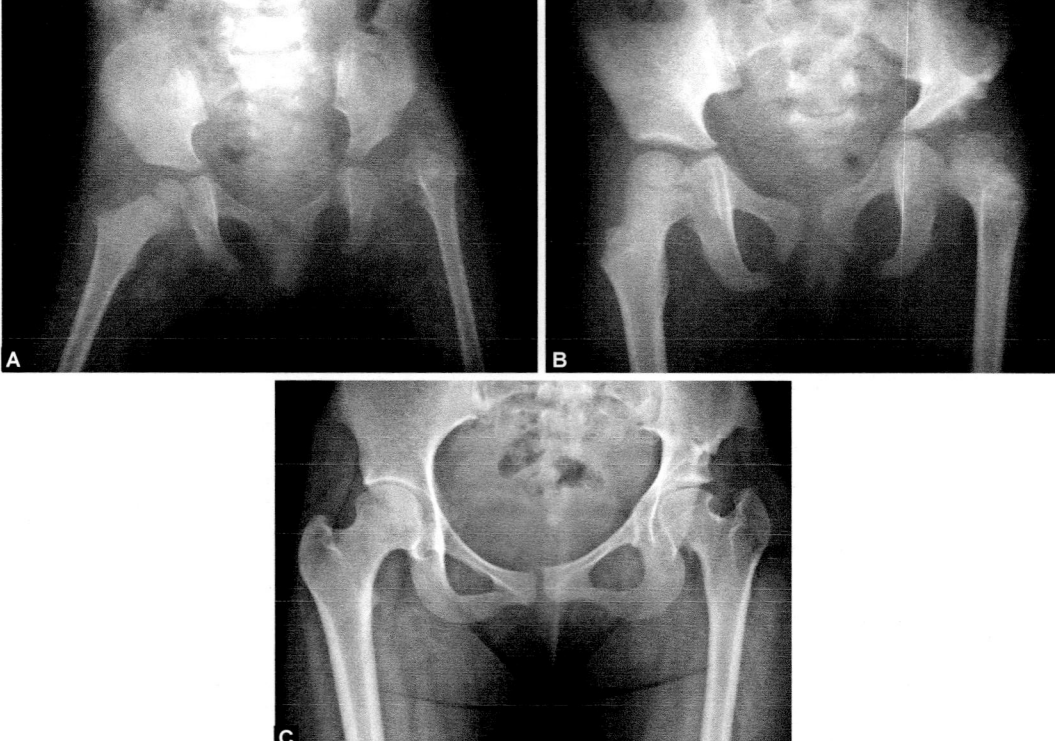

Figs. 8.4A to C: (A) X-rays of a walking child with developmental dysplasia of left hip; (B) Hip joint was reposed by open operation, concomitant innominate osteotomy; (C) Appearance at maturity shows nearly normal hip with full function.

Children above the Age of 6 Years

One can attempt to do open reduction in children between the age of 6 and 10 years. One may succeed to repose the femoral head into the acetabulum after an extensive surgery including stripping of gluteal muscles and capsule from the outer surface of iliac bone, up to the superior lip of acetabulum, opening of hip joint, adductor tenotomy at the pubic bone, tenotomy of ilio-psoas at its insertion on lesser trochanter, excision and/or double-breasting of redundant capsule, excision of hypertrophied ligamentum teres and transverse acetabular ligament, concentric reduction of femoral head deep into acetabular socket, insertion of a K-wire (one or two) to hold the reduction in position, concomitant innominate osteotomy; Salter's in children <4 years, or Pemberton's or newer modifications **(Figs. 8.5 and 8.6)**. Currently many surgeons would perform innominate osteotomy for most of the cases to improve the stability. **In long standing cases**, the proximal femur has developed coxa-valga and anteverted femoral neck, one may require an upper femoral osteotomy to ensure

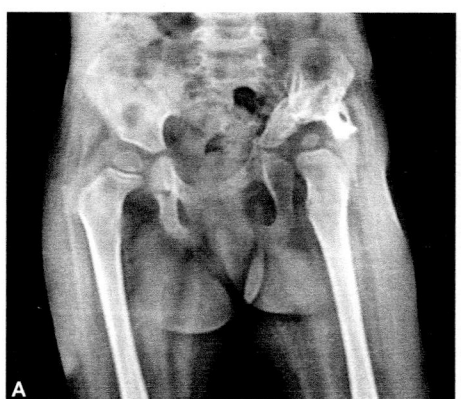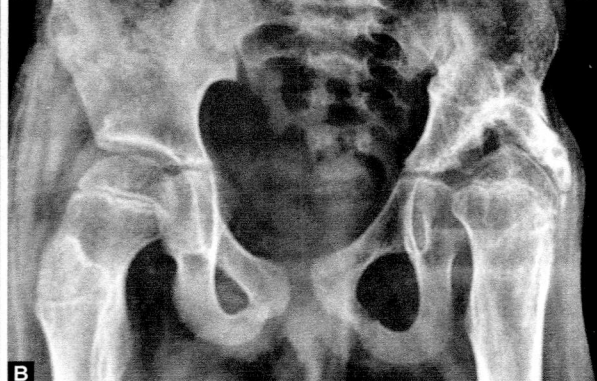

Figs. 8.5A and B: An operation to repose the femoral head into the acetabulum failed in this patient because the bones of the left pelvis were very thin and hypoplastic. Innominate osteotomy did not provide any coverage. Bank-bone was used to create a shelf. One can appreciate the development over a follow-up of 7 years.

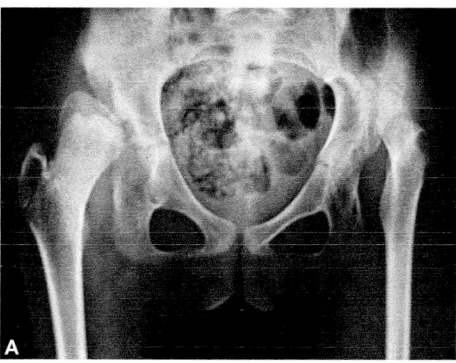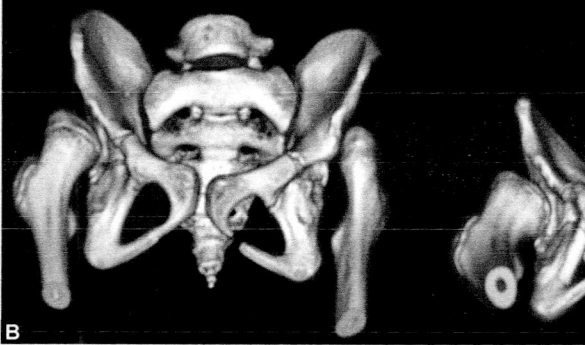

Figs. 8.6A and B: Developemental dysplasia of hips: (A) X-ray appearance of a neglected case of bilateral developmental dysplasia of hips in a 10-year-old walking girl; (B) It is the 3-dimensional CT-scan. Note empty and hypoplastic acetabulum, deformed femoral head and neck and attempt at formation of "secondary acetabulum" superior to the original acetabuli.

concentric positioning of femoral head. After femoral osteotomy, the upper fragment is positioned into internal rotation and varus, held by plate and screws. In difficult cases and grown up children a few centimeters of femoral shortening may be required to achieve adequate reduction of femoral head. These procedures are best undertaken in centers with special expertise. Approximately 30% of such patients may need further treatment/operation for avascular necrosis, instability, and stiffness of the joints. The chances of failure are higher if dislocation is a part of generalized conditions (syndromic) like arthrogryposis or neuromuscular imbalance.

CONGENITAL CLUBFOOT

Broadly speaking, there are three types of clubfeet; primary idiopathic, arthrogrypotic and neurogenic, generally associated with spinal dysraphism. Arthrogryposis multiplex congenita is associated with multiple "rigid" deformities of hip, knees, feet, elbow, hands, shoulders, temporomandibular joints and practically all joints of body. In addition to deformities of bones and joints, the musculature is also poorly developed. The basic principle of deformity correction is to obtain a plantigrade foot.

The treatment should start soon after birth: Different components of deformities should be corrected in a sequence—the fore-foot adduction first, the inversion next, and the equinus last, whether treated by corrective manipulations or corrective plaster or operative procedures, all corrections must be made gently; forceful correction of deformities may achieve cosmetically normal looking foot, but functionally the foot will not be supple.

Up to 4 weeks, the foot should be corrected by gentle manipulations, 10–15 excursions 3–5 times a day. From approximate **4 weeks to 3 months** after corrective manipulation, strap the foot by adhesive plaster extending from foot to leg. From **3 months to 3 years,** manipulate the foot into correction either under sedation or light anesthesia and hold the correction in best corrected position by moulded plaster, change the plaster every month to achieve more correction. In most of the patients, you will be able to achieve a corrected foot in 4–5 manipulations. Maintain the correction by suitable orthotics and corrective exercises. If one is doing corrective plasters under anesthesia, one may perform percutaneous tendo-Achilles lengthening to achieve correction of equinus deformity (Ponseti technique).

Ponseti's Technique

Ponseti's technique of conservative method of correction of clubfoot deformities (1963, 1992) is now popular. The philosophy comprises of gentle manipulations to correct the deformities and moulding the plaster cast to hold the correction achieved. Start with passive stretching soon after birth. Hold the corrected position by plaster cast starting usually at three weeks of age. The **first "Ponseti cast"** is considered an important step: the foot in supinated with an upward pressure over the first metatarsal. Usually the deformity looks exaggerated in the plaster cast. The subsequent plasters are done at about 3 weeks intervals. The hindfoot varus, forefoot inversion and adduction deformities are corrected simultaneously by manual shifting of navicular, cuboid and calcaneum laterally. This is achieved by the basic principle of 3 point corrective pressure. The manual pressure medially is countered by pressure on the anterolateral aspect of talar-head (rather than the calcaneocuboid joint). Start with passive stretching in the earliest stage soon after birth. After 3–4 weeks follow the corrective manipulations with serial casting. While applying the corrective plaster (the below-knee plaster cast applied first) hold the foot in the best corrected position. Once the below-knee cast has "set", the plaster is extended to above the knee (upto the grown with knee at 90 degrees of flexion) and hyperabduction of foot. Once the heal varus is corrected, the equinus deformity may be corrected by percutaneous lengthening of tendo calcaneus.

The percutaneous tenotomy is needed in about 80% of cases. The tenotomy is performed from medial to lateral side (to minimize neurovascular injury) with the tendon held in tension (taut). The skin is infiltrated with local anesthetic, complete tenotomy is performed about one cm proximal to the calcaneal tuberosity. The completeness of tenotomy is suggested by a "popping sound" and increase in the dorsiflexion at the ankle joint. The bleeding at the site of percutaneous tenotomy is easily controlled by local pressure for a few minutes. An above the knee plaster cast is applied with full correction of deformity for about 3 weeks.

Foot abduction brace: Having achieved full correction, a foot abduction brace is continued for 3–4 years. The bar length is equal to the child's shoulder width and the corrective shoes or boots are attached at the ends of the bar. The shoes and the bar are constructed in a way that the corrected foot (or feet) is held in dorsiflexion and 70 degree of external rotation. The bace is worn full time for about 3 months, then at night and naptimes, at least for 10 hours per day for 3–4 years. During the follow-up continue the stretching exercises when the child is out of the brace, observe the feet for recurrence of deformity, which may require surgical correction at a later stage.

Joshi's External Stabilization System (Ligamentotaxis)

Joshi's external stabilization system (JESS) is another method of achieving correction of difficult clubfoot deformities. The principle is the same of gradual ligamentotaxis. The basic assembly consists of three sites of pin hold (tibial, calcaneal, metatarsal) and three pairs of connections of which tibiocalcaneal and calcaneometatarsal are distractors, tibiometatarsal are connecting rods. After inserting all the K-wires under general anesthesia (3 each in tibia, calcaneum, and metatarsals) try to reduce the deformities by Ponseti method. The reduction achieved is maintained by the use of distractors placed on both sides between tibial-calcaneal and calcaneal-metatarsal attachments. On 3rd or 4th postoperative day distraction is started (almost like Ilizarov's principles) 0.25 mm 6 hourly on the medial (concave) side, while 0.25 mm 12 hourly on the lateral (convex) side in hospitalized patients. After discharge from the hospital the parents are asked to do the distraction at the rate of one mm on the medial side and 0.5 mm on the lateral side, once a day for convenience. Differential distraction on the medial side is twice the rate on the lateral side. The distraction on the lateral side prevents crushing of the articular cartilage and permits normal growth of the physeal plate. Having achieved correction by this method of differential distraction lasting for 3–6 weeks the assembly is held in static position for further 3–4 weeks to allow soft tissues to mature in elongated position. The assembly is now removed and plaster cast is applied in position of maximum correction. The children are allowed to ambulate full weight bearing in plaster for 3–6 weeks. There after appropriate orthosis is worn throughout the growing phase of bones. The prime factor for success by this process of ligamentotaxis is, the patient's attendants co-operation and participation.

OPERATIVE CORRECTION

A small number of patients cannot be fully corrected, or they come back with recurrence of deformity, or the patient presents for treatment after the age of walking. Scope and extent of operations in such patients vary widely depending upon the severity of deformity. Z-shaped lengthening of tendo-calcaneus and capsulotomy of posterior capsule of ankle joint and of talo-calcaneal joint would correct the equinus deformity; medial capsulotomy of tarsometatarsal joint, talo-navicular joint, talo-calcaneal joint would correct the adduction and inversion deformity; lengthening of tibialis posterior tendon may be needed for correction of adduction and inversion; and in neglected cases percutaneous plantar fasciotomy at its posterior attachment would correct the element of cavus deformity. After releasing all tissues, one should be able to swing the foot into corrected position, bring the heel down, and the foot is now put in a padded plaster cast with the best possible correction. Ideally one should aim at about 10 degrees of over correction at the time of operation or during subsequent change of plaster.

If a plantigrade foot is not achieved by soft tissue release by the age of 5 years, one may have to resort to bony procedures. Between 5 and 12 years, selective enucleation of cuboid, calcaneus and tarsal bones may he helpful. In very rigid clubfeet, especially those associated with arthrogryposis **(Figs. 8.7A and B)**, one may obtain a plantigrade foot by excising the talus, permitting tibia to articulate on the upper surface of calcaneum. Above the age of 12 years, correction can be obtained by dorsolateral wedge resection (from talus, calcaneum, cuboid). In severe deformities, wedge resection is generally combined with fusion of talo-calcaneal, talo-navicular and calcaneocuboid joints. The corrected foot may be held in position with the help of a few K-wires inserted across the talo-navicular and subtaloid joints and plaster cast. The plaster cast should be changed around 6 weeks after the corrective operation, one may be able to add more correction of deformities, remove the K-wires, put the foot in corrective plaster cast again, encourage the patient full weight-bearing for another 6 weeks.

After the full correction, the foot must be exercised and a suitable orthotic boot is worn till almost the maturity, 12–15 years of age. The foot must be examined periodically to detect any tendency for relapse of the deformity.

Correction of deformities must be done in the above mentioned order. Correction of equinus before correction of other deformities almost breaks the foot in mid-tarsal region resulting in "rocker bottom foot". For clubfeet deformities, which are **resistant, relapsed** or **recurred** or **neglected**, operative intervention is mandatory. The optimum time for operation in childhood is considered 1 year of age; the foot is of reasonable size for

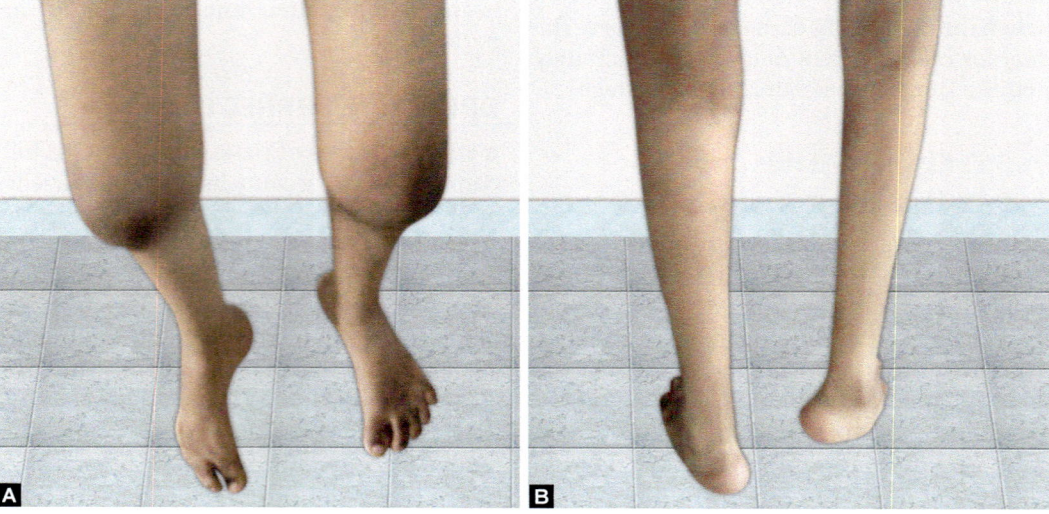

Figs. 8.7A and B: Clubfoot deformity in arthrogryposis multiplex congenita: Despite standard soft tissue release, the deformity (equinus and inversion) in this 9 years child persisted. Decancellation and talectomy may achieve a plantigrade foot.

comfort while operating. Having achieved the correction, the patient should be encouraged to walk with corrective plaster and corrective orthosis. Forces during walking help maintain the correction obtained. It is wise to continue stretching exercises and corrective orthosis till the maturity of patient.

Difficult cases: For late presenters, relapsed cases, and very rigid deformities, supplementary procedures are justified in addition to the standard posteromedial soft tissue release. Decancellation or enucleation of cuboid, calcaneum, or osteotomy of calcaneum to correct the varus and inversion of heal, split transfer of tibialis anterior tendon to base of fourth metatarsal, transinterosseous transfer of tibialis posterior to the dorsum of 3rd metatarsal (in cases of neurogenic clubfeet), and calcaneofibular ligament release are useful procedures for difficult cases.

LOCAL CONGENITAL DEFECTS

Congenital Pseudarthrosis of Tibia (Fig. 8.8)

This rare congenital condition is a non-uniting fracture of tibial shaft at the junction of middle and lower third of the diaphysis. A child may be seen with a "pre-pseudarthrosis" where the X-rays show sclerosis of bone with convexity anterolaterally. Despite protection, the tibia may fracture and lead to pseudarthrosis. This condition, if associated with neurofibromatosis or multiple café-au-lait patches, the prognosis is worst. This is one of the most intractable conditions to achieve the union. Many operative procedures involving local bone grafting, bypass bone grating, excision of the pseudarthrosis and telescopy on Ilizarov's principles have been tried with negligible success. One of the practical methods worth trying is intramedullary nailing and repeated bone grafting. In some patients, the condition stabilizes after skeletal majority **(Figs. 8.9 to 8.11)**.

Congenital Bowing of Tibia

Congenital fibular deficiency is generally associated with anterior convexity of tibia, and deficiency of the lateral side of ankle and foot. The stability of ankle can be improved by centralization of tibia, the deformity and shortening can be improved by corrective osteotomy **(Figs. 8.11A to C)**.

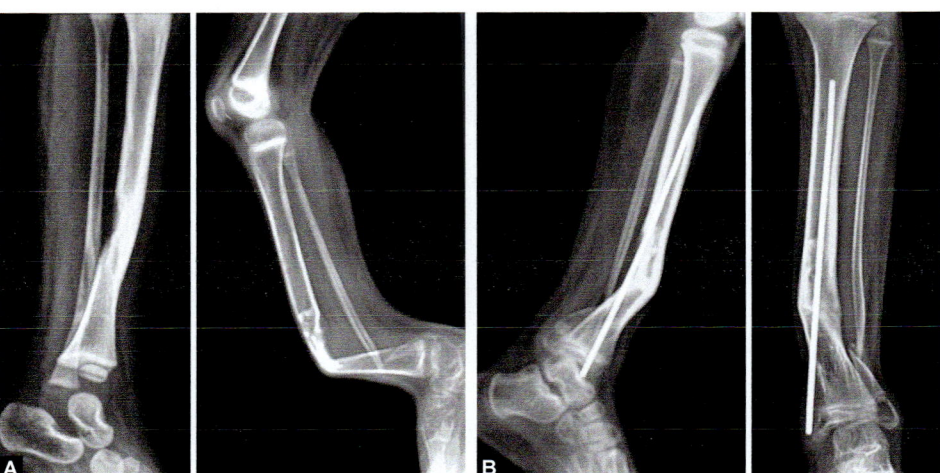

Figs. 8.8A to D: Congenital pseudarthrosis of tibia: (A) One can observe pseudoarthrosis of tibia and fibula. (B) The defect in tibia has healed by intramedullary nail and bone grafting.

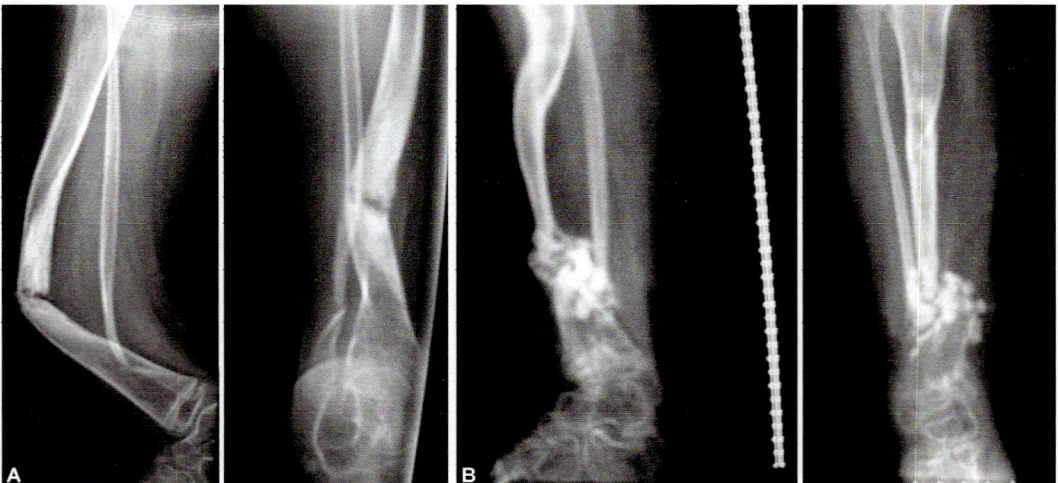

Figs. 8.9A and B: X-rays of a typical case of congenital pseudarthrosis of tibia (A) shows the resorption of attempted bone grafting (B).

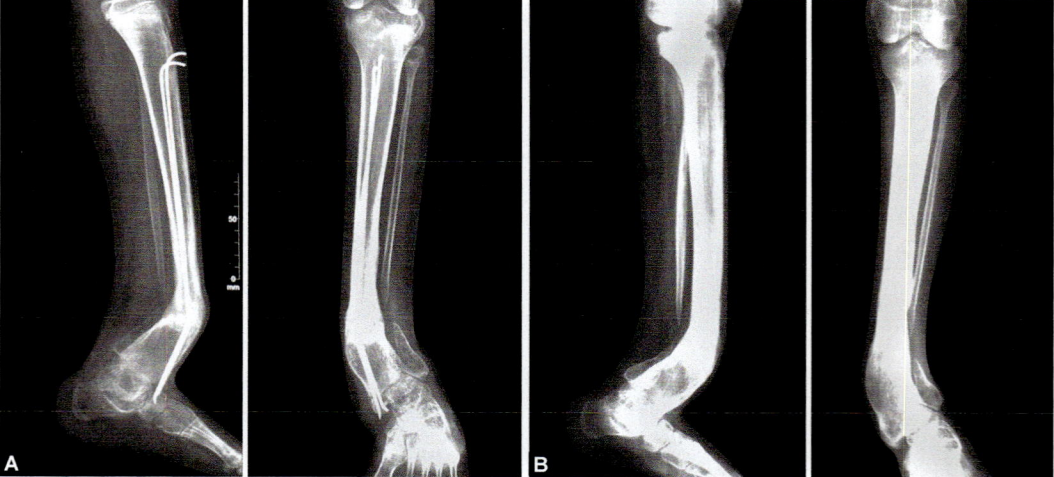

Figs. 8.10A and B: Congenital pseudarthrosis of tibia: One of the practical methods of treatment is intramedullary nailing and (repeated) bone grafting. This patient was operated 4 times, the fracture united though with some angulation.

Resistant Clubfoot Deformity

It may be associated with arthrogryposis multiplex congenital defect. These patients need multiple operations to achieve a plantigrade foot, in some cases one may have to do talectomy to correct the foot deformity.

Spina Bifida (Dysraphism)

This is a congenital defect in the walls of the spinal (vertebral) canal because of lack of union between the laminae of the vertebrae. The commoner site affected is lower lumbar spine. As a result of the bony defect, the membranes of the cord herniate through the opening, some of these patients may have neural tube defect. In its most severe form, the condition is associated with major neurological complications and sphincter involvement. In the mildest form (spina bifida occulta), there is a midline defect and nothing more. Many patients on local examination

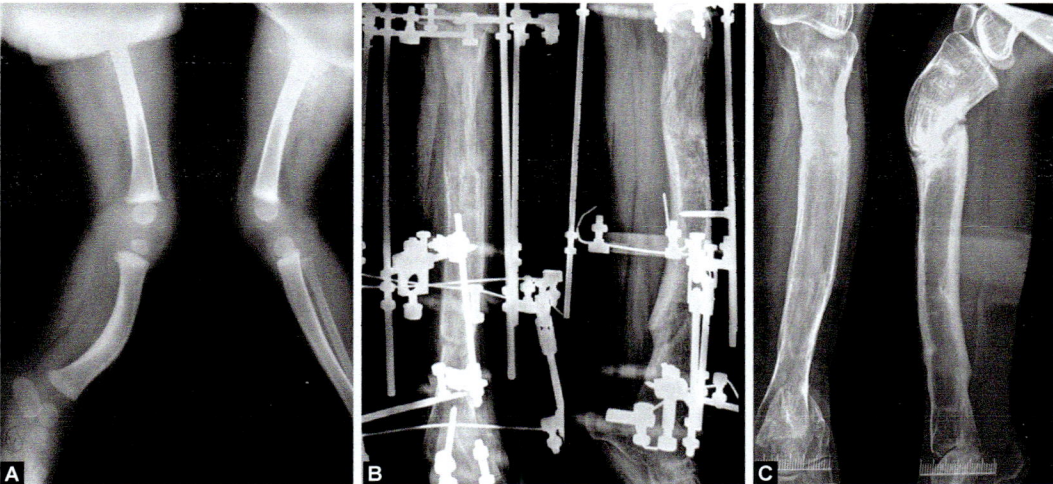

Figs. 8.11A to C: Congenital absence of fibula with anterior convexity of tibia: Tibia has been centralized and its length has been gained through Ilizarov's technique.

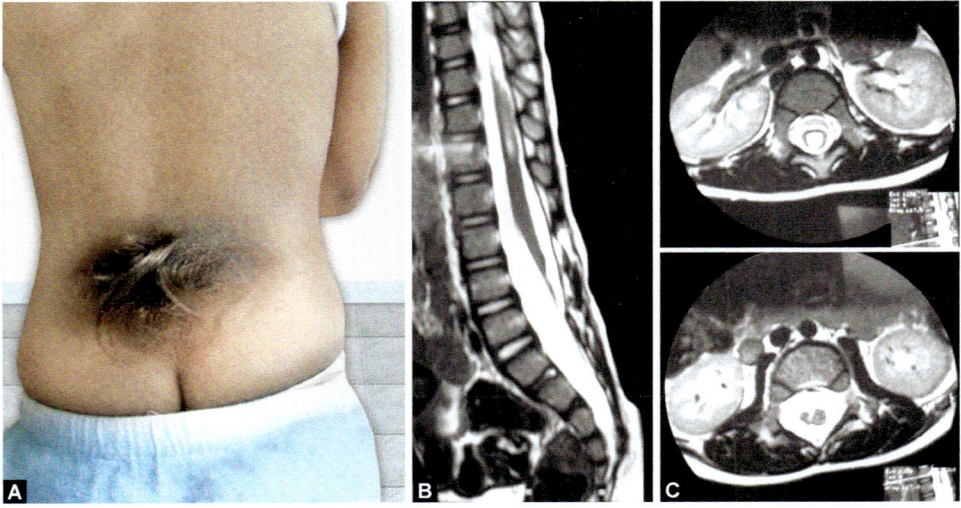

Figs. 8.12A to C: Hairy tuft (A) at lumbosacral spine in a child with spinal dysraphism. MRI (B) shows a low tethered dural sheath. Note the tethering at lumbar 5 level; (C) The axial cuts show extensive syrinx in lower cord and the split cord.

would show tell-tale defects in the skin such as a dimple, a lipoma, a hairy tuft, or pigmented patch. Patients with neural complications need to be treated in dedicated centers. Many patients with neural complications will never be functionally normal **(Figs. 8.12A to C)**.

Consumption of folic acid by the expectant mothers in the preconception period has been suggested to reduce the incidence of spinal dysraphism by 90%.

SUGGESTED READINGS

1. Ponseti IV, Smoley EN. Congenital clubfoot: the results of treatment. J Bone Joint Surg. 1963; 45(2):134-41.
2. Turco VJ. Resistant congenital club foot-one-stage posteromedial release with internal fixation. A follow-up report of a fifteen-year experience. J Bone Joint Surg Am. 1979;61A:805-14.
3. Fern ED, Stockley I, Bell MJ. Extending intramedullary rods congenital pseudarthrosis of the tibia. J Bone Joint Surg Br. 1990;72B:1073-5.
4. Ponseti IV. Treatment of congenital club foot. J Bone Joint Surg Am. 1992;74A:448-54.
5. Joseph B, Mathew G. Management of congenital pseudarthrosis of the tibia by excision of the pseudarthrosis, onlay grafting and intramedullary nailing. J Pediatr Orthop B. 2000;9:16-23.
6. Bor N, Coplan JA, Herzenberg JE. Ponseti treatment for idiopathic clubfoot: minimum 5-year follow-up. Clin Orthop Relat Res. 2009;467:1263-70.
7. Jowett CR, Morcuende JA, Ramachandran M. Management of congenital talipes equinovarus using Ponseti method: a systematic review. J Bone Joint Surg Br. 2011;93B:1160-4.
8. Sadana A, Pal CP, Dinkar KS. An assessment of the results of controlled fractional distraction by Joshi's external stabilization system in club foot. J Foot Ankle Surg (Asia-Pacific). 2015;2:13-6
9. Holt JB, Oji DE, Yack HJ, Morcuende JA. Long-term results of tibialis anterior tendon transfer for relapsed idiopathic clubfoot treated with the Ponseti method: a follow-up of thirty-seven to fifty-five years. J Bone Joint Surg Am. 2015:97A:47-55.

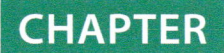

CHAPTER 9

Common Orthopedic Tumors

For any swelling consider it can be traumatic, congenital, infective, inflammatory, tumors, tumor-like conditions, and cystic conditions present with many similarities to the clinician. A few tables and diagrams are helpful in understanding possible care of such cases **(Table 9.1)**. Benign tumors are quite common, malignant tumors are rare. The commonest malignant tumor located in the skeleton is a metastatic deposit. In reality it is not a tumor of origin from the skeletal system (mesenchymal). The commonest

Table 9.1: Common primary tumors and tumor-like lesions of the skeletal system.		
Source	**Benign**	**Malignant**
Cartilage	• Osteochondroma • Chondroma benign • Chondroblastoma • Chondromyxoid fibroma	Chondrosarcoma
Osseous	• Osteoid osteoma • Osteoblastoma • Ivory osteoma	Osteosarcoma
Fibrogenic	• Nonossifying fibroma • Desmoplastic fibroma • Fibrous dysplasia	Fibrosarcoma
Marrow tumor (Hematopoietic)		• Ewing's sarcoma • Myelomatosis • Lymphoma
Neural tissues	• Neurofibroma • Neurilemmoma • Schwannoma	• Malignant–Schwannoma • Chordoma
Vascular tissues	• Hemangioma • Aneurysmal bone cyst • Glomus tumor	Angiosarcoma
Giant cell tumor	Benign osteoclastoma	Malignant osteoclastoma
Lipogenic tumor	Lipoma	Liposarcoma
Synovial lesions	• Synovial chondromatosis • Pigmented villonodular synovitis (PVNS) (can also occur in synovial sheaths of tendons)	Synovial sarcoma
Uncertain and miscellaneous	• Eosinophilic granuloma • Simple bone cyst • Hamartoma	Adamantinoma

primary malignant tumor of the skeleton is myeloma (arising from marrow cells).

CLINICAL FEATURES

Many benign tumors remain asymptomatic for long. Malignant tumors too, many remain silent if there is room for inconspicuous growth (e.g., cavity of pelvis). Age may be a useful factor in diagnosis. Many benign tumors occur in childhood and adolescence; however, Ewings sarcoma and osteosarcoma also occur during young age. Chondrosarcoma and fibrosarcoma occur in old age (fourth to sixth decade). Myeloma the commonest of all primary malignant tumors of skeleton (from marrow cells) generally occurs after sixth decade. In patients over 70 years of age, metastatic bone lesions are more common than all primary tumors together.

Pain: Progressive and unremitting pain is a sinister symptom associated with a malignant tumor or an aggressive neoplasm. The typical night-time pain of osteoid osteoma (a benign lesion) gets significant pain relief by use of salicylates. Paget's disease of bone also presents more pain at night.

Swelling

Generally, the patients seek advice only when a lump becomes palpable or painful. The source of origin may help in diagnosis. Discrete clear borders suggest a benign lesion; diffuse ill-defined borders suggest malignant or aggressive tumors, pulsatile swelling may be an aneurysm or a highly vascular tumor. Swelling of the neighboring joint may be an effusion, regional lymph node enlargement may be present in rhabdomyosarcomas, epithelioid sarcomas, and synovial sarcomas. A malignant tumor always shows progressive enlargement. Any growing swelling >5 cm should be suspected to be malignant until proved otherwise.

Pathological Fracture

This may be the first clinical signal to suggest the presence of a cystic lesion (nonossifying fibroma, unicameral bone cyst during growing age) or a metastatic deposit in the elderly.

Neurological Symptoms

Neurological symptoms (paresthesia or numbness or paralysis) may be caused by a tumor pressing on a neighboring nerve. Spinal lesions whether benign or malignant often cause pain and stiffness in the back, and there may be painful scoliosis and neural deficit.

INVESTIGATIONS

X-rays

X-rays are still the most useful of all imaging modalities. Ask for X-rays of the involved limb as well as the contralateral asymptomatic limb, and an X-ray of chest. The X-rays may show cortical thickening, irregularity of surface, a discrete lump, a cystic lesion, a deformity or ill-defined destruction. We learn where is the lesion: metaphyseal, diaphyseal or epiphyseal. Are the margins well-defined and sclerotic (biologically containable benign lesions), or the margins are ill-defined (aggressive or malignant tumors). Careful examination can show the health of surrounding soft tissues. Look for "sunrays", "onion peel", "Codman" triangle and calcification in the soft tissue swelling or mass: All these suggest possibilities of a malignant tumor; however, similar picture can be seen in some infections. The X-rays are less informative for soft tissue tumors or lump; however, careful examination may show the mass (of a long standing) scalloping effect on the underlying bone, phleboliths in a vascular hamartoma, calcification in a synovial sarcoma, or a fat density of a lipoma (**Figs. 9.1A and B**). In general

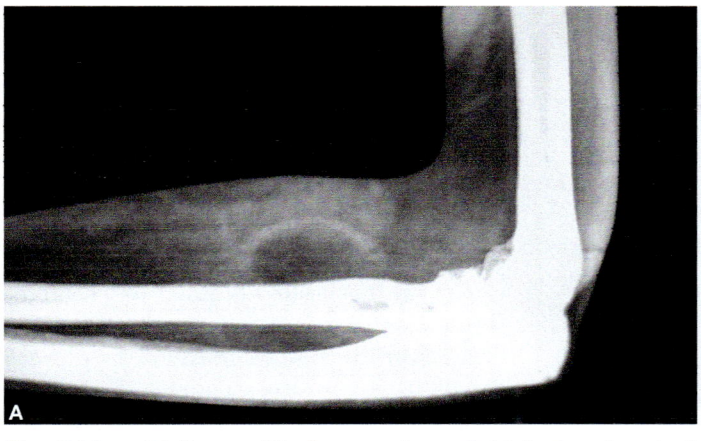
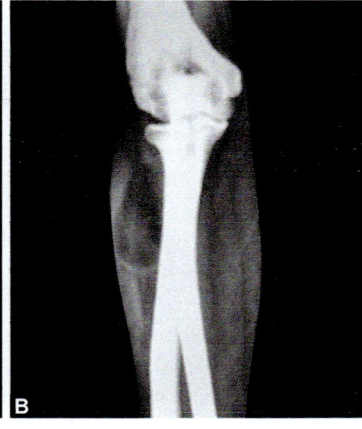

Figs. 9.1A and B: X-rays of the forearm show a light shadow deep to the muscles of forearm, excision of the lesion proved it to be a lipoma. Radiological density of subcutaneous tissue is that of fat.

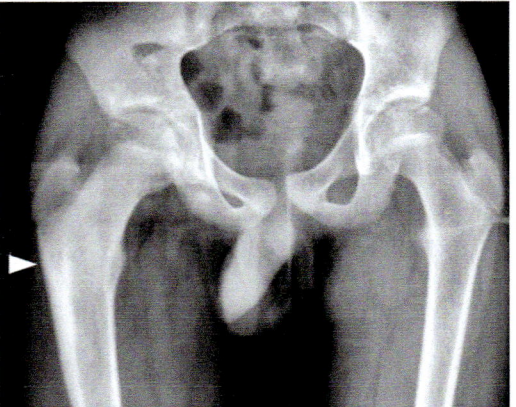

Fig. 9.2: Osteoid osteoma: Note a small lytic lesion surrounded by dense bone; situated in the lateral border of upper femur.

recommendations today are that a tumor or a lump deep to the deep fascia, larger than 5 cm should be suspected to be malignant and should be excised extracapsularly for further investigations. With all the information provided by X-rays, it is rarely (e.g., in osteochondroma, nonossifying fibroma, osteoid osteoma), that one can reach a definitive diagnosis **(Fig. 9.2)**. In most of the cases, other investigations are mandatory before one can reach the definitive diagnosis. CT scan and MRI should be done before doing a biopsy, which itself may adversely distort/disturb the images.

Isotope Bone Scan

Isotope bone scan would show nonspecific hot areas (metabolically active) due to any pathology including degenerative disorders; however, it helps to suspect tumors (osteoid osteoma, subclinical metastatic deposits) in difficult (inaccessible) areas not clearly seen in X-rays. In a multicentric disease (myeloma, metastatic deposit), this investigation also guides the surgeon for the most easily accessible site for biopsy.

CT Scans

CT scans essentially extend the information obtained by conventional X-rays, extra-osseous extension of tumors, and lesions in inaccessible sites. It is also a reliable method of detecting pulmonary metastases.

MRI Scans

MRI scan has the greatest value in the assessment of tumors' spread: (i) Within the bone, (ii) into a nearby joint, (iii) into soft tissues. MRI is also useful in assessing soft-tissue tumors, cartilaginous lesions and the tumors in the spine. Pigmented villonodular synovitis (PVNS) at present can be diagnosed by MRI scans; deposits of hemociderin crystals in synovial membrane are exhibited as irregular dark shadows.

PET Scan or PET-CT

It is a very sensitive test showing the areas of high metabolic activity which typically occurs in malignant cells. It helps in mapping the primary and metastatic foci in the body, is also useful in staging of disease, to detect the response to therapy and possible recurrence during follow-up. Unfortunately in countries where tuberculosis is prevalent, this infection may also show local or disseminated foci of high metabolic activity. Before treating a lesion as "malignant" the clinician must have a robust proof of malignancy by semi-invasive or open biopsy procedures.

Laboratory Investigations

Laboratory investigations including blood tests are necessary to exclude other conditions like infections, metabolic bone disorders, hyperparathyroidism (brown tumor). Serum electrophoresis for myeloma protein, and Bence Jones protein in urine may help diagnose myeloma. A raised serum acid phosphates and prostate specific antigens may suggest prostatic carcinoma.

Biopsy

Any drastic procedure or a mutilative operation for the tumor must be preceded by the study of biopsy material. We must obtain adequate amount of representative tissue for histological investigations. Ideally, open biopsy gives most reliable information. In expert hands a large bore, Jamshidi or a Trucut needle may provide adequate representative material. Biopsy should be carried out by the surgeon who is going to do the definitive treatment or a specialist well-versed with the surgical intervention that may be needed in future for excision, resection-reconstruction, limb salvage procedure or ablation. Ideally, if possible, a block of tissue about 1 cm^3 should be removed from the boundary zone (junctional area) to include the abnormal and normal tissue. The material should reach the histopathology service without much delay and without crushing of the tissues. For tumors suspected to be malignant, it is a good practice to send the request for opinion on histology to two centers. For "tumors" that are almost certainly benign (unicameral bone cyst, fibrous dysplasia), an excisional biopsy or thorough curettage with concomitant compact bone grafting is permissible. The patient and the attendants must, however, be explained a possibility of a change in diagnosis after the availability of the histology report on the tissue obtained by curettage. While dealing with tumors that could be malignant, do not be tempted to perform the biopsy in a hurry. Biopsy must be done only after all imaging modalities have been completed. Biopsy should be performed through a planned axial incision which may be used for possible ultimate operative treatment.

Pitfalls

Pitfalls are in plenty especially when dealing with malignant or aggressive tumors. Adequate consultations between orthopedic surgeon, pathologist and oncologist would help minimize serious errors. Patient, his parents or attendants must be fully informed about the pros and cons. All this is not possible at district level hospitals. Such patients are best taken care of in specialized centers. Even in the best of centers, the options depend upon the age of patient, the location of lesion, the pathological nature and staging of the tumors and accessibility to various modalities of treatment. In addition to surgical treatment like curettage, excision, amputation, limb salvage and reconstruction, adjuvant treatment using radiation-therapy and chemotherapy have a role to play to make the patient free from disease, and in a patient with metastatic disease to minimize pain and preserve function for a few more years **(Table 9.2)**.

Many patients who have been reported to have long-term survival after histological diagnosis of "osteosarcoma" probably need to revise the diagnosis according to current criteria. The outcome of frankly malignant tumors even today is abysmal. Once the patient develops generalized metastasis irrespective of the treatment, the average survival is < 2 years **(Table 9.2)**.

BENIGN "TUMOR-LIKE" LESIONS

Nonossifying Fibroma (Fibrous Cortical Defect)

It is one of the commonest benign lesions of bone. Almost all the patients are children, most often the lesion is detected on an incidental finding on X-rays. Metaphyseal region is the usual location. X-ray of the pelvis is advised as a rule to exclude any additional lesion. X-rays reveal an oval lytic area surrounded by thin sclerotic margins. The "cystic cavity" is full of fibrous tissue.

Small subcortical lesion is called "fibrous cortical defect" and some of them may heal spontaneously. Large central defects involving more than one-third of the diameter or those who report with pathological fracture require to be treated by intralesional thorough curettage and compact bone grafting. Recurrence and malignant change are extremely rare.

Polyostotic Fibrous Dysplasia

Polyostotic fibrous dysplasia is a developmental defect where the bone is replaced by multiple "cystic areas" filled by fibrous tissue. The defect may be in a single bone, single limb, or generalized in most of the skeleton. The patients generally present in childhood or adolescence with pain, limp, local swelling, gradually developing deformities or a pathological fracture. Rarely the skin may show café-au-lait patches. X-rays show radiolucent cystic areas filled up with hazy ground-glass material, the cortices are thin, weight-bearing bones show deformities and typically upper ends of femora show coxa vara with lateral convexity of shaft producing "Shepherd's crook" deformities. At operation, the cavities are full of fibro-osseous tissue which feels coarse and gritty because of specks of calcified material it contains **(Figs. 9.3A and B)**.

Table 9.2: Average survival after diagnosis of metastatic deposits despite all treatment.

Source of metastasis	Average survival in months
Thyroid	26
Breast	19
Prostate	18
Gastrointestine	10
Kidney	10
Lungs	10

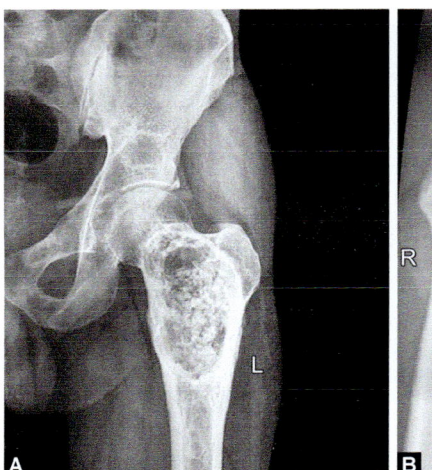
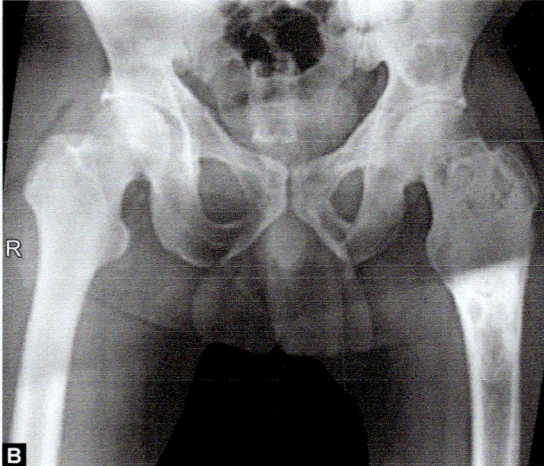

Figs. 9.3A and B: Fibrous dysplasia: Cystic lesion in the upper end of femur treated by curettage and bone grafting. Note another lesion above the acetabulum.

Treatment

Large, painful areas, threatening to deform or fracture the bone should be curetted and compactly packed with allogenic bank bone. Autogenous bone graft would generally fail because these are inherently dysplastic. The author has observed a case where both autogenous fibulae were used to fill a large defect in the femur; the grafts resorbed completely within a year. There are less chances of resorption of allogenic bank bone. Gross deformities may be helped by careful osteotomies. The osteotomies and fractures would need to be fixed with intramedullary nails along with bone grafting. Large recurrence of cavities or gross deformities may require repeat operations. These lesions on operation do bleed profusely, adequate replacement must be available.

Simple Bone Cyst (Unicameral Bone Cyst)

This is a cystic lesion in the metaphyseal area of bones (during childhood), most commonly in upper end of humerus or femur at metadiaphyseal junctional area. It may be an incidental finding on X-rays, or the patient may present with pain, moderate swelling or a pathological fracture. The bone would show a moderate swelling and thinning of cortex. The differential diagnosis during childhood would be from nonossifying fibroma, aneurysmal bone cyst and central chondroma. A CT-guided aspiration of the "cyst" would show straw-colored (serous) fluid from a simple cyst (without fracture), and blood from an aneurysmal bone cyst. Cysts near the physis are likely to grow in size (active cysts). With bone growth, the cyst moves away from the physis, and there are less chances of rapid increase in size **(Figs 9.4A to C)**.

Treatment

Small cysts may not need operative intervention, these can be left alone for occasional observation. Large cyst may be treated by aspiration and instillation of methyl prednisolone or autogenous bone marrow or bisphosphonates. If the cyst is enlarging or there is a pathological fracture, the cavity should be opened, curetted and compactly filled with bone grafts. Follow-up after treatment is essential, about 5% may need a second operation for recurrence.

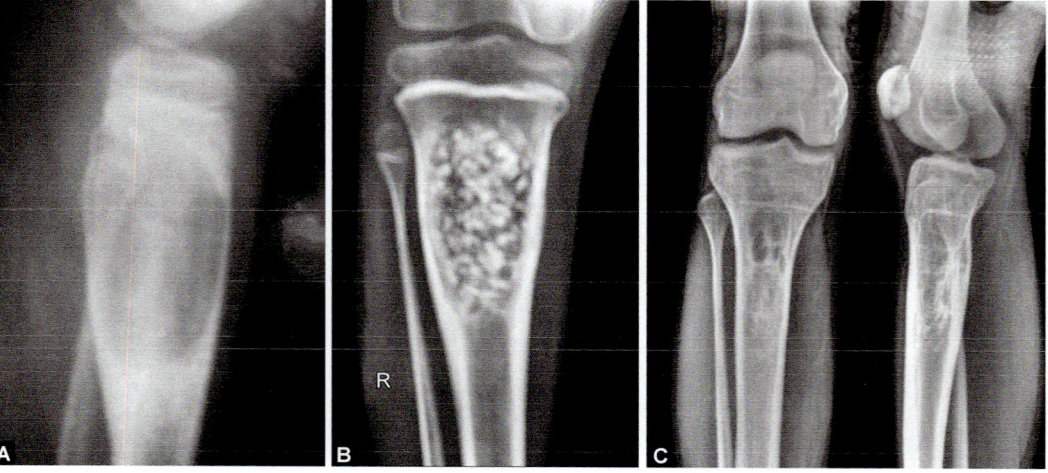

Figs. 9.4A to C: (A) A typical solitary simple bone cyst in a child (unicameral bone cyst) as a cavity in the upper part of tibia without much expansion of bone; (B) Soon after compact allogenic bank bone grafting; (C) 4 years follow-up after grafting.

Aneurysmal Bone Cyst (Figs. 9.5A to C)

This lesion may be encountered at any age from childhood to old age. Any long bone may be involved. Vertebral involvement may occur rarely. Usually it exists as a spontaneous pathology; however, about 20% may be associated with another pre-existing lesion. The patient presents with an expanding lesion with moderate pain. X-rays show a radiolucent cyst with trabeculations and usually an eccentric ballooning. According to the age and location of the cyst, differential diagnosis is needed from giant cell tumor and simple bone cyst. The cyst is filled up with blood, which may be clotted as a thick fleshy lining on the walls or collected in the cavity. Considerable bleeding is expected while curetting the cyst, blood transfusion may be needed for large tumors.

Treatment

The essential treatment should entail carefully opening a window, thorough curettage, cleaning the cavity with hydrogen peroxide and ethanol, and compact packing with abundant bone grafts. If adequately followed, the recurrence observed within 5 years is about 10% which would need reoperations **(Figs. 9.6A to C)**.

BENIGN BONE TUMORS

Solitary osteochondroma (exostosis): This is a bony tumor arising from the surface of a long bone, it has a cartilaginous cap covering the top. The cartilage is inherently from the cells of the neighboring growth plate. The size of osteochondroma increases due to the activity of the cartilage cap, it stops growing when the growth of the parent bone is complete. Common sites are the lower end of femur, upper end of tibia and upper end of humerus. The exostosis usually have a narrow bony pedicle; however, sometimes it has a broad base attached to the bone—sessile exostosis **(Figs. 9.7 to 9.9)**.

The marrow of the pedicle of an osteochondroma is continuous with the marrow of the parent bone. With growth the osteochondroma moves away from the physis of origin. Many osteochondromas have cauliflower-like appearance. The cartilage cap of exostosis differentiates the same way as the growth plate from which it was derived. All cartilaginous tumors have pale glistening surface.

Multiple Osteochondromatosis

This is a hereditary growth disorder (usually autosomal dominant) due to a disturbance

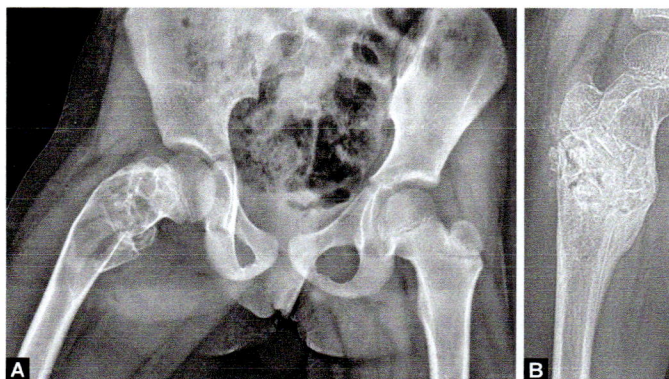
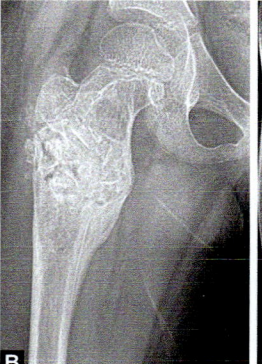
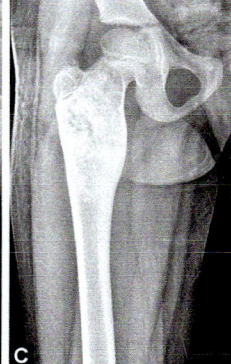

Figs. 9.5A to C: Aneurysmal bone cyst (ABC): (A) A cystic lesion at meta-diaphyseal junction with pathological fracture. (B) The lesion healed after curettage and impaction bone grafting, (C) Complete healing.

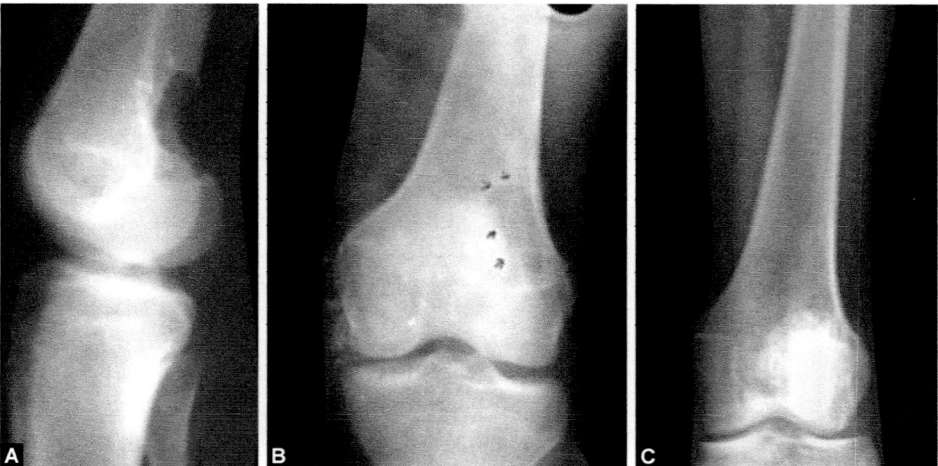

Figs. 9.6A to C: Fibrous cortical defect (non-ossifying fibroma): (A) Essentially a lytic lesion at (B) metaphyseal–diaphyseal junction of femur; (C) Healing took place by compact filling with bone grafts after thorough curettage.

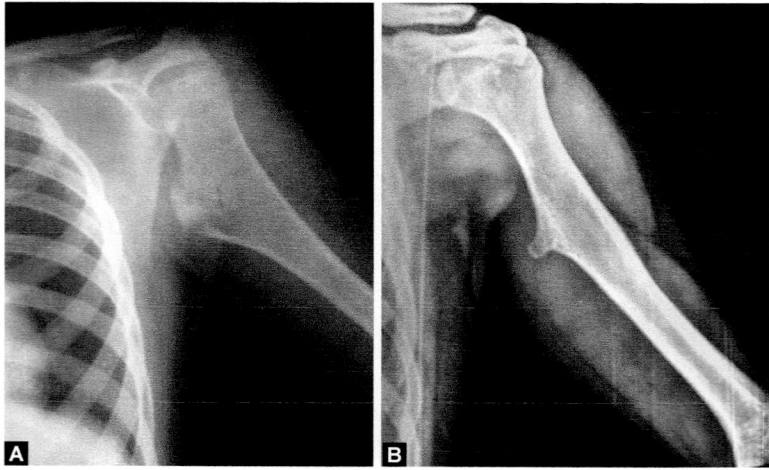

Figs. 9.7A and B: A solitary osteochondroma. (A) Near the proximal humeral metaphysis. (B) With growth the exostosis shifts towards diaphysis away from their growth plate of origin. The exostosis stops growing in size with the end of the growth of the bone (proximal humerus here).

of endochondral ossification. The patient presents with multiple exostosis near the growing ends of long bones, scapula, ribs and pelvis. There is a disturbance of growth and remodeling of bones, resulting in deformity.

With growth, the exostosis (solitary or multiple) move away from the metaphyseal area and the cartilage cap gradually gets directed towards diaphysis. With fusion of the physis of the parent bone, the cartilaginous cap also gets ossified and no further growth of the exostosis takes place. The defect is usually cosmetic but sometimes the large size interferes with movements of joints or tendons. In multiple osteochondromatosis, X-rays may show defective remodeling and shortening of bones.

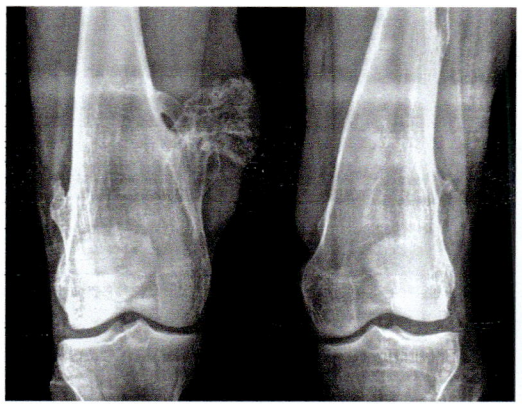

Fig. 9.8: Multiple osteochondromatosis: Note multiple osteochondromas (a genetic disorder autosomal dominant) with deformities of bone.

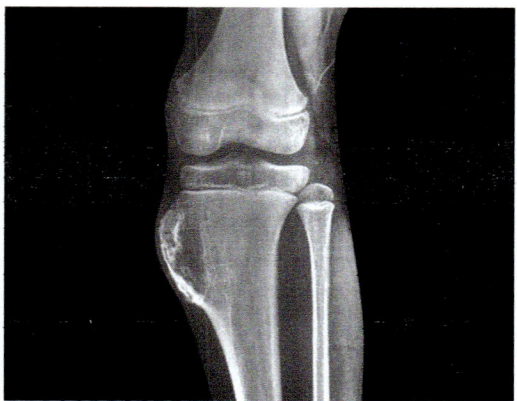

Fig. 9.9: An osteochondroma: Note a sessile base.

Treatment

Every exostosis does not require to be excised. Excessively large tumor or the one interfering with the function of joints, tendon or nerve, or fracture of the exostosis, are the indications for operative removal from the base.

The incidence of **malignant transformation** has not been clearly assessed, it is generally quoted as 1% for solitary lesions and 3% for multiple exostosis. Maximum predilection is for the cartilaginous or osteocartilaginous lesions situated in pelvic and shoulder girdles.

Enchondromatosis (see Chapter 7)

This is a nonhereditary disorder in which multiple cartilaginous tumors appear throughout the skeleton **(Figs. 9.10A and B)**. The tumors may result in swelling (mostly short bones), growth deformities in limbs and rarely in malignant transformation (around pelvic and shoulder girdles).

Ivory Osteoma

It is a benign tumor presenting as a small (1 cm+) rounded swelling usually arising from the cortical layer of flat bones of the skull. The tumor is ivory hard and slow growing, it is generally symptomless except when it presses upon a cranial nerve.

Osteoid Osteoma

It occurs generally in persons younger than 30 years of age and presents as a localized pain in the bone. The pain increases in course of time, it is worse at night and typically responds to salicylates. Gradually, a tender bony swelling develops at the site of tumor with no clinical signs of inflammation. A tender swelling would be palpable if the tumor is located on the superficial bone (e.g., medial surface of tibia). Males are affected more commonly. X-ray would show a small osteolytic lesion generally <1 cm in diameter in the subperiosteal region surrounded by a dense sclerotic area. When the tumor is located in a cancellous bone, the lytic area (nidus) may contain a dense spot in the center; however, the surrounding sclerosis is not prominent. CT scan is now considered a standard investigation for diagnosis of osteoid osteoma in any location of skeleton. Osteoid osteoma is generally <2 cm, and osteoblastoma is >2 cm. Differential diagnosis from Brodie's abscess must be entertained.

Treatment consisted of excision of the tumor with nidus along with a part of

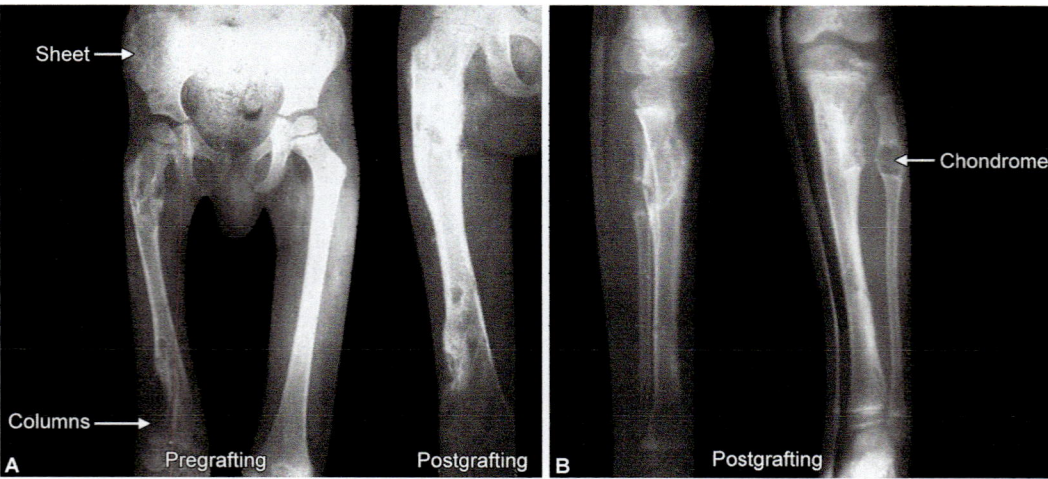

Figs. 9.10A and B: Enchondromatosis (dyschondroplasia) showing multiple cartilaginous deposits in the bones. The deposits are in the form of round—chondromes, columns, or sheets. Bones can show deformities. Fibula in Figure B was not grafted.

sclerotic bone. The excised bone specimen was X-rayed in the operating room to ensure complete removal of the nidus. If the tumor was located in a vulnerable area (e.g., femoral neck), one tried a longer course of salicylates (6–9 months taken at bed time) or try CT-guided radioablation. At present radiofrequency ablation (RFA) is considered the standard treatment for osteoid osteoma in any location of skeleton.

Osteoblastoma (Giant Osteoid Osteoma)

This tumor is similar to osteoid osteoma but it is larger than 1 cm and is more commonly situated in flat bones and spine. No malignant change has been observed in osteoid osteoma and osteoblastoma over the life time.

Giant Cell Tumor of Bone (Osteoclastoma) (Figs. 9.11A to D)

The exact origin of this tumor is still under debate. The tumor probably arises from the connective tissues stromal cells or the osteoclasts located within the bone. Giant cells reaction is seen in many other conditions like aneurysmal bone cyst, fibrous dysplasia, chondroblastoma, chondromyxoid fibroma (all collectively addressed as giant-cell-variants), chondromatous lesions and also during the repair process of osseous tissues.

At present, giant cell tumor (GCT) is considered a locally recurring or aggressive tumor. The tumor occurs in patients in third and fourth decades after the fusion of the epiphyses of long bones. The commoner sites are lower end of femur, upper end of tibia, and distal end of radius. A skeletally mature patient presents with a slowly growing tumor at the end of a bone. The cortex of the tumor is firm at places, it yields in some areas giving the feeling of an egg shell crackling. The neighboring joint is not involved; however, a large tumor may lead to mechanical restriction of movements.

X-rays show an osteolytic lesion occupying the end of a bone with an eccentric expansion of the cortex. Trabeculations on the wall of the tumor exhibit as "soap bubble" appearance in the X-rays. The tumor abuts the subchondral bone but as a rule does not penetrate through the articular cartilage. Untreated large tumors may report with pathological fracture (10–15% in the Indian subcontinent)

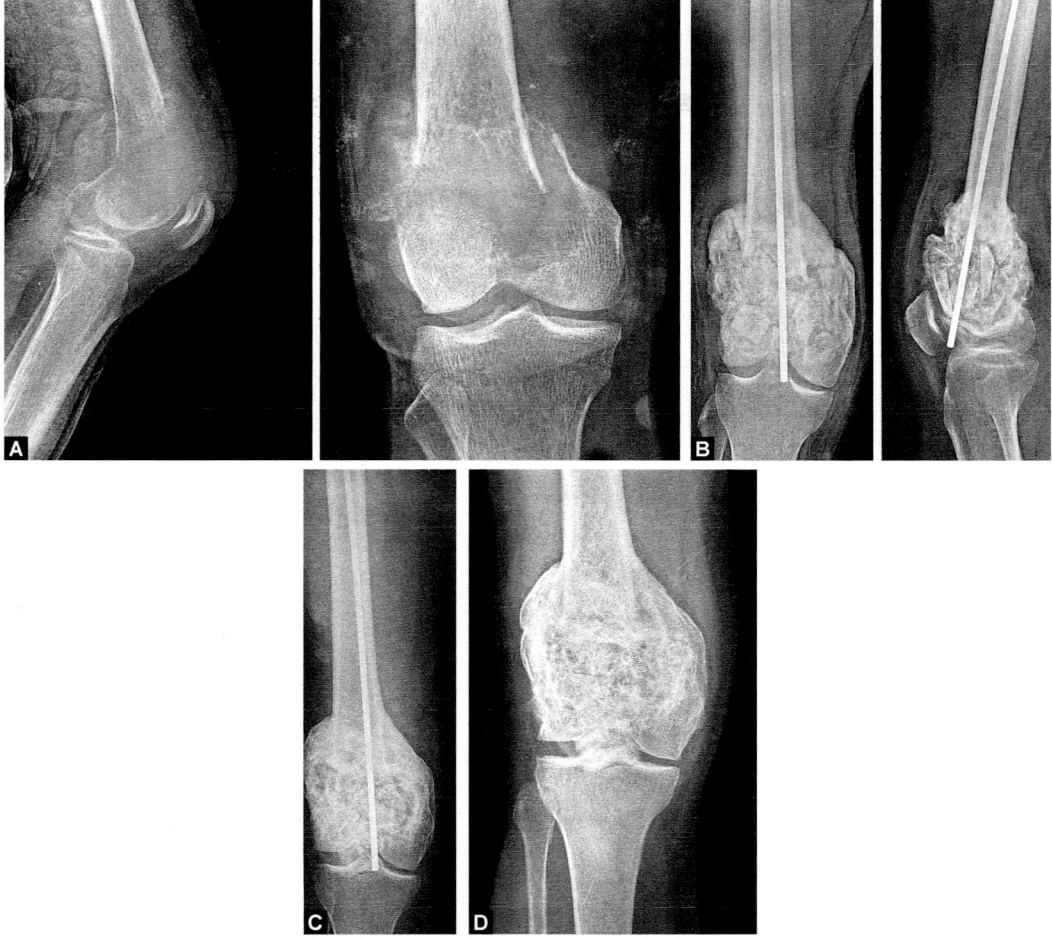

Figs. 9.11A to D: Giant cell tumor (GCT). (A) Distal end of femur showing a GCT with pathological fracture (Campanacci III). (B) Soon after curettage and bone grafting, (C) Showing healing with incorporating bone grafts, (D) Complete healing, 9 years follow-up.

(Figs. 9.12 to 9.14). Campanacci classifies, GCT as grades = I—completely intraosseous, II—presence of cortical erosion (break-up), III—cortical destruction with pathological fracture with extra-osseous presence of tumor.

Treatment

En bloc resection is probably the best treatment for easily resectable tumors like those located in distal ulna, proximal fibula and distal radius. The resection of distal radius can be satisfactorily reconstructed/replaced by a fibular graft. Tumors located in major weight-bearing bones like femur and tibia would need more complicated procedures for reconstruction after en bloc resection. The first treatment accepted for such tumors is thorough intra-lesional curettage using burrs and gouges, application of hydrogen peroxide and ethanol to clean the cavity, and compact packing with copious bone grafts. More aggressive or recurrent tumors require to be treated by resection with reconstruction or prosthetic replacement. Tumors at difficult sites, e.g., vertebral column are difficult to

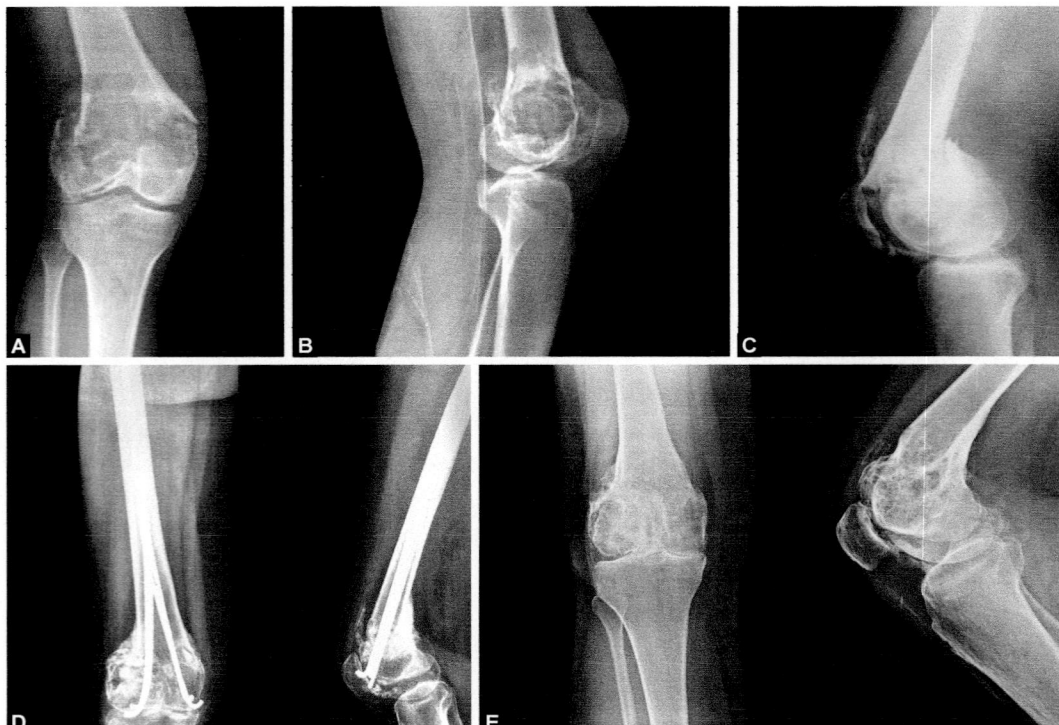

Figs. 9.12A to E: Giant-cell tumor (osteoclastoma): (A) Lytic cystic lesion in a mature skeleton abutting the joint margin (distal end of femur Campanacci grade II). Despite a (B and C) pathological fracture, an intralesional curettage, compact bone grafting and stabilization using elastic nails, the tumor healed. The implants were removed. (D) Shows the healed status 12 years after operation. (E) Full extension to 90 degrees flexion.

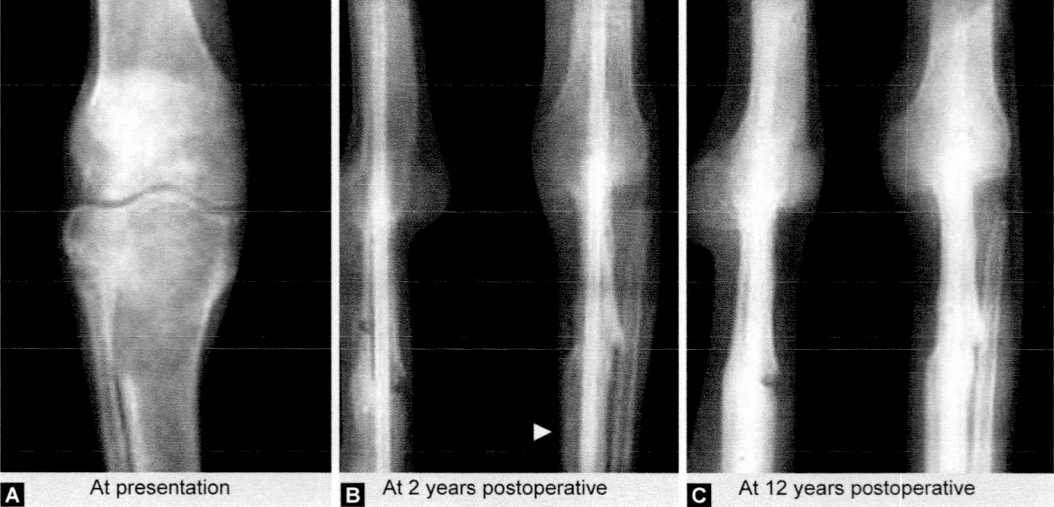

Figs. 9.13A to C: Giant-cell-tumor: Abutting upper end of tibia. It was treated by en bloc resection and structural bone graft sacrificing the knee joint. Note the hypertrophy of the bone graft according to Wolff's law.

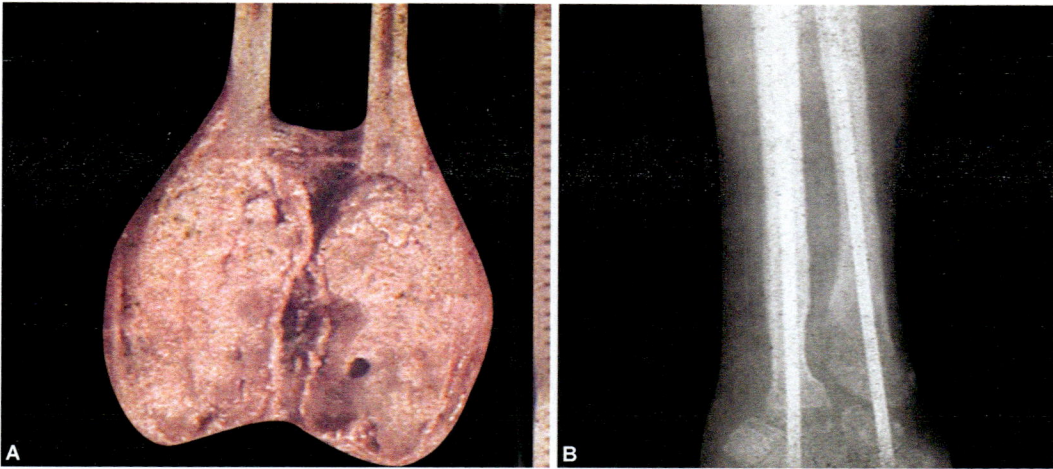

Figs. 9.14A and B: (A) Giant cell tumor of distal radius. The tumor typically occurs in a mature bone and it abuts the subchondral end of the bone. (B) Upper end of autogenous fibula was used for reconstruction after en bloc resection of the tumor.

eradicate, after possible curettage, radiation therapy is recommended. In general if these patients are followed for 5 years or more after the primary treatment, the recurrence rate after en bloc resection is about 5%, and 20% after intralesional curettage and bone grafting. Malignant transformation is extremely rare, most likely such tumors are giant cell rich osteosarcomas from the onset, or malignant giant cell tumor.

MALIGNANT BONE TUMORS

Osteosarcoma

This is a highly malignant tumor arising from bone. Of all the malignant tumors of bone, osteosarcoma constitutes about 50%. The tumor arises from the multipotent mesenchymal cells situated within the bone, therefore, the tumor, is constituted by osteoblastic, chondroblastic and fibroblastic tissues in various proportions. Highest incidence is between the ages 10 and 20 years, with male preponderance. Generally, the patient presents with progressively increasing constant pain in the initial stages, followed by the appearance of a swelling. The commonest location is the metaphyseal area of lower end of femur and upper end of tibia. Once the swelling is palpable, it is bony hard, has diffused margins, warm, and tender on palpation. The swelling and symptoms progressively increase, patient develops loss of weight, cachexia and anemia. In a large tumor of long-standing, the central part may show softening because of tissue necrosis and a pathological fracture may occur. Blood examination may show a raised ESR and alkaline phosphatase. By the time a patient in clinically diagnosed as osteosarcoma, the presently available investigations reveal the presence of micrometastasis in the lungs, advising osteosarcoma to be treated as a systemic disease.

Radiological Features

The tumor arises from the metaphyseal region, there may be generalized enlargement of bone or an eccentric expansion. There are mottled areas of rarefaction and new bone formation in the initial stages. As the size increases, the periosteum gets lifted up along with the blood vessels running at right angles to the underlying bone. New bone is laid along these blood vessels creating a picture of "sun-burst", ("sun-rays"), and subperiosteal bone laid parallel to the involved bone gives an appearance of "onion-peels". At the proximal and distal margins of the elevated periosteum, a triangle shaped subperiosteal new bone forms called "Codman's triangle". The subperiosteal changes may also be seen in other rapidly growing tumors and rarely in chronic osteomyelitis. In neglected cases, the bony cortex is broken and the tumor mass involves the soft tissues. Most of the cases would show a mixture of osteosclerosis and osteolysis, one predominant than other.

On presentation of the patient, chest X-ray is mandatory to exclude metastatic deposits. About 10% of patients have radiologically visible pulmonary metstasis at the time of first visit. Whenever a neoplasm is suspected the diagnosis must be established by histological examination of a representative biopsy material. Adequate amount of biopsy material should be obtained from the growing peripheral part of the tumor.

Histologically, the tumor has to be differentiated from chondrosarcoma, reticulum cell sarcoma, fibrous dysplasia, and repairing fracture callus.

Treatment

The conventional treatment has been to amputate the limb well above the limit of tumor. Amputation like hind-quarter or forequarter may be needed for tumors situated near the hip or shoulder joints. Amputation even as a palliative measure would relieve the pain and avoid the miseries of fungation of the tumor. Even today amputation at a suitable level has the least chances of local recurrence, less uncomfortable for postoperative survival years, easy for rehabilitation and most cost-effective.

During the last two decades, oncological therapies are trying limb saving modalities using multiple neoadjuvant chemotherapy, radiation therapy and custom made endo-prosthetic replacement after resection of the tumor. The average survival after such therapies is about 50%, at 5 years follow-up. There is a fairly high complication rate, such as wound breakdown, infection and implant failure. These modalities are highly expensive, time consuming and can be carried out only in highly specialized centers after elaborate counseling with the families.

Variants of Osteosarcoma

There are a few varieties of possibly less aggressive sarcomas of the bone; "parosteal sarcoma" is considered to arise from the periosteum, and "periosteal osteosarcoma" is considered to arise from the superficial part of bone. The clinical behavior is relatively less aggressive, the basic principles of treatment are the same as for osteosarcoma.

Paget's disease is uncommon in the Indian subcontinent, the sarcomatous transformation is a rare complication, which may occur after the age of 50 years. Most of these patients have pulmonary metastases by the time of diagnosis of malignant changes. palliative treatment using radiation therapy and chemotherapy may be a wiser option.

Chondrosarcoma

The incidence of chondrosarcoma is almost half of that of osteosarcoma. It may be arising from the center (medullary area) of the bone called "central chondrosarcoma", or it may arise from the periphery of a bone called "peripheral chondrosarcoma". The tumor may arise de novo or it may be a malignant transformation of a pre-existing cartilaginous tumor, central chondroma or exostosis. Common locations for this tumor are ends of femur, upper end of tibia or humerus, pelvis, shoulder, or ribs, more common in rhizomelic areas. The patient generally presents with a swelling between 30 and 40 years of age. The swelling is preceded by a history of vague pain for a few months. The swelling feels lobulated and is moderately tender on deep palpation. Clinically, the clearest sign of malignancy is progressive enlargement of an osteochondroma or a central chondroma after the fusion of physis of the host bone.

Radiologically, the tumor presents with a lobulated fluffy appearance with flecks of irregular calcification **(Fig. 9.15)**. In central chondrosarcoma, there would be expansion of bone with patchy destruction, and in peripheral tumor one may be able to appreciate the bony pedicle. MRI is the best modality to show the size and expansion of the cartilaginous elements.

Macroscopically, the tumor looks lobulated, covered at most of the places by bluish-white cartilage. In tumors of long standing, there would be areas of soft myxomatous degeneration. If the cartilage cap is >3 cm, suspect malignant change. Confirmation of malignant changes is essentially based upon histological appearance of tissues from different parts of the tumor.

In general, these tumors are nonresponders to radiation as well as to chemotherapy. The treatment of choice is amputation at suitable level. In some cases, wide resection and prosthetic replacement may be possible. Long-term follow-up of these patients is essential because recurrence or metastasis may present even 10 years after the primary treatment.

Multiple Myeloma

This is a highly malignant tumor arising from the plasma cells of the bone marrow. The common locations are the vertebral column, skull and ribs. It may start as a solitary lesion called solitary "plasmacytoma" or as multiple myelomas. Most of the cases of solitary plasmacytoma ultimately become multiple myelomas.

The common age of presentation is after 40 years, most of the patients complain of pain in the back, generalized vague pains, weakness, loss of appetite and weight. This tumor originates essentially from the plasma cells which are associated with production of serum globulins. Serum electrophoresis in such patients would show "M-protein", and urine examination may reveal Bence Jones proteins in about 50% of cases. Blood examination may show low hemoglobin, raised ESR, high creatinine, and hypercalcemia. Marrow obtained from sternum or iliac crest may show typical "myeloma-cells" and plasmacytosis **(Fig. 9.16)**.

X-rays may show generalized osteoporosis of the spine and skeleton. The typical lesions are multiple punched out osteolytic areas present in the skull, pelvis and proximal femur. The vertebrae may show compression

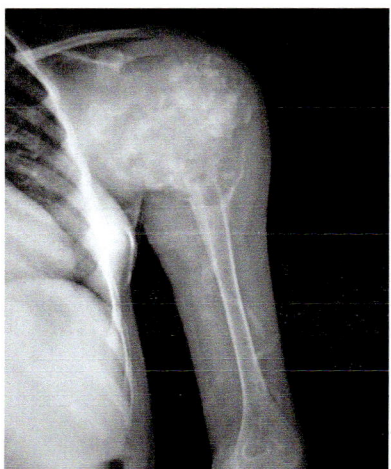

Fig. 9.15: Chondrosarcoma arising from upper end of left humerus. Note the rhizomelic location, fluffy swelling with flecks of patchy calcification.

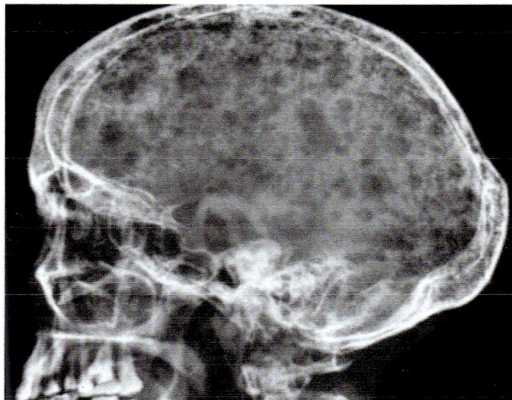

Fig. 9.16: Classical appearance of multiple punched out areas in the skull in a case of multiple myeloma ("pepper-pot").

fracture, which requires to be differentiated from senile osteoporosis, metastatic deposits and tuberculosis. For a fracture in the trochanteric region in an elderly patient, the clinician must exclude the possibility of myeloma or metastasis.

Treatment

The aim of treatment is to keep the patient mobile with suitable braces. Pathological fractures in extremities may get relief of pain by intramedullary fixation or by less extensive procedures. Neural complications would require cord decompression with stabilization of the column. Multimodal chemotherapy, intermittent use of steroids and radiation therapy along with the general supportive measures may help relieve the pain, keep the patient mobile for the surviving years after the diagnosis and treatment. Conventional chemotherapeutic agents and thalidomide are used in combination with dexamethasone. Treatment is recommended to be carried out in specialized centers. Approximate survival time is 2–7 years in generalized disease.

Ewing's Sarcoma

It is an uncommon highly malignant sarcoma of bone, probably arising from the endothelial cells of the bone marrow. Typically the tumor occurs in children between the age of 10 and 20 years, involving the diaphyseal segment of tibia, femur, other long bones, pelvis and vertebrae. The patient presents with pain and progressively increasing swelling. The swelling breaks through the bony cortices and invades the surrounding soft tissues. The swelling is warm and tender, and there is accompanying pyrexia suggesting the diagnosis of subacute osteomyelitis.

X-rays usually show an area of destruction of diaphyseal segment of bone with surrounding soft tissue swelling. The bony swelling may show mottled appearance, "sun-ray" appearance, "onion-peel" appearance and Codman's triangles, not unlike the picture in osteosarcoma **(Figs. 9.17A and B)**.

Histology of the biopsy material is essential to make the diagnosis and to differentiate it from other sarcomatous lesions and osteomyelitis. An incision for biopsy may show a liquid material resembling pus, brain tissue or reddish jelly. The characteristic cells are small rounded cells arranged in sheets without any ground substance.

Treatment at present consists of neoadjuvant chemotherapy and radiation therapy. In accessible favorable location, excisional

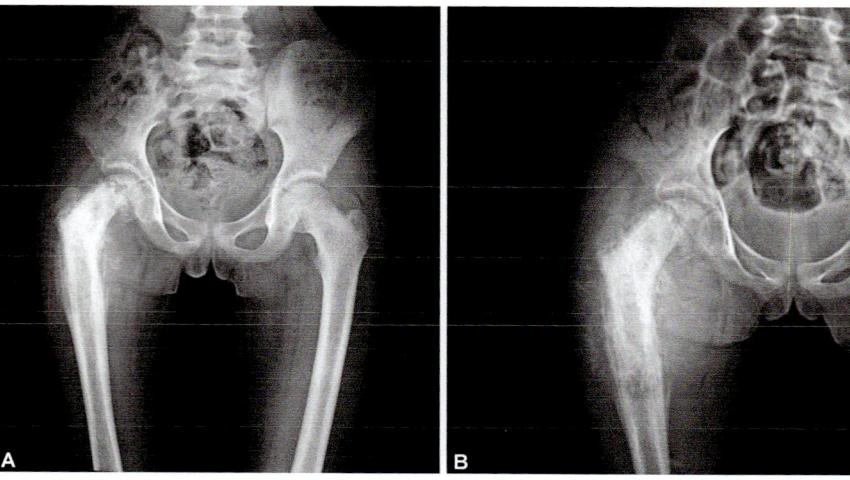

Figs. 9.17A and B: Ewing's sarcoma arising from upper shaft of femur in a child. Note maximum involvement of a segment of diaphysis, pathological fracture of femoral neck, "sun-burst" appearance on the medial side and "onion-peel" appearance on the lateral side.

surgery is being tried. The long-term prognosis is still very poor, 5 years survival rate is about 50%.

RETICULUM-CELL SARCOMA OF BONE (NON-HODGKIN'S LYMPHOMA)

This rare tumor clinically and histologically has some resemblance with Ewing's sarcoma. Like Ewing's tumor, it is a round cell tumor; however, each cell is surrounded by reticulum fibrils. Clinically, it is a slow growing tumor and prognosis is better than Ewing's sarcoma. The tumor is generally located in femur, tibia, humerus and flat bones. In most of the cases, there is involvement of regional lymph nodes. The usual age of presentation is 25–45 years.

X-rays show mottled appearance with patchy areas of bone destruction and new bone formation. Usual treatment is a combination of radiation and chemotherapy. Easily resectable tumors may be resected after local radiation therapy.

Metastatic Bone Deposits

The skeleton is the most common site for metastatic deposits from carcinomas and sarcomas, and metastatic malignancy is the most common malignancy affecting the skeleton. Sometimes the secondary deposit may be the first clinical feature while the source of the primary focus is still subclinical. The malignant cells reach the skeleton through the arterial or venous circulation. Batson's vertebral venous plexus provides a free vascular communication between the pelvic, portal and caval system; this permits the spread of malignant cells from the viscera to the vertebrae without passing through the lungs. The common sources of metastatic deposits in the skeleton are from prostate, breast, kidney, lungs, thyroid, bladder, gastrointestinal tract and neuroblastoma. Despite all investigations in about 10% of patients, the primary tumor cannot be detected. In patients over 50 years of age, metastatic malignancy is commoner than all primary malignant tumors put together. In a patient with a carcinoma, even in remote past, a new discovered bone lesion is mostlikely a metastasis **(Fig. 9.18)**.

Clinical Features

The main clinical features of a metastatic malignancy are bone pain, local swelling and a pathological fracture. Pain in the back with girdle radiation or neural deficit may occur due to deposits in the vertebral column. Generally, bone secondaries are not seen distal to the elbow and knees. Deposits located in these areas are mostly from a primary in the lungs.

Imaging and radiological features: The metastatic deposits are usually osteolytic, those from prostatic cancer are generally osteoblastic; however, concomitant osteolytic lesions may also be present. The metastatic deposits are located where red marrow is present. The usual location is vertebrae, ribs, pelvis, skull, proximal ends of femur and humerus (rhizomelic areas). The deposits gradually grow in size, destroy the bone, invade the soft tissue and cause a pathological fracture. MRI scanning of vertebral column and radioisotope whole body scanning are most sensitive methods for

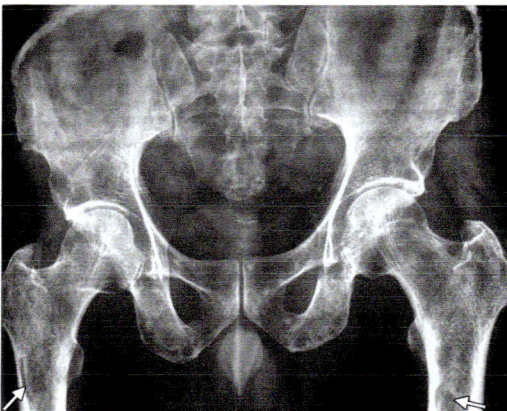

Fig. 9.18: Metastasis from prostate malignancy would in general exhibit a combination of sclerotic and lytic deposits.

detecting the "silent" deposits and those in difficult areas. Once metastasis is diagnosed, average survival (despite all treatment) in months is: Thyroid 26, Breast 19, Prostatic 18, Gastrointestine 10, Kidney 10.

Laboratory Findings

The ESR is raised and the hemoglobin level is low. Serum alkaline phosphatase is elevated in general, and in prostatic carcinoma acid phosphatase is also raised. Patients with breast cancer and those with prostatic cancer may show elevation of cancer-associated antigen markers.

Treatment

By the time a patient is diagnosed with a metastatic deposit, the prognosis for long-term survival is poor; 6 months to a few years. The treatment in majority of patients is essentially symptomatic. The patients must be made comfortable for the remaining part of their life.

Occasionally more vigorous treatment for deposits from renal cells, breast, thyroid and prostate is rewarding. The treatment in such cases would consist of radiation therapy, chemotherapy, hormone therapy and selective ablative surgery. Prophylactic intramedullary nailing is justified for impending fracture of the shaft of femur, tibia or humerus, if the metastatic lesion (or myeloma deposit) is involving more than 50% of the diameter of the shaft. Major shaft fractures need to be fixed with intramedullary nails and one may have to settle for less extensive procedures. Vertebral deposits threatening the neural functions may need early decompression and stabilization of the spine. Any surgical intervention must be done after elaborate counseling with the family and patients.

NEOPLASMS: PITFALLS ARE IN PLENTY

With the availability of modern imaging modalities like MRIs, CT scans, Isotope bone scans and PET scans, imaging features of certain normal reactive benign tumors, inflammatory, traumatic and degenerative processes may mimic malignant neoplasms. Misinterpretation of the imaging findings especially when isolated from clinical findings and clinical behavior can lead to inappropriate clinical management. When in doubt, it may be safer to treat the lesion as a benign tumor rather than as a "malignant one". Before labelling and treating a lesion as "malignant" the clinician must have a robust proof of malignancy by semi-invasive or open biopsy procedures.

At present, with availability of modern diagnostic facilities and therapeutics enbloc intercalary resection of tumor bearing bone followed by reconstruction is being tried. A few conditions for such trials have been chondrosarcoma, malignant giant-cell-tumor, a solitary (isolated) metastatic deposit from carcinoma (breast, prostate, thyroid). Endoprosthetic reconstruction has been tried using sterilization of the resected bone (autoclaving, boiling, radiation or chemical sterilization) or by employing biomimetic prosthetics, mega-endoprosthetics, or allogenic bone grafts.

Risk-benefit-ratio however must be considered. Survival of such therapies is about 50% at 5 years postoperative follow-up.

SUGGESTED READINGS

1. Tuli SM. Bridging of bone defects by massive bone grafts in tumorous conditions and in osteomyelitis. Clin Orthop Relat Res. 1972;87:60-73.
2. Tuli SM, Varma BP, Srivastava TP. Giant-cell tumour of bone: a study of natural course. Int Orthop (SICOT). 1978;2:207-14.
3. Goel SC, Tuli SM, Singh HP, Sharma SV, Saraf SK, Srivastava TP. Allogenic decalbone in the repair of benign cystic lesions of bone. Int orthop. 1992;16:176-9.
4. Crawford AH, Schorry EK. Neurofibromatosis in children: the role of the orthopaedist. J Am Acad Orthop Surg. 1999;7:217-30.

5. Capanna R, Campanacci D. The treatment in metastases in the appendicular skeleton. J Bone Joint Surg Br. 2001;83B:471-81.
6. Grimer RJ, Briggs TWR. Earlier diagnosis of the bone and soft tissue tumors. J Bone Joint Surg Br. 2010: 92B:1489-92.
7. Bus MPA, Dijkstra PDS, van de Sande MAJ, Taminiau AHM, Schreuder HWB , Jutte PC, et al. Intercalary allograft reconstructions following resection of primary bone tumors: A nationwide multicenter study. J Bone Joint Surg Am. 2014;96A:1-1.
8. Pretell-Mazzini J, Murphy RF, Kushare I, Dormans JP. Unicameral Bone Cysts: General characteristics and management controversies. J Am Acad Orthop Surg. 2014: 22:295-303.
9. Mak IWY, Evaniew N, Popovic S, Tozer R, Ghert M. A translational study of the neoplastic cells of giant cell tumor of bone following neoadjuvant denosumab. J Bone Joint Surg Am. 2014;96A:1-8.
10. Ippolito E, Farsetti P, Boyce AM, Corci A, Maio FD, Collins MT. Rdiographic classification of coronal plane femoral deformities in polyostotic fibrous dysplasia. Clin Orthop Relat Res. 2014;472:1558-67.
11. Capanna R, Scoccianti G, Frenos F, Vilardi A, Beltrami G, Campanacci DA. What was the survival of megaprostheses in lower limb reconstructions after tumor resections? Clin Orthop Relat Res. 2015;473:820-30.
12. Tuli SM. Allogenic Decal-Bone Grafts: A Viable Option in Clinical Orthopedics. Bone Grafting - Recent Advances with Special References to Cranio-Maxillofacial Surgery. Intech Open; 2018.
13. Rose PS. What's New in Musculoskeletal Tumor Surgery. J Bone Joint Surg Am. 2021;103A;2251-60.

CHAPTER 10

Common Neuromuscular Disorders

POLIOMYELITIS

While assessing a child for neuromuscular disorders the orthopedic clinician has to give a little extra-time to make the child more comfortable to arrive at the truly representative findings and possible diagnosis. A normal growing child holds up the neck at about 3 months, sits up on his own at about 6 months and begins walking at about 1 year. If a child cannot sit unaided by 4 years, and those who cannot walk by 8 years are unlikely to walk independently. Only common neuromuscular disorders are mentioned in this chapter.

Poliomyelitis is an acute infectious viral disease which spreads by oropharyngeal route. The organisms multiply in the alimentary tract and spread to central nervous system. In the spinal type, anterior horn cells of cervical and lumbar enlargements are most commonly affected. Infection in the bulbar type leads to respiratory paralysis and is generally fatal. The virus localizes in the anterior horn cells causing death of the cells by chromatolysis. There is also pericellular (perineural) edema. The death of cells is responsible for permanent paralysis, whereas resolution of edema explains the recovery of some paralyzed muscles. The viruses have varying virulence and in countries where preventive vaccination is practiced, it has become a rare disease, however, the effects of post-polio residual paralysis are still with us. It was generally held that the extent and pattern of motor weakness was firmly established to be static by 2 years after the acute attack, however, now it has been observed that about 20% of patients may show reactivation of the virus about 15 years after the onset of disease. The reactivation may result in weakness of both old and new muscle groups. This condition has been addressed as post-polio syndrome (PPS), the treatment is symptomatic. One must however exclude other medical causes for symptoms.

Acute Stage

Acute stage is characterized by sudden onset of fever with symptoms of meningeal irritation and gastrointestinal symptoms. On the second or third day, there is sudden onset of flaccid paralysis of the muscles and trunk. The paralyzed muscles are tender on palpation. The treatment of this stage is essentially supportive for pyrexia, meningeal irritation and nutrition. The paralyzed limbs are supported in the best functional position with the help of splints. Contractures and deformities are prevented by gentle exercises.

Stage of Convalescence or Recovery

About 2 weeks after the onset, acute symptoms subside, muscle tenderness disappears and paralyzed muscles begin to recover power. The stage of recovery lasts for about 2 years, however, maximum recovery takes place within 6 months. The aim of treatment is to prevent deformities by the use of orthotic appliances, and to help recovery of muscle power by remedial exercises. The progress of a case can be assessed by recording the grading of muscle power according to Medical Research Council (MRC grading). Remedial exercises are aimed at elimination of contractures and deformities, and improvement of power in the muscles. The child can be helped by doing exercises in exercise pools (Hubbard tanks) and cycling. As various muscle groups recover suitable appliances are used for walking.

Stage of Residual Paralysis (Fig. 10.1)

No further recovery of muscles power is expected at the end of 2 years, after the onset. The aim at this stage is to make the best use of available muscle power and make the patient ambulatory. A neglected patient may present with deformities. If conservative methods like passive stretching do not achieve correction, selective operations are performed. The aim of the operations should be: (1) To make the patient fit for wearing an appliance for walking; (2) To reduce the size of appliance the patient is using; (3) To eliminate the necessity of an orthotic appliance.

Hip, Knee and Foot

Marked flexion contracture of hip is corrected by release of contracted tensor fascia late and tight muscles from anterior part of iliac crest. Flexion contracture of the knee can be corrected by division of iliotibial tract near the knee joints and lengthening of hamstrings. Gross equinus deformity of foot can be corrected by lengthening of tendo-Achilles provided the combined muscle power of ipsilateral quadriceps and gluteus maximus is more than 5 MRC grading. If this power is less than MRC-5, the patient has acquired the equinus deformity with extension of knee to stabilize the limb. Plantar flexion (equinus) plus knee extension work as "couple" to enable the patient to walk.

Prerequisite for planning correction of equinus must ensure presence of good power in hip and knee extensors. Botulinum (toxin) injection may help judge the efficacy of planned surgical release of contracted tendons. Tendo-Achilles lengthening in such a case may convert the patient to be a non-walker or dependent on a long above knee appliance, or use **"a hand to knee"** gait for walking. Muscle balance may be improved by surgical redistribution of available muscle power. As an example, quadriceps weakness may be minimized by transferring biceps femoris tendon and gracilis tendon to the weak quadriceps muscles. After the age of 12 years, if some joints are unstable due to loss of power, function can be improved by arthrodesis of joints in best functional position. The commonest example is triple arthrodesis of the foot.

Triple Arthrodesis of foot

In this operation, talocalcaneal, talonavicular, and calcaneocuboid joints are fused after excising the articular cartilage and subchondral bone with appropriate wedge resection to correct fixed deformities, like equinus, varus, and valgus of the foot. If the ankle and foot are flail, pantalar fusion is advised, in addition to the triple fusion, perform the fusion of ankle joint as well. While performing pantalar fusion aim at fusion with 5 degrees of external rotation and 5 degrees of valgus.

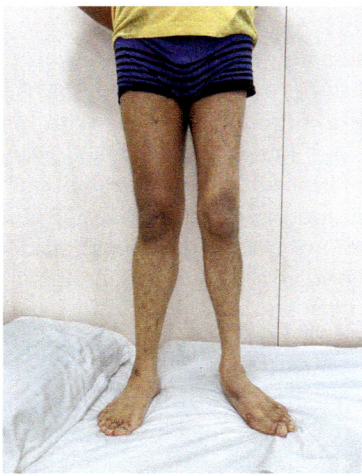

Fig. 10.1: Post-polio-residual paralysis (PPRP): Clinical picture showing marked wasting of muscles of thigh and calf, pes-plano-valgus in left lower limb.

The family, the patient and the medical profession often concentrate on the lower limbs because of the importance of ambulation, however upper limbs functions are also important for children who are dependent on walking aids.

Shoulder

For a weak or flail shoulder some function at the shoulder can be restored by arthrodesing the glenohumeral joint in "saluting position" (50 degrees abducted, 25 degrees flexed and 30 degrees internal rotation). Prerequisite for this operation is good power in periscapular muscles (e.g., trapezius, serratus anterior, rhomboideus). Gross weakness of serratus anterior becomes obvious by presence of winging of scapula.

Elbow, Forearm and Hand

Important function can be improved by transposing separable active muscles. Weakness of opposition of thumb can be overcome by transferring one of the flexor digitorum superficialis (FDS—usually of ring finger). The tendon is cut near its insertion on the middle phalanx, is wound around the insertion of flexor carpi ulnaris (on pisiform bone), threaded across the palm and fixed to the radial border of distal end of the first metacarpal. In gross deformity or instability of wrist, the function can be markedly improved by wrist arthrodesis in about 10 degrees of dorsiflexion. Active dorsiflexors or palmar flexors of the wrist can then be used to augment the finger functions.

Hip Deformities

Hip deformities are usually complex and difficult to manage. The problems get aggravated by concomitant paralytic scoliosis, tilting of pelvis due to scoliosis, imbalance of abductors of hip joint, maldevelopment of upper end of femur, and under development of acetabulum, all these increase the tendency to hip joints instability and dislocation. Basic guidelines to improve the function would require correction of paralytic scoliosis, minimize the pelvic tilt, correct upper femoral deformities (coxa valga, coxa vara), repose the femoral head into the acetabular socket, deepen the acetabulum by acetabuloplasty if it is hypoplastic. The judgment for the choice of procedures needs experience and understanding.

MUSCULAR DYSTROPHIES

This is a group of disorders of the muscles resulting in difficulties in locomotion. The exact etiology is not clear, however, most of these cases are hereditary and familial with recessive or dominant traits of transmission. It is a progressive degenerative disease of the muscles without any evidence of regeneration. Anatomically, the innervations of the muscles are intact, there is no sensory deficit. However with progressive disease, the muscle fibers get replaced by fibrous tissue and fat. The two least uncommon varieties are "pseudohypertrophic muscular dystrophy (Duchenne)" and "facioscapulohumeral dystrophy."

Duchenne muscular dystrophy (incidence 2–3 per 100,000 population) usually gets clinically noticed around the age of 5, and is more common in males. The child hesitates to walk or run and falls frequently. The mother notices that the child has difficulty in getting up from the squatting position on the grounds. The muscle weakness deteriorates and the child gets up by climbing upon his lower limbs and by supporting the body weight with his hands on his legs, knees and thighs (Gower's sign). The calf muscles show apparent hypertrophy (look enlarged in girth). The glutei and calf muscles are involved early, shoulder girdle muscles are involved at a later stage. The child walks with waddling gait and exaggerated lumbar lordosis. By the age of 10 years, most of the children become dependent in a wheelchair. Involvement of muscles of the trunk and chest lead to cardiopulmonary failure ultimately leading to death by about 30 years of age. The author has observed a family of four affected male siblings, the eldest aged 11 crawling on floor and the youngest aged 3 years running around the home. The diagnosis is usually based upon clinical features and family history. The laboratory confirmation is achieved by the estimation of serum creatine phosphokinase (CPK) levels which are higher by 200–300 times of the normal values. Muscle biopsy would reveal replacement of muscle fibers by fibrous and fatty tissues. The weakest accessible muscle with about 50% of strength is most likely to give a useful information.

Family counseling is important: by the time the first child is diagnosed, in about 20% the family already has younger affected sibling. Unfortunately, at present, there is no clinically effective medical treatment for muscular dystrophies.

Limb Girdle Muscular Dystrophy

Limb girdle muscular dystrophy is characterized by weakness of pelvic and shoulder girdle muscles. It represents a heterogeneous group of conditions with an autosomal recessive inheritance pattern affecting both sexes. Symptoms usually start around adolescence.

Facioscapulohumeral Muscular Dystrophy

Facioscapulohumeral muscular dystrophy is an autosomal dominant condition with very variable expression. In general, males are more severely involved than females. Characteristically muscle weakness is first seen on facial muscles followed by involvement of scapular muscles.

ARTHROGRYPOSIS MULTIPLEX CONGENITA (AMYOPLASIA)

These children are born with multiple nonprogressive soft tissue contractures and restriction of joint movements. The condition may be generalized affecting all the joints of body, or may be localized to one limb or even a part of limb as 'congenital clubfoot'. It is believed that there are 2 distinct varieties 'neuropathic' and 'myopathic', however mostly both features may coexist in the same patient. The incidence is said to be one in 3,000 live births. Intellect is generally not affected. The author has observed an affected boy who underwent multiple corrective operations, attended a normal school despite his short stature and is a school level champion in the game of chess. Clinically, the limbs are held in flexion at hips and knees, and the feet may be in gross equinovarus deformity. The involved limbs appear smooth, tubular, and tapering, giving a shapeless appearance. Abnormal facial features (whistling face) may be present in generalized involvement. In some patients, soft tissue webs may be identifiable on the flexor aspect of knees and elbows (pterygium syndrome). The hips often show congenital dislocation, and the involved joints show restriction of movements.

Treatment

The deformities require to be treated by exercises, stretching of contractures, splinting and appropriate operations for dislocation of hips, contracture of joints and clubfeet deformities. Sustained treatment will give reasonable functional outcome, however, additional operations may be needed for recurrence of deformities till skeletal growth is completed. Some cases may require talectomy to achieve a plantigrade foot. Upper femoral osteotomy may be needed in some for improving the stability of the hip joints.

CEREBRAL PALSY (LITTLE'S DISEASE)

The global incidence is about 2 in 1,000 live births. The patient would generally present during childhood with spastic paralysis of one or more limbs. Generally it is associated with premature babies, those born after difficult labor and those of multiple births. The cause is deficient development of upper motor neurons predominantly in prefrontal brain cells due to prenatal cerebral anoxia or birth trauma. Similar paralysis may follow damage to these cells as a sequelae to encephalitis in early childhood.

Topographic Distribution

The spasticity may involve one half of body (hemiplegia) or may involve both sides of the body (diplegia) generally showing more involvement of both lower limbs and mild involvement of upper limbs. Severe involvement of all the four limbs (quadriplegia) generally with concomitant intellectual involvement is addressed as total body involvement. Rarely only one limb may be affected (monoplegia) usually the upper limb with minimal abnormalities in remaining parts of body.

Clinical Features

Clinical features depend upon the degree of damage to the brain cells. The disability may be mild, moderate, severe or crippling. Involvement of prefrontal part of brain would produce 'spastic type', however, concomitant involvement of basal ganglia and cerebellum would add on elements of athetoid and ataxic movements. The diagnosis is suspected when the child's milestones are delayed, there is a clumsiness in the movements of limbs and unsteadiness while walking. Mild cases are detected by the presence of spasticity in lower limbs, spasm in the adductor muscles of hips, equinus spasm in the feet, extensor plantar response (lasting beyond the age of 2 years), exaggerated knee and ankle jerks, and there may be patellar and ankle clonus. In moderately severe cases, the stance and gait are characteristic; both feet are in equinus, knees are in slight flexion and legs cross each other while walking creating a "scissoring" gait. With steady pressure on the feet, the spasm of the calf muscles may be overcome and the feet may be brought to normal position. In neglected cases, however, there may be fixed equinus and adductor contractures **(Figs. 10.2A and B)**.

If upper limbs are affected, the shoulder is held in internal rotation, the elbow in flexion, forearm in pronation, wrist in flexion, thumb is drawn in flexion or "thumb in palm position" and fingers are flexed at metacarpophalangeal joints.

Mental development and power of speech may be affected to varying degrees. Diagnosis of cerebral palsy does not always imply poor intellect. The author has observed some of these children having succeeded in the

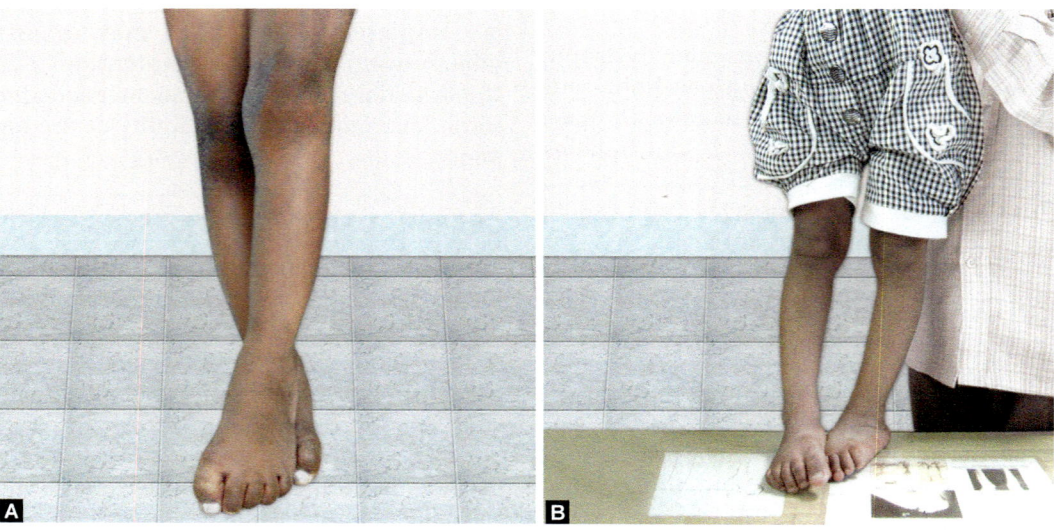

Figs. 10.2A and B: A child with cerebral palsy attempting to walk. Severe adductor spasm leads to scissoring, which makes it difficult to take steps, picture of two children.

most competitive disciplines. In very severe cases due to neuromuscular incoordinations, there is dribbling of saliva and incontinence of urine. In the severest from, the children are bedridden and totally dependent for their activity of daily living (ADL) including personal hygiene. A child, who is not walking by the age of 6 or 8 years, is unlikely to do so despite all efforts. Some ambulation may be possible with (motorized) walkers.

Treatment

In mild cases, with good mental functions, the deformities can be corrected by physiotherapy and appropriate operations, and the patient can be made fit for near normal life.

In moderately severe cases who are educable and trainable, corrective exercises and appliances, and surgical correction of deformities would help them to get education in special schools. Most of these children can achieve vocational training to become socially productive and earn a livelihood in trades like knitting, embroidery, stitching, carpentry, and shop assistance.

Surgery plays an adjuvant role in the total management of such children. Active and passive stretching exercises, use of orthotics for ambulation and working, and night splints to maintain correction must continue throughout the life of such patients. The aim of surgery in cerebral palsy is to correct deformities, improve motor function, and in adults to stabilize the joints. A few common and useful operations are as follows: Severe flexion deformity of knee in a patient who is able to stand may be corrected by lengthening of medial hamstrings (medial head of biceps femoris) and gracilics tendon. Care must be taken to avoid doing too many operative procedures in one sitting. Best time to plan operations is when the child has reached the age of 6–8 years. Earlier operation may be called for if the hip joint threatens to dislocate.

A few useful musculotendinous procedures: The tendons planned to be lengthened must be identified during pre-operative physical examination. When the child is under anesthesia the "spasmodic elements" of deformity would vanish or resolve, though the "mechanical" shortening or contracture would persist. Most useful lengthenings in clinical scenario have been tenotomy of *adductor longus* near its origin at superior pubic ramus for adductor spasm of thigh or for scissoring gait.

Hamstring tendons lengthening; biceps femoris just proximal to insertion at fibular head, semitendinosus near its insertion on medial tibial tuberosity, for severe flexion deformity at knee joint.

Gastrosoleus release at musculotendinous junction for tendo-calcaneal lengthening for equinus deformity.

Tibialis posterior tendon transfer to mid-dorsal foot—'*through the interosseous membrane*' for correction of equinus and inversion deformity of foot.

Pronator teres may be released from its insertion on lateral border of radius; may be transferred to dorsum of radius or the forearm extensors through the interosseous membrane for severe pronated forearm deformity.

Lengthening of Contracted Tendons

Tendo-Achilles lengthening for equinus deformity of foot, and adductor tenotomy if passive abduction is less than 20 degrees for scissoring gait. Gastrosoleus release by inverted-V (^) or Y-shaped incision at musculotendinous junction is preferred option for correction of equinus deformity.

Tendon Transfer Operations

Tibialis posterior to dorsum of foot, pronator transfer to extensors of wrist may help improve the function.

Partial Neurectomy

Partial neurectomy of obturator nerve for severe adductor spasms at hip joints may be considered in nonambulant patients for better perineal care.

Stabilization of Joints

Stabilization of joints to improve the function of the limbs in adults (triple arthrodesis of foot and arthrodesis of wrist) are very helpful to improve the function in lower limbs, however, not so beneficial in the upper extremity. Planning the management of gross deformities of spine in nonwalker children is a moral dilemma. The aim here is to make the sitting of the child in a wheelchair more comfortable. Adaptations in the wheelchair and spinal braces may help. Where surgical expertise and special facilities are available and the families have been counseled, spinal stabilization has been advocated. It is an extensive operation fixing the spine from thoracic region to pelvis (with bone grafting) and it carries a high complication rate of wound healing, implant failure and neurological defect.

Medical Treatment

Anticonvulsants for seizures (when present) have to be continued with modulation of doses. Other drugs, like benzodiazepine, trihexy-phenadryl, baclofen, botulinum toxin have been tried in conjunction with physiotherapeutic measures and selective operations. The efficacy of these drugs however has seldom been assessed in isolation. Overall doses and duration of use must be kept within safe limits.

LEPROSY (HANSEN'S DISEASE)

Leprosy is a chronic mildly infectious disease, spread by prolonged contact with an infectious case of leprosy. The causative organism is *Mycobacterium leprae* which is an acid-fast organism. By the time obvious deformities of foot, hand and face are detected the disease has been in the patient's body for a few years. The management of problems should include not only the treatment and rehabilitation of the presenting patient but also the elimination of the disease from the family and society. Traditionally the disease has been classified as: (1) "Tuberculoid": neural, noninfective associated with moderate decrease in cell-mediated immunity (CMI); (2) "Lepromatous": infectious type and associated with gross decrease in the CMI; (3) "Intermediate" or mixed type. Peripheral nerves are always affected in leprosy, cutaneous nerves as well as major nerves may thus be involved. The affected nerves get thickened by various extent of granulomas and hypertrophy of epineurium and perineurium. Hypopigmented skin patches with impaired sensibility and mucosal ulcerations in nasopharynx develop in all types of leprosy. Thickened cutaneous nerves and thickened nerve trunks may be visible. Thickened nerve trunks are palpable, especially where they cross a bone, e.g., ulnar nerve behind the medial epicondyle of humerus and common peroneal nerve (lateral popliteal nerve) around the neck of fibula. Damage to the nerves leads to trophic ulcers, progressive destruction of the affected parts in the hands and feet, and typical deformities of hand and feet due to nerve involvement. Any peripheral nerve can be involved, however, the commonest ones are ulnar nerve behind the elbow and at the wrist, common peroneal around the fibular neck, posterior tibial nerve behind the medial malleolus and radial cutaneous nerve at distal third of radial border of forearm.

Gross involvement of nerves lead to chronic nonhealing ulcers, neuroarthropathies, especially in weight-bearing joints and typical deformities of feet (foot drop) and hands—partial claw hands due to ulnar nerve involvement, and complete (total) claw hand due to combined involvement of ulnar and median nerves. In atypical or early case, or in countries where the disease is not common, diagnosis may have to be confirmed by scrapings from the skin and mucosa, or nerve biopsy and serological tests. In countries, where the disease is common, a person may present with tuberculous lesions along with leprosy. The author has seen such patients while working in Varanasi (India).

Drug Therapy

Multidrug therapy is considered the main stay of treatment. The choice of drugs would depend upon the response and reaction of patient. Generally, dapsone 100 mg daily and clofazimine 50 mg daily is given for one to 2 years. Most specialists at present would combine rifampicin 600 mg once a month or as a daily dose for one to 2 years. Periodic nonsteroidal anti-inflammatory drugs (NSAIDs) or prednisolone may be required for acute inflammatory episode (so called reactions). Cleanliness, and supportive therapy are important and integral part of treatment.

Operative Interventions

Surgical decompression of the nerve trunks is sometimes required when the related neural signs are deteriorating despite the use of multidrug therapy. Common operations involve anterior transposition of ulnar nerve at the elbow, "tunnel release" of median nerve at the wrist and that of posterior tibial nerve behind the medial malleolus. Release the epineurium by giving a long incision along the length of the involved segment. Stripping and excision of the epineurium is not recommended. Intraneural cold abscesses should be surgically evacuated. These procedures minimize the neural deterioration and may help in restoration of some lost functions.

Trophic changes in feet and hands can be prevented to a large extent by awareness of the patient, hygienic care of feet and hands, attention to cracks, fissures, boils and ulcers, and proper footwear.

Trophic Ulcers

Walking on anesthetic sole with clawing of toes results in ulceration of skin, fungation and foul-smelling discharge. This leads to destruction of soft tissues and bones (phalanges, metatarsals and other bones) not unlike the changes in advanced diabetic neuropathies. Rest to the part, control of infection, special footwear for insensate sole, and elevation of feet when not walking help in the healing process.

Foot Drop

In an established case of foot drop ankle-foot orthotic appliance with 5–10 degrees ankle dorsiflexion may suffice. In late cases, tibialis posterior (almost always available in leprosy) transfer through the interosseous space to the dorsum of foot at 3rd metatarsal is indicated. In fixed deformities of foot, a triple arthrodesis is helpful.

Any tendon transfers must be preceded by active and assisted exercises of the involved joints. Postoperative active exercises are required for re-education of the transferred tendons to perform the new function.

Total Claw Hand

This is due to the involvement of both median and ulnar nerves. The deformity produced is also called intrinsic minus hand because of total loss of intrinsic muscles of the hand. There is wasting of hypothenar and thenar eminences, hollowed out appearance of the thumb web space and intermetacarpal spaces, the thumb lies flat in an ape thumb-position and fingers are held in extension at the metacarpophalangeal joints and flexion of the interphalangeal joints.

In ulnar claw hand, the little and ring fingers are held in extension at metacarpophalangeal (MCP) joints and flexion at interphalangeal joints.

The deformities and movements lost due to intrinsic muscle paralysis can be improved upon by a number of tendon transfer operations. These procedures are however worth trying where the facilities for preoperative preparation and postoperative physiotherapy and rehabilitation are available.

Many tailed tendon transfers were developed by Paul Brands where extensor carpi radialis longus (ECRL) is detached from its insertion (second metacarpal) and used as a motor. Free tendon graft is taken from the palmaris longus tendon, it is split into 4 strips taken separately into the palm through the dorsum of interosseous (intermetacarpal) spaces, attached distally to the lateral margin of extensor expansion of each finger, proximally attached to the dorsally situated distal end of ECRL which would act as the motor. The operation currently favored by most surgeons is the "lasso operation" of Bunnell and Zancolli, in which, the tendon of flexor digitorum superficialis (FDS of ring finger) is detached from its insertion, split into four slips and one slip each is attached to the radial side of extensor expansion of fingers to provide flexor function to the MCP joints.

Transfer for Opponens Palsy of Thumb

The flexor digitorum superficialis (FDS) of the ring finger is detached near its insertion, pulled into the forearm proximal to the wrist and routed around the insertion of flexor carpi ulnaris proximal to the pisiform bone, threaded across the palm and fixed to the radial side of the first metacarpal or inserted into the lateral margin of its extensor expansion. All tendon transfers need cooperation of the patient for doing postoperative active exercises and physiotherapy for a long time.

Wrist Drop

Wrist drop is due to the injury of radial nerve at the elbow or upper arm. If the cause is an open injury the nerve should be explored and repaired as soon as possible. In closed injuries observation for spontaneous recovery is justified for about 6 months. If recovery does not start nerve must be explored and repaired according to the intraoperative observed damages. If recovery does not occur, the disability can be compensated by tendon transfers: pronator teres to extensor carpi radialis brevis, flexor carpi radialis to the long finger extensors, and palmaris longus to abductor pollicis longus.

PERIPHERAL NERVES

Seddon's classification (1942) of peripheral nerve injuries is a very useful clinical method to classify the damage and to project the prognosis.

Neurapraxia

It is a reversible physiological nerve block (with intact axons) leading to diminution of sensation and partial motor weakness. If the insult to nerve is not repeated and the limb is given rest in the functional position, most of these patients recover within a few days or weeks. Commonest clinical examples are "Saturday night palsy" due to the arm hanging on the edge of bed after alcohol consumption, or axillary "crutch palsy" or tourniquet palsy.

Axonotmesis

It literally means that there is damage to the axons but the neural tube is intact. The biological repair of the damaged axons starts soon after the stoppage of the damaging factors or the insult on the peripheral nerve. The speed of repair proximodistal is about 1–2 mm per day. If the neurologically damaged or affected or paralyzed area does not get re-innervated within 2 years, there are no chances of recovery.

Axonotmesis may be associated with closed fractures or dislocations. The more proximal is the injury lesser are the chances of spontaneous recovery.

Neurotmesis

Literally neurotmesis means physical transection of the peripheral nerve occurring in open fractures or dislocations or rarely iatrogenic. Sometimes the nerve may appear to be intact however, the damage has been done due to fibrosis of a long segment of the nerve (traction injury or intraneural injection). Endoneural tubes are transected or damaged over a long segment of the nerve, the damaged or destroyed segment of nerve gets replaced by fibrous tissue. End-to-end repair of the transected nerve or use of nerve grafting (for large defects) to replace or repair the damaged segment is advised and practised, however the quality of recovery is poor in patients with more proximal damage. Some sensations and motor functions recover, however it is never a complete recovery.

In a case of long-standing damage to the nerve, or while attempting repair in proximal areas of the peripheral nerve it may be helpful to use Galvanic stimulation of the paralyzed muscles to minimize the loss of "neuromuscular junctions" pending the regenerative process reaching to end-organs.

Tinel Sign

It is a clinical test where the peripheral nerve is percussed by tapping along its course. The tapping causes tingling or tickling (dysesthesia) distal to the tapping along the course of nerve. A positive Tinel sign is a reflection of damage to the nerve. During periodic clinical examination (2-3 monthly) if the Tinel sign is shifting distally, it is an indication of recovering nerve. However, if the location does not proceed distally, it is a sign of non-recovering nerve damage, the damaged nerve may show a swelling (neuroma) due to proliferation of neuraxons and Schwann cells.

Peripheral Nerve Entrapment Syndrome

Wherever a peripheral nerve passes through a fibro-osseous tunnel, there is a risk of compression of the nerve. The contents of the neural tunnel may be swollen due to rheumatoid inflammation, during pregnancy or in hypothyroidism or diabetes. The osseous wall of the tunnel may become irregular causing irritation of the traveling nerve due to malunited fracture, infection or gross deformity. Rarely there may be a ganglion, exostosis or an osteophyte from the osseous wall, or a deformity (cubitus valgus for ulnar nerve).

Commonest sites for nerve compression are carpal tunnel syndrome deep to the flexor retinaculum (median nerve), ulnar tunnel syndrome in the cubital tunnel posterior to the medial humeral epicondyle, tarsal tunnel syndrome behind the medial malleolus deep to the deltoid ligament (pressure on posterior tibial nerve).

Commonest symptoms of compartment syndromes are tingling and dysesthesia in the sensory distribution of nerve, Tinel sign may be present on tapping or percussing over the nerve. There may be diminution of sensations and muscle wasting in long-standing causes.

Symptoms are exaggerated during sleeping time (median nerve), prolonged flexion of elbow (ulnar nerve), prolonged walking (posterior tibial nerve).

In early case of entrapment syndrome use of splints and local steroid injection into the entrapment compartment can reduce the swelling and symptoms. However, if symptoms persist and there is muscle wasting, operative decompression is mandatory.

SUGGESTED READINGS

1. Rang M, Wright J. What have 30 years of medical progress done for cerebral palsy. Clin Orthop Relat Res. 1989;247:55-60.
2. Sharan D. Orthopedic surgery in cerebral palsy: Instructional course lecture. Indian J Orthop. 2017;51:240-55.

SECTION 2

REGIONAL ORTHOPEDIC CONDITIONS

Section Outline

11. Disorders Related to Neck
12. Shoulder
13. Elbow and Forearm
14. Wrist and Hand
15. Back Pain and Spine
16. Hip
17. Knee and Leg
18. Ankle and Foot
19. Atlas of Rare Conditions

CHAPTER 11

Disorders Related to Neck

CLEIDOCRANIAL DYSOSTOSIS

While taking care of a patient for cervical spine disorders, the commonest useful investigation is an X-ray of cervical spine. One may be able to see occipitocervical fusion (atlanto-occipital assimilation). In a normal cervical spine one should note that hyoid bone is at the level of C3± vertebral body, thyroid cartilage is at the level of C4± vertebral body and cricoid cartilage is at the level of C5± vertebral body. The prevertebral space between the air shadow and the anterior surface of vertebral bodies is about 5 mm proximal to the thyroid cartilage, the space is about 15 mm distal to the thyroid cartilage. Any increase in these distances may suggest an infective lesion, or traumatic hematoma or a neoplastic lesion. Lateral view in "flexion-extension" would show any mechanical instability, however this is not advised in cases with recent trauma or with neural signs.

In a normal adult and a standard X-ray of cervical spine, the anteroposterior diameter of mid-cervical canal, the distance from the posterior surface of vertebral body to the base of it's spine should not be <11 mm.

MRI scans are very helpful for lesions in the cervical spine, however, 20% of asymptomatic adults above the age of 40 years may show abnormalities like disc bulge or desiccation of disc and osteophytes. All images must be interpreted in relation to the clinical picture.

TORTICOLLIS

Congenital torticollis may be caused by irregular segmentation of the cervical vertebrae or segmentation defects at cervicodorsal junction. Such patients are kept under observation for neurological complications during the growing period.

Acquired torticollis (wry neck) is most commonly caused by fibrofascitis of the soft tissues in the neck. Such cases are generally relieved of symptom by the use of non-steroidal anti-inflammatory drugs (NSAIDs), local heating and gentle exercises of neck, within 5–10 days. Infection of cervical spine (tuberculosis or pyogenic), cervical lymphadenitis, rheumatoid inflammation, and injury to cervical spine may also present as wry neck.

Rarely an adult may present with **"spasmodic torticollis"** characterized by repeated apparently uncontrolled spasm of muscles, acting on cervical spine (focal dystonia). There is marked psychogenic bases for this condition. In addition to the standard treatment for fibrofascitis-induced wry neck, psychiatric help would relieve this condition.

BRACHIALGIA

Brachialgia or brachial neuralgia is the counter part of "sciatica" in upper limb. The behavior and etiological factors are similar to those causing sciatic pains. Brachialgia, however, is less common than the presentation of "sciatica". The pain usually starts from the neck or shoulder and travels down the arm, many a times up to fingertips. Irritation of nerve roots of C5 or C6 would present as pain along the radial side of forearm and index finger and thumb. Irritation of C8 or T1 nerve roots spreads along the ulnar border of forearm up to the fifth and fourth fingers. Every case of brachialgia is not necessarily due to a prolapsed cervical disc, in fact majority of cases of "brachialgia" are caused by non-discogenic causes or enthesopathy.

A few common causes are acute or chronic strains on cervical spine and shoulder, occupational or postural stress due to long hours in a desk-job (computers and internet), inflammatory or infective cause (rheumatoid inflammation or infections), degenerative changes in the cervical vertebrae (osteoarthrosis and spondylosis), and cervical disc prolapse. Rare causes must, however, be kept in differential diagnosis: old injury to cervical vertebrae, tuberculosis, metastatic deposits, tumors of cord and nerves, syringomyelia are a few examples. Lesions of shoulder (inflammatory, infective, tumorous, degenerative) may also cause brachialgic pains. Subdiaphragmatic lesions may sometimes cause referred pains in the shoulder area.

Clinical examination, laboratory investigations, X-rays and MRI are able to reach the basic cause of brachialgia. Appropriate treatment would relieve the symptoms.

For nonspecific cases, rest to the limb by arm-pouch sling when shoulder pathology is suspected, or soft cervical collar if suspected pathology is in cervical spine, NSAIDs, gentle exercises for the neck and shoulder, use of local heating or ultrasonotherapy relieve the pain within a few weeks in most of the cases.

CERVICAL SPINE DISC PROLAPSE

One of the common causes of brachialgic pains is prolapse of the intervertebral disc in the lower cervical spine. The symptoms are generally preceded by a history of sudden jerk and sprain of the neck, the patient presents with painful restrictions of neck movements and radiation down the arm to the tips of fingers. The commonest level of prolapse is the C5–C6 disc, which irritates the C6 nerve root, and causes dysthesia along the outer border of forearm and thumb. Prolapse of C6–C7 disc irritates the C7 nerve root and causes dysthesia mostly in the index and middle fingers.

Radiological examination may show narrowing of the affected disc space. In long standing cases, there may be sclerosis of the paradiscal borders with or without osteophyte formation. In patients with history of repeated attacks or severe symptoms, MRI investigations are justified. MRI provides information about the exact location and the size of the disc prolapse, and also the health of the spinal cord **(Fig. 11.1)**.

Treatment

In acute stage, the patient must be put to rest for 7–10 days and given anti-inflammatory drugs. Any essential mobility especially to toilet may be permitted wearing a cervical collar. In younger patients (<30 years), cervical traction with 6–8 kg weight for 1–2 weeks may relieve the symptoms. Cervical traction may be of use in persons younger than 30 years of age when the disc is hydrated. Continuous traction for 2–3 weeks, or intermittent traction: 30 minute 2–3 times a day may be helpful in young patients. Once the pain has subsided, the patient should do gentle neck exercise and shoulder bracing exercises to prevent further attack of brachial neuralgia. Massive disc prolapse with objective neural signs, and recurring attack of severe pains would need removal of the offending disc through the standard anterior approach to the cervical spine. Up to 2 prolapsed discs (adjacent levels) can be removed through the anterior approach without disturbing the spinal cord. In younger people, one may insert a snug fitting bone graft (preferably autogenous) between the adjacent vertebral bodies. More extensive, anterior procedures may be associated with increased incidence of complications like the injury to recurrent

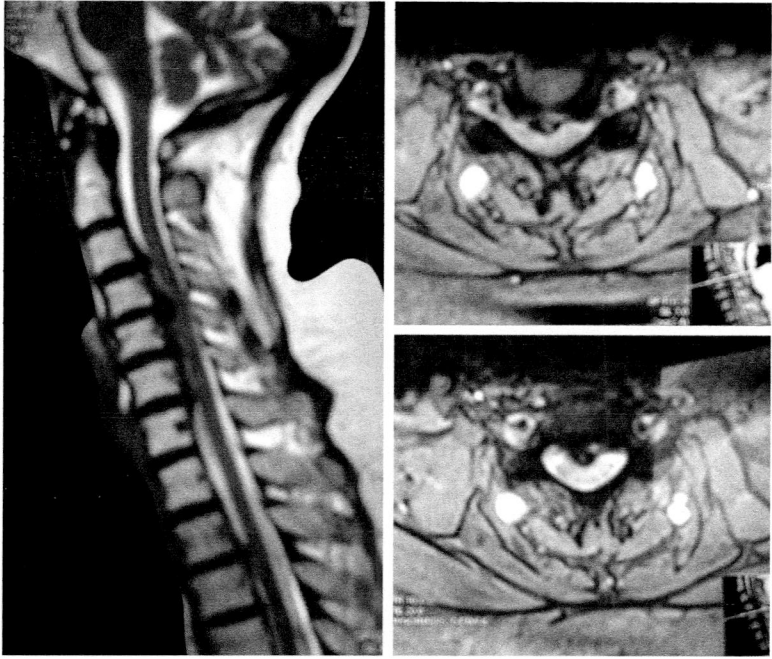

Fig. 11.1: Classical case of ossification of posterior longitudinal ligament (OPLL) from C4 to C6. Axial views are showing posterior bulge of hypertrophied OPLL.

laryngeal nerve, postoperative dysphagia and dyspnea. In multilevel extensive fusion, there is predisposition to accelerated degeneration of the adjacent level. Vertebral column in senior citizens is seldom frightfully unstable, and less extensive procedures are preferred. Fusion may be indicated if preoperative flexion-extension X-rays reveal mechanical instability or in the presence of concomitant infection or neoplasm.

CERVICAL CANAL STENOSIS AND MYELOPATHY

Sagittal diameter of the mid-cervical spinal canal is measured on plain lateral X-ray from the posterior surface of the vertebral body to the base of spinous process. This distance varies considerably in human beings, however, anything <11 mm is suggestive of canal stenosis. Symptomatic canal stenosis may be associated with skeletal dysplasias (e.g., achondroplasia), multiple level disc degeneration, thickening of ligamentum flavum, ossification of posterior longitudinal ligament (OPLL) and vertebral displacement. In cases of severe canal stenosis, patient may develop neurological signs and symptoms. The neurological symptoms are due to mechanical compression (which can be relieved by decompression), and also due to ischemic changes in the neural elements, which seldom recover completely despite decompression **(Figs. 11.2 and 11.3)**.

Symptomatic cervical canal stenosis may be caused by age related changes (degenerative osteophytosis), diffuse idiopathic spinal hyperostosis (DISH) or fluorosis. The vertebral column in such conditions is mechanically stable, a standard laminectomy without bone grafting or implants is adequate.

Ossification of posterior Longitudinal ligament (OPLL): OPLL was once considered to be a disorder mainly in Japan. However, with awareness of the disease and facilities (X-rays and MRIs) for diagnosis, it is recognized as a widespread disorder in all countries. Imaging modalities show ossification of posterior longitudinal ligament in cervical spine.

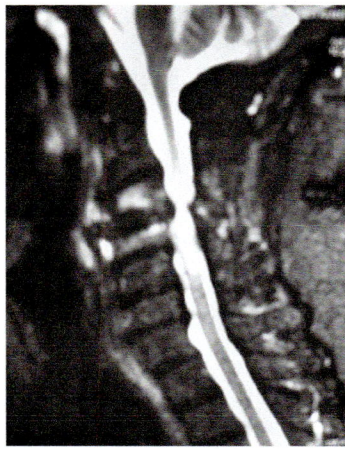

Fig. 11.2: MRI of a neglected case of cervical spondylotic myelopathy, one can see a long segment of the cord (C3–C6) showing myelomalacia.

However, generalized survey frequently show concomitant associated features of DISH, fluorosis, and various forms of rheumatoid and metabolic disorders.

CONGENITAL TORTICOLLIS DUE TO THE CONTRACTURE OF STERNOCLEIDOMASTOID (SCM) MUSCLE

In contracture of the right-sided muscle as an example, the chin is tilted to the left side and upwards, the occiput is tilted to the right side and downwards. The right ear approaches the right shoulder. In neglected cases brought to the clinic at the age of 3 or 4 years, one can observe the facial asymmetry, the face on the

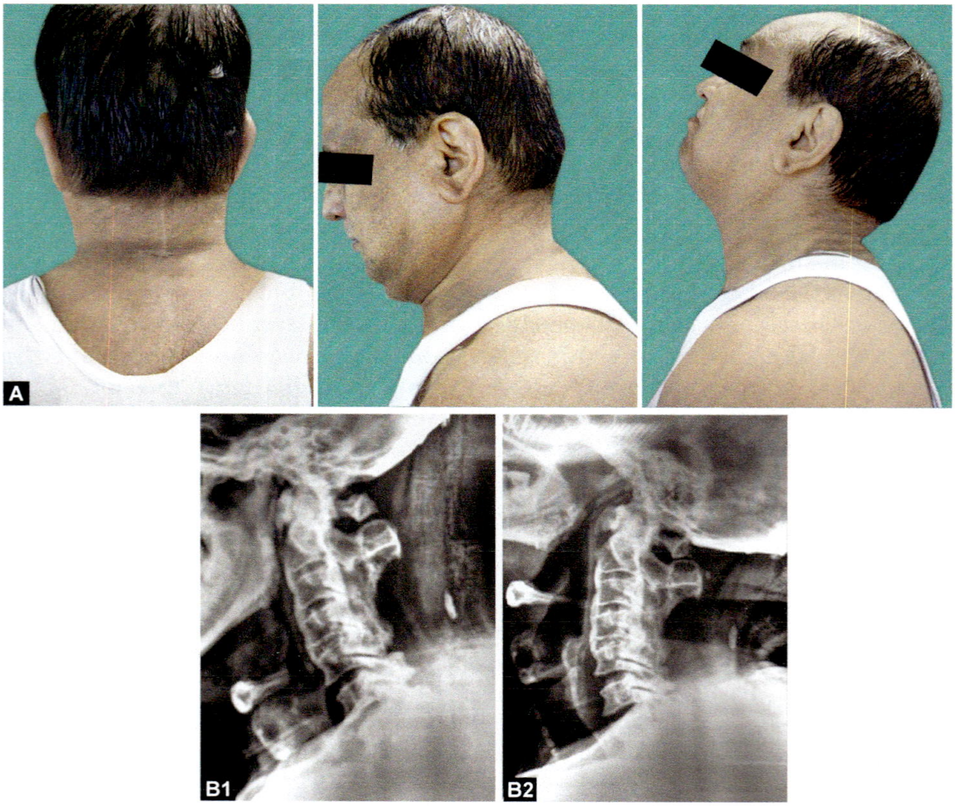

Figs. 11.3A and B: (A) Human spine starts showing progressive osteoarthrosis of all the joints of vertebrae above the age of 50 years. Osteophytes form around all articulating surfaces giving mechanical stability though at the cost of mobility. X-rays (B1) and (B2) show follow-up 20 years after standard laminectomy for symptomatic ossification of posterior longitudinal ligament (OPLL). The patient maintained neural recovery, neck mobility and stability.

right side would appear less developed as compared to the left side. If the deformity is left uncorrected up to the age of 12 years or more a new macula develops in the fundus of eye to level the vision in the tilted position of the neck and face. Congenital torticollis must be differentiated from the deformity produced by inflammatory, infective or traumatic causes. Before considering any operative correction of "torticollis", cervical spine X-rays must be obtained to exclude irregular segmentation of the cervical vertebrae.

Pathology of Congenital Torticollis

The sternocleidomastoid is contracted, shortened and fibrotic on one side. The contracture may be a part of congenital myelodysplasia, or fibrosis of the muscle or a result of healing of birth trauma, intramuscular hematoma, or ischemia generally in the lower half of the muscle. In some cases, one can palpate a localized swelling, or a fibrotic area, however the SCM in general is short, prominent, and fibrotic **(Figs. 11.4A and B)**.

Treatment

In the newborn, the deformity should be corrected by passive movements of the neck by undoing the deformity. If the patient presents after the age of 3 years, the treatment is mainly operative. The lower end of SCM is divided transversely ensuring the division of clavicular and sternal heads. The contracted cervical fascia is also divided to obtain full correction of the deformity. In neglected cases, or those with severe deformity or contracture, the proximal attachment of SCM at the mastoid process is also sectioned transversely for obtaining full correction. This is called bipolar release of SCM muscle. The proximal attachment of SCM is cut transversely at the tip of mastoid process to avoid damage to the spinal accessory nerve. Generally, the spinal accessory nerve traverses behind the SCM diagonally, distally and posteriorly emerging into posterior triangle of neck at the junction of upper and middle third of SCM; however, possibility of an anomalous route must be kept in mind while cutting the upper pole of SCM.

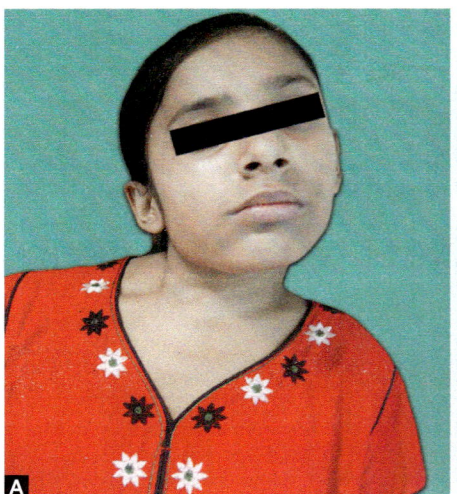 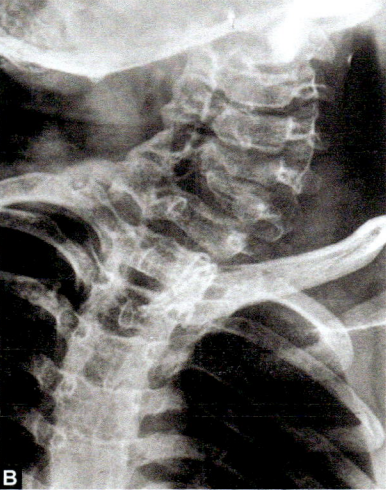

Figs. 11.4A and B: (A) Picture of a untreated case (age 12 years) of congenitally short right sternocleidomastoid muscle: Note chin rotated to left side, neck flexed to right side, less development of right side of face (had relatively small right eye); (B) Adaptive changes due to a long standing deformity have produced a scoliotic deformation of the cervical vertebrae.

Postoperatively the neck is held in corrected position for 2–3 days by a soft sling traction; corrective active and assisted exercises are initiated on the 2nd or 3rd day after surgery. If the patient has been trained to do corrective exercises preoperatively, it is easy for the patient to do repetitive corrective exercises without much discomfort. Bipolar release even at mature age can give a satisfactory outcome.

Infections of Cervical Spine (See also Chapter 2)

Broad outlines for care of infective lesions of vertebral column are given in Chapter 2. In the Indian-subcontinent majority of spinal infections are caused by tuberculosis, however pyogenic infection (e.g., *Staphylococcus aureus*) should also be considered as a possibility if there is a short history with severe pain and high fever. Insidious onset with low-grade fever, and night pains is more likely to be tuberculous infection. In addition to imaging modalities, blood culture, examination of the infected tissues may help to reach the correct diagnosis. Treatment of spinal infections is mainly nonsurgical, antibiotics and use of orthotics. Operative intervention might be needed if neural compromise does not resolve (anterior decompression) or infection does not come under control (debridement).

Secondary torticollis: Torticollis like deformity may be secondary to infection, inflammatory disorders, or neoplastic lesion in the neck area. X-rays and MRIs help us reach the appropriate diagnosis.

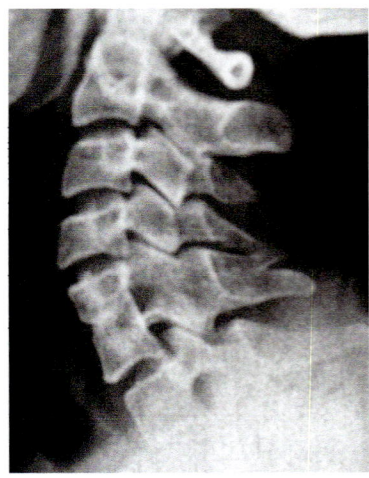

Fig. 11.5: Congenital synostosis: C5 and C6 are showing fused vertebral bodies and spinous processes.

Klippel–Feil syndrome: It is a rare congenital disorder showing fusion (synostosis) of 2 or more cervical vertebrae. The patient may present with short neck and low hairline. Clinically there may be pain due to stress on the neighbouring segments, as a compensatory attempt at hypermobility. The fused segments may show a dumbbell shaped appearance (wasp-waist appearance) and fusion of spinous processes. Patients should be advised to continue normal activities and exercises, avoid head-loading and vigorous contact sports. Posterior neural decompression may be needed if patient develops neural signs **(Fig. 11.5)**.

SUGGESTED READINGS

1. Fredrickson BE, Baker DR, McHolick WJ, et al. The natural history of spondylolysis and spondylolisthesis. J Bone Joint Surg. 1984;66A:699-700.
2. Law MD, Bernhardt M, White AA. Evaluation and management of cervical spondylotic myelopathy. J Bone Joint Surg. 1994;76A:1420-33.
3. Lim KS, Shim JS, Lee YS. Is sternocleidomastoid muscle release effective in adults with neglected congenital muscular torticollis? Clin Orthop Relat Res. 2014;472:1271-8.

CHAPTER 12

Shoulder

INTRODUCTION

The shoulder is characterized by a shallow glenoid cavity, and a large humeral head which gives the freedom of mobility to the joint. The stability is essentially maintained by the shoulder capsule that is surrounded by layers of muscles; anteriorly—the subcapularis, superiorly—the supraspinatus, and posteriorly—the infraspinatus and teres minor. The tendons of these muscles are closely attached to the capsule all around the joint to form the musculotendinous cuff or 'rotator cuff'. The rotator cuff is covered by the deltoid muscle with intervening subdeltoid bursa, and the acromion with intervening subacromial bursa. Degenerative changes in the rotator cuff (calcific tendinitis or rupture of tendons), inflammatory changes in the bursal sheaths or traumatic inflammation of these structures would lead to painful restrictions of the shoulder joint. Immobilization of the shoulder for any injury of the upper limbs in persons above the age of 40 may also result in the stiffness of shoulder. Patients with diabetes, myocardial ischemic pains are more prone to develop periarthritis of the shoulder. After the availability of MRI and arthroscopic visualization, many subclassifications have been introduced. However, broadly speaking, a large number of patients can be relieved by exercises, physiotherapy, nonsteroidal anti-inflammatory drugs (NSAIDs) and local injections of long-acting steroids.

Normal acromiohumeral space plays an important role in normal scapulohumeral rhythm. Dystrophic calcification of a part of rotator cuff (degenerative calcification), gross diminution of acromiohumeral space due to damage of rotator-cuff, leads to painful restriction of shoulder movements.

Fresh lesions of rotator cuff would show in the MRI-T2 shadows as fluid filled area, in chronic cases these get replaced by granulation tissue, fibrous scarring and later on as fluffy osteophytes. 'Sourcil' sign or sclerosis on the undersurface of the acromion is a better radiological sign for diagnosing chronic "rotator cuff lesions".

Periarthritis of shoulder is one of the common causes of stiffness and diffuse pain in shoulder spreading down to the arm. Stiffness of shoulder may occur in a variety of conditions—age-related arthrosis, a consequence of generalized rheumatoid inflammation, or shoulder stiffness may be associated with cervical spondylosis, or it may be a part of reflex sympathetic dystrophy (RSD). Most of the cases of RSD are initiated by an injury or fracture around the wrist and hands: trophic and vasomotor changes in the hand may also be associated with painful stiffness of shoulder (hand-shoulder syndrome). Having excluded the presence of active infection and a recent fracture or a neoplastic condition, the treatment is essentially conservative.

PAINFUL SHOULDER: COMMON PATHOLOGIES

Commonest of causes of pain around shoulder is disorders of "rotator cuff". Rotator cuff is almost like a conjoint tendon inserting into greater and lesser tuberosities at upper end of humerus. The conjoint tendon is composed of supraspinatus, infraspinatus, teres minor and subscapularis, it passes beneath the acromioclavicular arch (under surface of acromion and coracoacromial ligament). Subacromial bursa is present between the coracoacromial arch and the rotator cuff, deep surface of the cuff slides over the shoulder joint capsule and the tendon of long head of biceps. Rotator cuff pain syndrome may be caused by tear of the cuff, inflammatory tendinitis or bursitis or calcific tendinitis or degenerative changes (age related).

Gross limitations of shoulder movements have been addressed as "adhesive capsulitis", or "frozen shoulder". Compressive loading of the shoulder in flexion plus abduction position can damage the glenoid labrum superiorly, anteriorly and posteriorly (addressed as SLAP-lesion, superior labrum, anteriorly, posteriorly).

Mostly the painful conditions of shoulder without gross destruction of bones and joints and without instability can be treated for relief of pain with the help of NSAIDs, pendulum exercises and physiotherapy, and rarely by local steroids instillations. In some patients residual restriction of external rotation may persist.

In advanced cases or those who do not get relief, **arthroscopic procedures** are accepted as a preferred operative technique for repair of rotator cuff tears, debridement of coracoacromial arch, removal of intra-articular loose bodies, repair of glenoid labrum, arthrolysis, synovectomy, debridement for unresolving inflammation, infection, or neoplastic lesions.

Tuberculosis rarely occurs in shoulder (<5%), with standard antituberculosis drugs most of these patients achieve a painless status. Motion at the glenohumeral articulation depends upon the stage of disease at the onset of treatment, with early disease near normal range, may be achieved.

Hyperostosis of Bones Near the Shoulder

The patient may present with irregular thickening of bones with moderate discomfort. Most of the patients are above the age of 40 years. The bones involved may be clavicle (medial or lateral end), sternoclavicular joint, acromioclavicular joints and costosternal articulations. X-rays may show irregular thickening of bones, histological changes are nonspecific and no specific microorganisms have been identified. Active exercises, NSAIDs help resolve symptoms within a few weeks.

Joint Disorders

- Glenohumeral arthritis
- Acromioclavicular arthritis
- Infective arthritis
- Rheumatoid inflammation
- Osteoarthrosis

Osseous Lesions

- Sequel of fractures around shoulder
- Osteomyelitis of upper end humerus
- Tumorous or metastatic lesions
- Osteonecrosis

Rotator Cuff Disorders

- Tendinitis
- Tendinous ruptures
- Frozen shoulder

Referred Pains

- Cervical spondylosis
- Mediastinal pathology
- Cardiac ischemia
- Subdiaphragmatic lesions

Post-traumatic

- Fractures
- Dislocation
- Sudeck's dystrophy (Complex regional pain syndrome or RSD)

A patient would visit an orthopedic clinic commonly for pain, stiffness, instability or weakness of shoulder. Common conditions responsible for pain and stiffness are inflammation in the rotator cuff, rheumatoid inflammation, infection or a sequel of fractures around the shoulder joint. Common conditions are shown in the table. Rarely even a minimum trauma to the hand or upper limb if protected over-zealously may lead to painful stiff shoulder; the severest form is addressed as complex regional pain syndrome (CRPS—Sudeck's atrophy or RSD) and 'hand-shoulder syndrome'. Stiffness around the shoulder is often associated with diabetes, cardiac disease, hemiplegia or a history of prior trauma **(Fig. 12.1)**.

Supraspinatus tendinitis or calcification or its partial rupture would typically produce 'painful arc syndrome'; on abduction the range between 60 to 90 degrees is very painful and rest of the movements above or below have minimal pain or are practically painless. X-rays may show an area of calcification above the greater tuberosity. Most of the patients of painful arc syndrome would resolve by use of an arm pouch sling for 2–3 weeks, use of NSAIDs and graduated active exercises **(Fig. 12.2)**.

Any injury or inflammation of the rotator cuff leads to localized or generalized edema and swelling. Early and mild swelling is self-limiting and may resolve in a few weeks. Repetitive insults especially in middle-aged people would lead to impingement and adhesions between the rotator cuff and adjacent structures like coracoacromial arch, acromioclavicular arch, subdeltoid bursa and the shoulder capsule. Many conditions associated with the **pathology of rotator cuff** have been loosely addressed as 'supraspinatus tendinitis', 'painful arc syndrome', 'periarthritis', 'adhesive capsulitis', and 'frozen shoulder'. With the availability of MRIs and arthroscopic facilities, many pathological lesions have been detected, e.g., tears or degeneration of superior labrum anteriorly and posteriorly (SLAP lesion), erosion or small fragmentation of anteroinferior lip of glenoid rim. Exclusion of active infection of shoulder is mandatory before you put the patient on vigorous exercises or manipulations **(Figs. 12.3A and B)** or local steroids instillation.

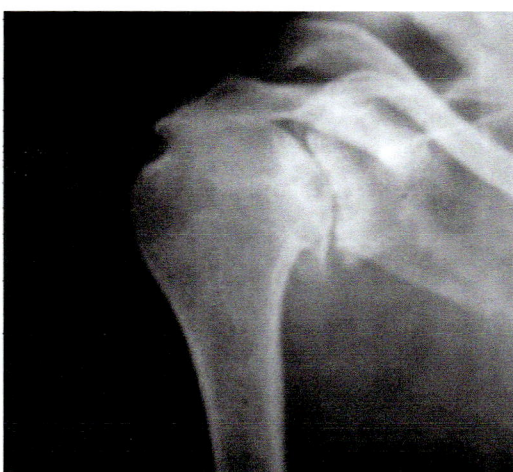

Fig. 12.1: Primary osteoarthrosis of non-weight bearing joints is extremely rare. This X-ray shows the classical picture of diminished joint (cartilage) space, sclerosis of articular margins, osteophytes and subchondral cysts, probably as a sequel of old-healed infection (secondary osteoarthrosis).

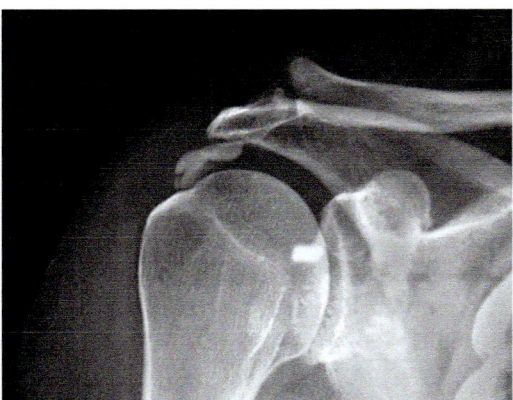

Fig. 12.2: Calcific tendinitis: X-ray of shoulder shows a typical band of calcification at insertion of supraspinatus tendon, the rest of the joint looks normal.

Treatment

Most of the rotator cuff disorders can be treated conservatively. Active and assisted exercise is the most important modality. The pain can be reduced and range of motion improved under the influence of short course of NSAIDs and local ultra-sonotherapy. If all these procedures fail instill 2 or 3 injections of

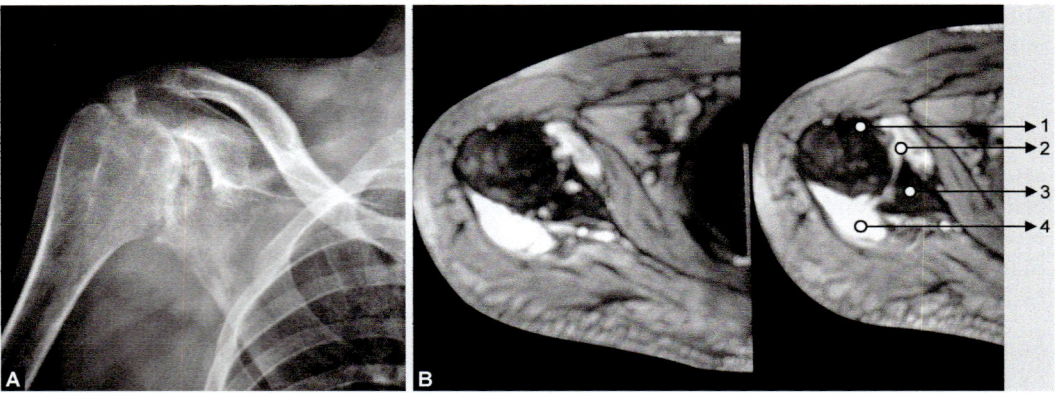

Figs. 12.3A and B: Advanced tubercular arthritis of shoulder. (A) Note gross obliteration of the joint space and destruction of bone on both sides of the joint; (B) MRIs show nonspecific changes of collection of fluid in the joint and irregular destruction of articular margins. ① humeral head, ② joint line, ③ glenoid cavity ④ synovial fluid.

long-acting corticosteroids in the subacromial space at one month intervals. The improvement achieved must be preserved by continuation of active exercise for life.

In refractory cases, manipulation under anesthesia may be considered. All manipulations must be done gently as there is a risk of fracture of neck of humerus, especially in the elderly and osteoporotic patients.

If symptoms do not subside after 3-4 months of semi-invasive techniques or there is a recurrence of symptoms or there is a complete rupture of supraspinatus tendon (in relatively younger persons), one may have to resort to surgery for decompression of the rotator cuff, release of pericapsular adhesions and repair of the torn cuff. Surgery can be done by open procedures or by arthroscopic techniques. Arthroscopy is a useful technique for rotator cuff disruptions, instability, and for intrasynovial (intra-articular) pathologies like rheumatoid arthritis, synovial pathologies and infections.

INSTABILITY OF SHOULDER

Most of the cases of shoulder instability are a sequel of an injury to the shoulder. However, one should be aware of cases of shoulder joint laxity as a part of generalized joint laxity or congenital habitual or recurrent subluxation or dislocation of the shoulder. Such cases are mostly treated conservatively by exercises and modification of physical activities. Operative procedures in such cases as a rule do not succeed.

Post-traumatic Instability

Recurrent anterior dislocation of shoulder usually follows a traumatic dislocation of humeral head. Generally the acute injury resulting in dislocation is where the arm is forced into abduction, extension and external rotation. About 25% of such patients develop recurrent dislocation or instability. Holding an overhead-bar while traveling in public transport, swimming or ball throwing may lead to recurrence of subluxation or dislocation of the shoulder.

Recurrent anterior dislocation of shoulder may cause loosening (detachment) of anterior glenoid labrum (Bankart's lesion) and erosion or loss of anterior bony glenoid margin. Similarly repeated abutting of anterior glenoid rim on the posterior aspect of humeral head would create an abutting depression (Hill-Sachs lesion).

Frequent recurrent dislocation in young active nonepileptic patient is an indication for operative intervention. Historically, there are

more than 2 dozens of operations described. Broadly speaking, these are 3 groups with many modifications and hybridization:
1. Repair the torn or loose glenoid labrum, reattach to the bone and anteroinferior capsule by conventional open surgery (Bankart procedure) or by arthroscopy.
2. Shorten the supposedly lax anterior capsule and muscles by double breasting (plication) the anterior capsule and overlying subscapularis (Putti-Platt's operation).
3. Create a bony buttress at anteroinferior part of glenoid rim to deepen the glenoid socket and to strengthen the anterior capsule. One may use a free graft abutting the capsule or use a pedicled bone graft based upon coracoid process with retained origin of short head of biceps and coracobrachialis (Bristow–Latarjet operation). These procedures can be performed by open operations or by arthroscopic techniques.

After any of these operations, there is still a significant recurrence rate (10–20%) usually following another trauma. Having tried almost all above procedures, the author's preference since 1972 has been to perform **glenoplasty** (resembling acetabuloplasty). Through an anterior approach perform a juxta-articular, extracapsular osteotomy of scapular neck, prize it open and insert a free bone graft buttress (5 × 5 cm) abutting the capsule. The recurrence as observed on patients with a follow-up of >10 years is <2% **(Figs. 12.4A to D and 12.5)**.

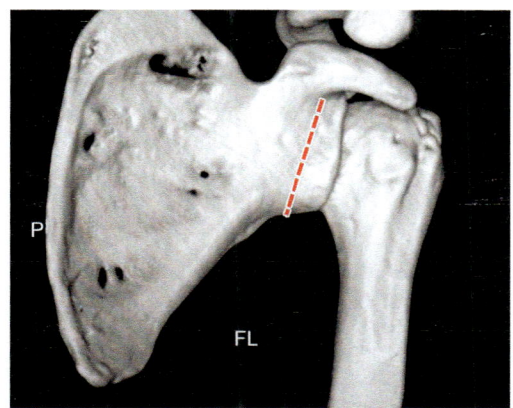

A. Anterior view scapular neck osteotomy. Superior 1 cm ± is left uncut to act as a hinge

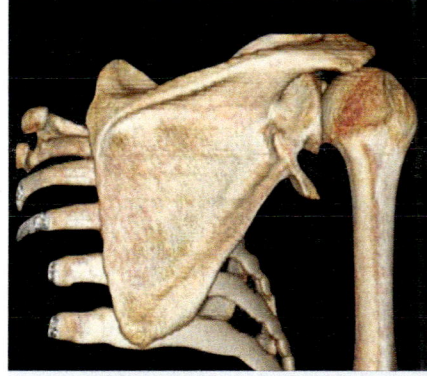

B. CT scan of glenoplasty (Rt). Posterior view 3D-reconstruction

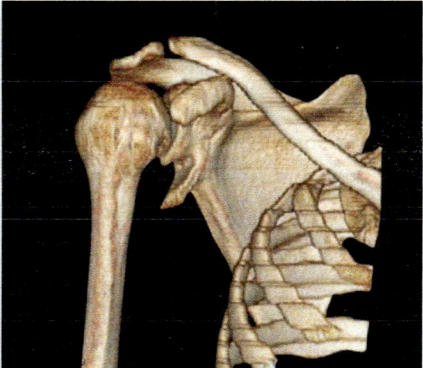

Follow-up 2 years, anterior view. 3D-CT reconstruction

Figs. 12.4A to D: *Continued*

Continued

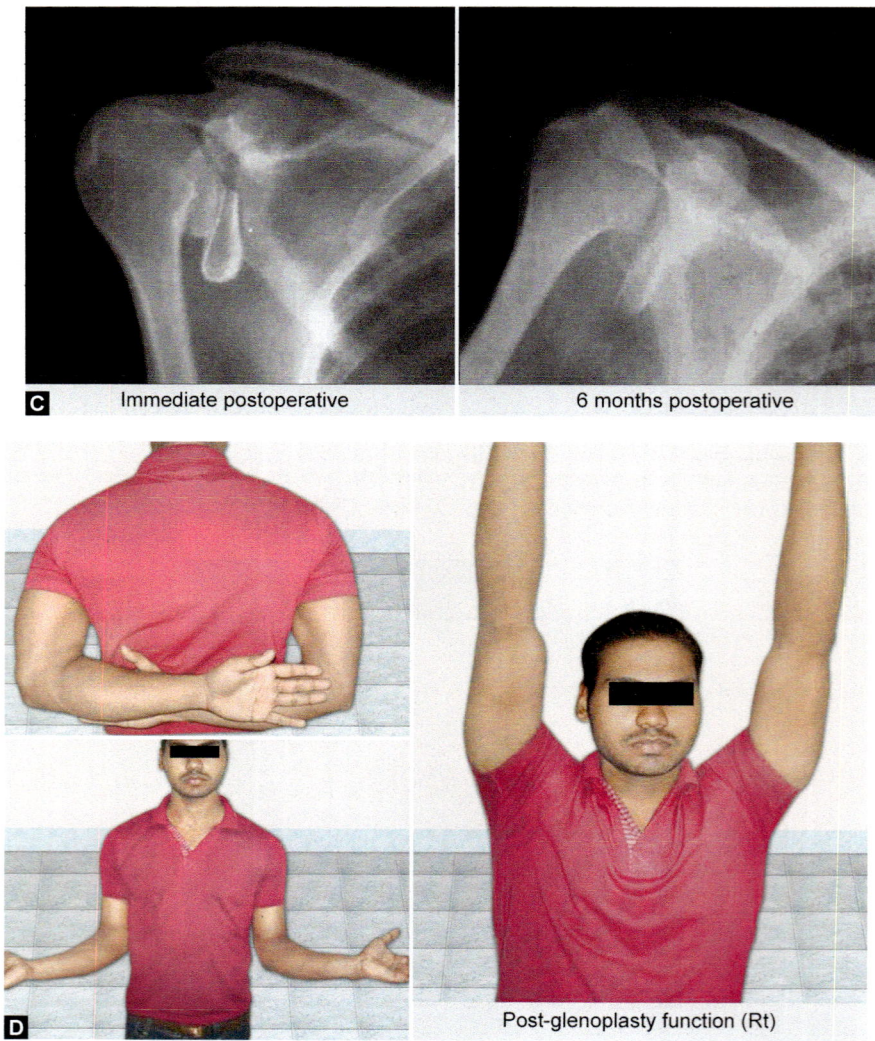

Figs. 12.4A to D: Recurrent anterior dislocation of shoulder treated by scapular neck osteotomy and buttress bone grafting (glenoplasty). (A) The line of osteotomy; (B) Postoperative CT scan shows the location of osteotomy and the bone graft; (C) Postoperative X-rays; (D) Functional outcome during follow-up 7 years after the operation.

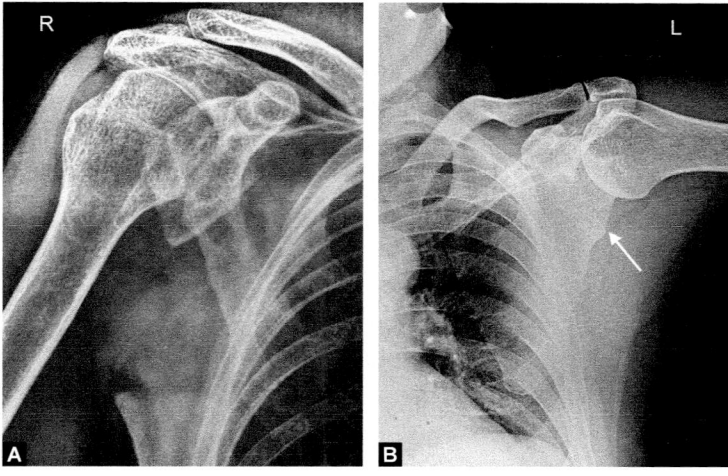

Figs. 12.5A and B: Buttress glenoplasty—2 patients: (A) 12 years post-operation, (B) 20 years after operation.

Bristow–Latarjet procedure is now gaining acceptance. Despite a large number of modifications described it involves transporting the osteotomized coracoid process along with the attached coracobrachialis and short head of biceps. Through a split in the subscapularis opposite to the scapular neck the coracoid process is fixed by 2 screws to the front of scapular neck near the anterior joint capsule. Whether performed by open procedure or by arthroscopy no difference has been found in the clinical outcome. The bone graft (the coracoid process) provides a buttress effect in front of the glenoid margin, the attached muscles (short head of biceps and coracobrachialis) probably act an dynamic stabilizers in front of the capsule, and the transplanted coracoid acts as a pedicled bone graft.

SUGGESTED READINGS

1. Tuli SM, Sharma SV. Long term follow-up of glenoplasty for recurrent anterior dislocation of shoulder. Indian J Orthop. 1990;24:186-8.
2. Shaffer B, Tibone JE, Kerlan RK. Frozen shoulder. A long-term follow-up. J Bone Joint Surg Am. 1992;74A:738-46.
3. Montgomery Jr WH, Wahl M, Hettrich C, Itoi E, Lippitt SB, Matsen FA. Anteroinferior bone grafting can restore stability in osseous glenoid defects. J Bone Joint Surg Am. 2005;87A:1972-7.
4. Bessiere C, Trojani C, Carles M, Mehta SS, Boileau P. The open Latarjet procedure is more reliable in terms of shoulder stability than arthroscopic bankart repair. Clin Orthop Relat Res. 2014;472:2345-51.
5. Longo UG, Loppini M, Rizzello G, Ciuffreda M, Maffulli N, Denaro V. Latarjet, Bristow, and Eden–Hybinette procedures for anterior shoulder dislocation: systematic review and quantitative synthesis of the literature. Arthroscopy. 2014;30:1184-211.
6. Cowling PD, Akhtar MA, Liow RYL. What is a Bristow–Latarjet procedure? Bone Joint J. 2016; 98-B:1208-14.

CHAPTER 13

Elbow and Forearm

On clinical examination with elbow flexed at 90 degrees, the tips of medial and lateral epicondyles and the tip of olecranon form an isosceles triangle. When the elbow is fully extended the three points make a straight line transversely. Interpretation of X-rays of elbow during the growing age is helped by remembering the MNEMONIC = CRITOE when the emerging secondary ossific centers appear (in years) = Capitulum-2, Radial head-4, Internal epicondyle-6, Trochlea-8, Olecranon-10, External epicondyle-12.

Affections of the elbow joints are the same as in any joints. The pain from the elbow may radiate to the forearm, and the pain felt in the elbow may be a referred pain from the neck.

TENNIS ELBOW (LATERAL EPICONDYLITIS)

This condition is characterized by acute pain over the lateral condyle of humerus. Though called tennis elbow, it does not necessarily affect the tennis players. It is often preceded by forceful extension of common extensors resulting in inflammation at the origin of common extensor group of muscles. Exact etiology is not clear, however, careful history and follow-up of such patients may show its association with evolving rheumatoid disorder like plantar fasciitis, tenosynovitis, and inflammation of other joints of the patient. The patient feels pain and a sense of weakness in lifting even small weights, local examination would reveal tenderness at or around the lateral epicondyle. The position of full extension of elbow, pronation of forearm, and flexion of ipsilateral hand and fingers causes maximum pain. Movements of elbow, pronation, supination, and X-rays of the elbow are normal.

Treatment

Rest to the elbow for a few days and use of nonsteroidal anti-inflammatory drugs (NSAIDs) may relieve the symptoms. On the other hand with the elbow fully extended and forearm pronated, repetitive flexion-extension at the wrist as a therapeutic exercise relieves the symptoms in most of the cases. A short course of ultrasound therapy may be required in some cases. In refractory cases, local injection of steroids into the painful area may be needed. Local steroids must be injected with standard aseptic precautious as close to the bone as possible. In patients with colored skin, one may get local discoloration of skin for a few months, if the injection was too close to the skin. Some workers have reported the use of lateral epicondylosis, and local injection, of autologous platelets.

GOLFER'S ELBOW

Golfer's elbow (medial epicondylitis) is a rarer condition similar to tennis elbow with symptoms around the origin of common flexor group of muscles. The area of pain and tenderness is around the medial epicondyle of humerus. The treatment is similar to tennis elbow.

CONGENITAL SLIPPING OF ULNAR NERVE

The ulnar nerve slips forward on flexion of elbow around the medial epicondyle of the humerus. In most of the cases, it is due to congenital absence of the fibrous roof over the ulnar tunnel or groove in which the nerve normally traverses. Hypoplasia of the medial epicondyle may be responsible in some cases. The patient presents with tingling and numbness in the distribution of ulnar nerve particularly on flexion of elbow or while resting the elbow on table during writing or for a desk-job. On examination, the nerve could be seen or palpated slipping anteriorly over the medial epicondyle when the elbow is slowly flexed. Resting the elbow on soft padding while doing the desk-job may relieve the symptoms. If symptoms are severe or there are objective neural signs, anterior transposition of the ulnar nerve placed in between the subcutaneous tissues and muscles would relieve the symptoms.

CUBITUS VALGUS

This is an exaggeration of the normal values of carrying angle present at the elbow. Normally the forearm deviates at the elbow by about 5 degrees in the males and a little more in the females. Cubitus valgus and varus deformities are best appreciated in full extended position of the elbow, flexion at the elbow masks the deformities. Valgus deformity may be the result of malunion of supracondylar fracture of humerus or destruction of lateral condyle of humerus due to infection during childhood, or premature arrest of lateral part of distal humeral physis (due to infection or injury), or neglected or inadequately treated fracture of lateral condyle of humerus **(Fig. 13.1)**. Moderate deformities are cosmetically acceptable; however, progressive deformity during growing age may lead to ulnar nerve involvement due to the stretching of nerve. Ulnar neuritis is treated by anterior transposition of the nerve.

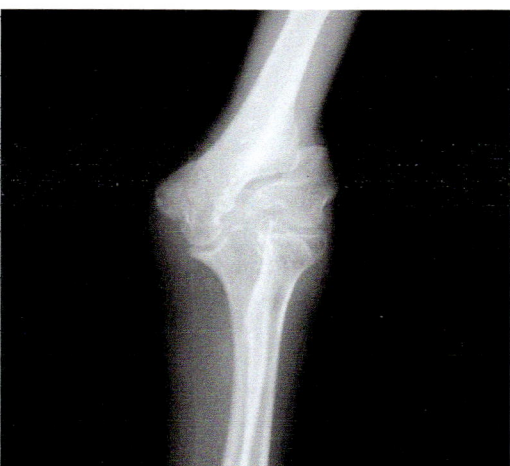

Fig. 13.1: Cubitus valgus: The commonest cause is damage to the lateral half of distal humeral physis or un-united lateral condyle fracture as in this X-ray.

Ulnar Nerve Transposition

Ulnar nerve compression or neuritis generally occurs at the elbow joint. Clinically one may find local tenderness of the nerve or recurrent slipping of the nerve over the medial epicondyle. The nerve may get irritated due to a malunited fracture at lower end of humerus or due to irregularity of the lower end as a result of osteomyelitis, or rarely due to involvement (thickening) of nerve due to leprosy. Depending upon the severity and duration of the defect the patient may present with dysthesia (paresthesias) in the sensory distribution of the ulnar nerve, i.e., the entire fifth finger and the dorsal and ulnar aspect of the ring finger. Weakness of flexor digitorum profundus of the ring and small fingers, abductor digiti minimi, interossei and adductor pollicis may be present. In patients with long-standing defect one can appreciate the wasting of the hypothenar muscles and the interossei.

Operative steps: The patient is placed supine on the table with the arm abducted 90 degrees on a padded hand table. The incision is made on the medial side of elbow, it extends approximately 10 cm proximal to the epicondyle about 8 cm distal to the medial epicondyle and passes about 2 cm anterior to the position of medial epicondyle. Continue the dissection through subcutaneous tissues to expose the ulnar nerve in the upper part behind the medial intermuscular septum. The septum is cut and released at the entry point of ulnar nerve. The nerve is separated from the surrounding tissues by careful dissection using blunt dissector and small knife or scissors. The entry point at the medial intermuscular septum must be released liberally, the nerve is freed from surrounding soft tissues from proximal to distal direction behind the humerus and medial epicondyle. The fibrous tissue behind the medial-epicondyle is like a thick band. Release the nerve upto it's entry, distal to the medial epicondyle between the origin of 2 heads of flexor carpai ulnaris. Throughout the dissection one would encounter many vessels surrounding the nerve and in the soft tissues. The nerve is freed and held in fine catheter loops, the bleeding is controlled using bipolar coagulation, ideally no vessel should be cut. Medial cutaneous nerve of arm arising from the ulnar nerve should be released (not cut) to permit anterior transposition of the ulnar nerve, short articular branches encountered in the retrocondylar area may be released or sectioned (if needed), however injury to the motor branches to flexor carpi ulnaris should be avoided. These branches are situated distal to the medial epicondyle between the two heads of flexor carpi ulnaris. The ulnar nerve is now mobilized and lifted from its original course and placed anterior to the humeral condyle. The nerve is inspected for any area of perineural fibrosis which must be released by a careful longitudinal incision. In a case of leprosy one may encounter an abscess or granuloma within the nerve sheath which may require decompression by making a longitudinal incision in the epineurium. When leprosy is suspected one of the articular branches and the tissue from the intraneural granuloma must be sent for histological examination.

Stitch the subcutaneous tissues to hold the nerve in the anterior position. Postoperatively splint the limb at 90 degrees of flexion for 2-3 weeks. Some surgeons prefer to hold the ulnar nerve deep to the origin of the pronator teres (flexor pronator tendon). Dissect and lift its origin from the anterior surface of medial epicondyle. Place the ulnar nerve anterior to the medial epicondyle, resuture the tendon to the bone anterior to the anteriorly transposed ulnar nerve. Cosmetically unacceptable valgus deformity may be corrected by supracondylar osteotomy and fixed with Kirschner wires (K-wires).

CUBITUS VARUS (GUNSTOCK) DEFORMITY

There is reversal of normal carrying angle, one can appreciate the medial deviation of the forearm at the elbow. The commonest cause is malunited supracondylar fracture of humerus in childhood. Deformity may be a sequelae of damages to the medial half of distal humeral physis due to trauma, infection, or iatrogenic injuries. Cubitus varus is cosmetically more disfiguring than the valgus deformity. Minimal deformities in children may get corrected by remodeling. Severe deformities need to be corrected by supracondylar osteotomy which is best done about 2 years before skeletal maturity **(Figs. 13.2A and B)**.

DISTAL HUMERAL OSTEOTOMY

Corrective osteotomy is indicated for unacceptable cubitus varus deformity, it should be performed only after the elbow has regained near complete extension and flexion, and ideally the patient is between 6 and 11 years of age. Distal end of the humerus is exposed through an 8 cm long lateral incision starting from lateral epicondyle and proceeding proximally almost along the lateral supracondylar ridge. Expose the site of osteotomy subperiosteally. Take care not to injure the radial nerve especially in the

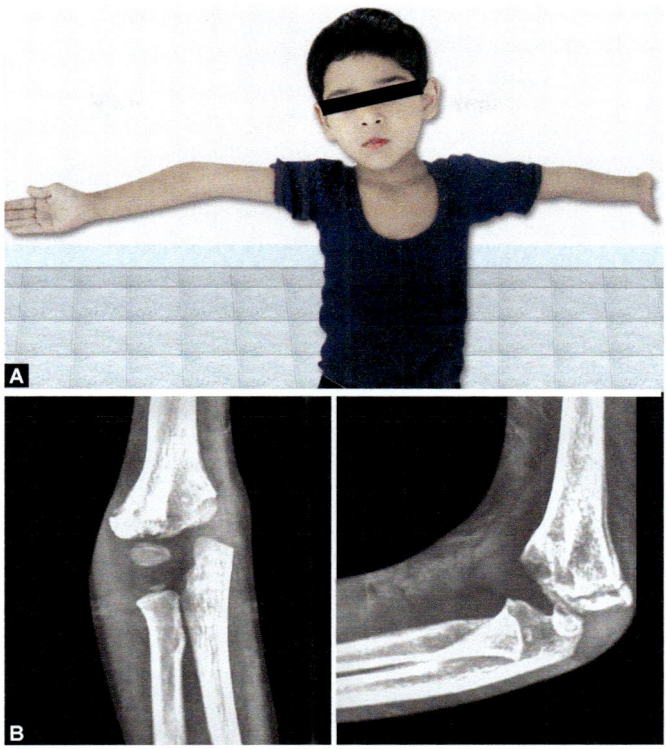

Figs. 13.2A and B: Classical picture of cubitus varus deformity (gunstock deformity) (A), The commonest cause is damage to the medial half of distal humeral physis as seen in these X-rays (B).

proximal part of incision. In cases with gross deformity and scarring or those who had previous surgery, it is wise to expose the radial nerve running between the brachioradialis (laterally) and brachialis (medially) muscles. Hold the radial nerve in a tape to keep it away from the operating field. Keep the elbow flexed 20–30 degrees to relax the anterior soft tissues. It is preferred to use low impact cutting of bone. The distal cut should be proximal to the olecranon fossa about 2 cm proximal to the lateral epicondyle, parallel to the joint line. The proximal line of osteotomy is dependent upon the base of wedge planned to correct the deformity, the cut is angled to meet the first cut medially. To make the process of osteotomy "gentle", make the outline of the proposed wedge using multiple drill holes first. With the help of a narrow sharp osteotome, complete the osteotomy, remove the wedge-shaped fragment, gently break the medial cortex at the apex of wedge and correct the deformity.

The size of the base of the wedge is determined depending upon the angle of varus to be corrected plus the physiological valgus angle of the normal contralateral elbow as judged in full extension. It almost works out to be 1 mm for 1 degree of correction to be achieved. In the growing age, some degree of correction may be negated by the epiphyseal growth, therefore, it is wise to add 3–8 degrees of additional correction. Having completed the osteotomy, correct the varus deformity and other associated deformities like medial rotation or displacements, fix the osteotomy with K-wires or contoured tubular plate or screws and wires. Some steps (mismatch) left at the osteotomy site get corrected by remodeling during the growth period.

Postoperatively use a posterior splint to hold the elbow in 90 degrees of flexion and mid-prone position. The splint is generally removed after 5–6 weeks and careful active exercises are started. No passive movements or local massage is permitted. Most of the patients gain the preoperative range of motion in the next 8–12 weeks. Unsightly prominence or steps visible after the removal of splint remodel within the next 1–2 years.

OLECRANON BURSITIS

Olecranon bursa is comparable with the prepatellar bursa at the knee. Inflammation of the bursa causes a painful, warm swelling at the olecranon tip. The condition was earlier known as "student's elbow" on the notion that students spent much of the time leaning on the elbows poring on the books. At present the condition is seen after an injury to the back of elbow or the bursal inflammation may be part of rheumatoid disorder or gout, or it may be an infected bursa. The bursal swelling may be aspirated and fluid sent for microscopic examination. Infected bursa requires to be treated by antibiotics. Anti-inflammatory drugs generally resolve the condition, and gout has to be treated accordingly. Non-resolving bursal swelling may need operative excision.

Pulled Elbow

Downward dislocation (or subluxation) of the radial head from the annular ligament is a fairly common injury in children under the age of 6 years. Generally, there is a history of the child being jerked or pulled by the arm followed by complain of pain and inability to use the arm. The diagnosis is essentially clinical, X-rays may be obtained to exclude a fracture. In childhood, the radial head gets subluxated or dislocated out of the envelop or noose of the annular ligament. When the child's attention is diverted, maintain pressure on the radial head, the elbow is quickly supinated and flexed, the radial head gets relocated with a snap.

STIFF ELBOW

Common causes of stiffness of the elbow may be due to the late effects of trauma (osteochondral fractures, old dislocation, heterotopic ossification), infection (pyogenic or tuberculous), rheumatoid inflammation, osteoarthrosis, arthrogryposis, osteochondritis dissecans (capitulum) or congenital synostosis **(Figs. 13.3A and B)**. Clinical assessment and investigations would help us to reach the diagnosis. Rarely one may encounter a neuropathic (Charcot's) joint of elbow (painless abnormal movements). X-rays would reveal 'destruction' of articular ends, 'displacement' (dislocation) of joint and 'debris' in the joint **(Fig. 13.4)**. Most of the activities of daily living (eating, brushing teeth, shaving) can be managed if the range of movements of elbow is retained; flexion from 30 to 130 degrees and pronation supination 50 degrees on each side. Most effective treatment for prevention of stiffness and for improvement of the range of motion is active exercises of elbow; aggressive passive manipulations and local massage are known to aggravate the formation of heterotopic ossification and stiffness of the elbow.

Failure to achieve a useful range of motion may be an indication for operative

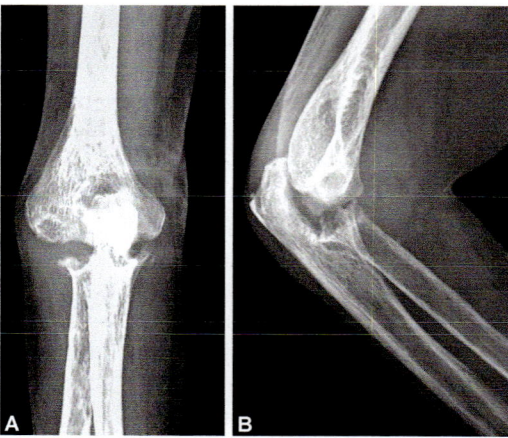

Figs. 13.3A and B: An advanced (stage IV) case of tuberculosis of elbow. Note soft tissue swelling, osteoporosis, destruction of upper end of ulna and lower end of humerus. Subperiosteal new bone formation can be appreciated on all the visible bones.

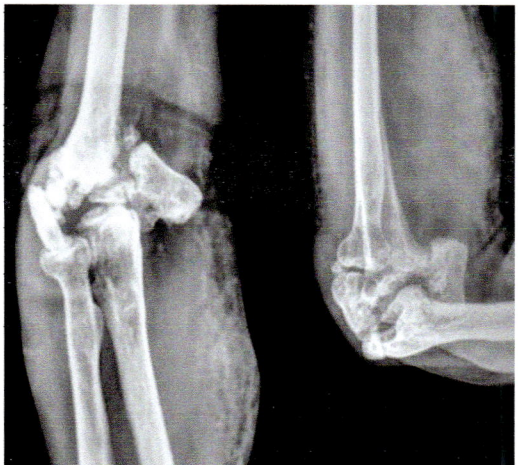

Fig. 13.4: X-rays of grossly destroyed elbow joint (Charcot's) with painless abnormal movements in a patient having syringomyelia of cervical cord.

intervention depending upon the patients' functional needs. The operation may be an arthrolysis and capsular release if there is no osseous incongruity. A bone block may need excision if it is causing mechanical obstruction. Myositis ossificans may be excised if it is blocking the movements. No operation on the heterotopic bone is advised unless it has reached the stage of "maturity". In cases of a gross ankylosis especially as a sequel of infection, an **excision-arthroplasty** of elbow may restore a useful range. Lower end of humerus is cut in an inverted V-shape and upper end of ulna (and radius) is trimmed carefully. Too liberal bone excision may lead to a flail elbow and too little may lead to reankylosis. Replacement arthroplasty may be justified in specialized hands, because of fragile bone stock and muscles, the success stories of hip replacement cannot be achieved. Elbow replacement procedures have a high rate of complications like wound failure, infection, dislodgement of implants and nerve palsies.

Radial Nerve Explorations

For any operation on the distal third of humerus and elbow it is wise to expose the radial nerve and hold it to safety throughout the operative procedure. Tedious dissection may be needed if there is scarring around the elbow due to previous operations, trauma or infection. Make a longitudinal incision (3–8 cm) along the lateral border of the biceps ending distally just proximal to the elbow flexion crease. Identify the lateral border of biceps, separate it by blunt dissection from the brachialis to allow for medial retraction of biceps muscle. Two muscles are separated by retracting biceps medially and the brachioradialis laterally. The radial nerve (can be palpated and visualized) lies between the brachioradialis (laterally) and brachialis (medially) anterior to the lateral condyle of humerus. The nerve is traced and dissected free from distal to proximal direction upto the penetration of the nerve through the lateral intermuscular septum.

CONGENITAL RADIOULNAR SYNOSTOSIS

Congenital radioulnar synostosis is a rare condition where there is fusion **(Fig. 13.5)** (fibro-osseous or osseous) of the superior radioulnar joint, sometimes the condition is bilateral. Elbow function is well-retained, the child compensates for loss of pronation-supination by rotatory movements at the

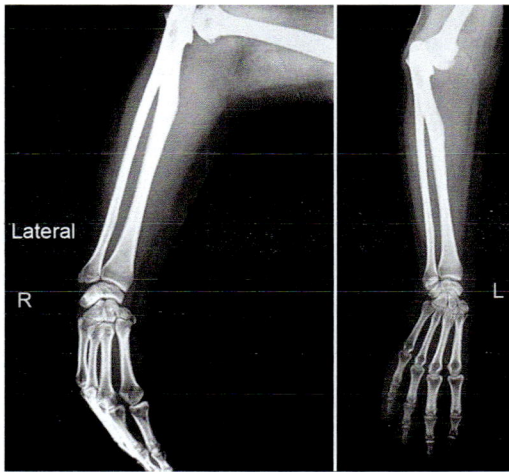

Fig. 13.5: Congenital synostosis in both forearms. Observe missing first ray in both hands.

shoulder, therefore often the disability is detected only after the age of 3–4 years. Both the elbows should be radiographed in full extension. Fusion of the superior radioulnar joints may be seen to an extent of 1–3 cm. Surgery to regain pronation-supination rarely succeeds as there may be other associated congenital defects like absence of supinator muscles and hypoplasia of other muscles. In cases of extreme deformity, the function may be improved by a rotational osteotomy performed at the middle of radius to bring the forearm to mid-prone position.

CONGENITAL ABSENCE OF RADIUS

Congenital absence of radius may occur alone or in association with visceral anomalies. The radius may be absent or hypoplastic. The forearm is short and bowed with convexity to the ulnar side, the hand is underdeveloped and markedly deviated towards the radial side (radial club hand), the thumb may be missing. In half the cases, the condition is bilateral. The treatment should start as soon as the diagnosis is made by repeated stretching and splintage to avoid soft tissue contracture. Many children are able to manage activities of daily needs. Centralization (radialization) of ulna may be performed at 2–3 years of age to minimize the deformity. The lower end of ulna is positioned at the place of lunate bone **(Figs. 13.6A to D)**. Prolonged postoperative splintage is still required to avoid recurrence of deformity. Radialization of ulna does improve the cosmetics of hand and forearm however full length, and complete function is seldom achieved because on the radial side in addition to the deficient radius the muscles, nerves and vessels are not fully developed.

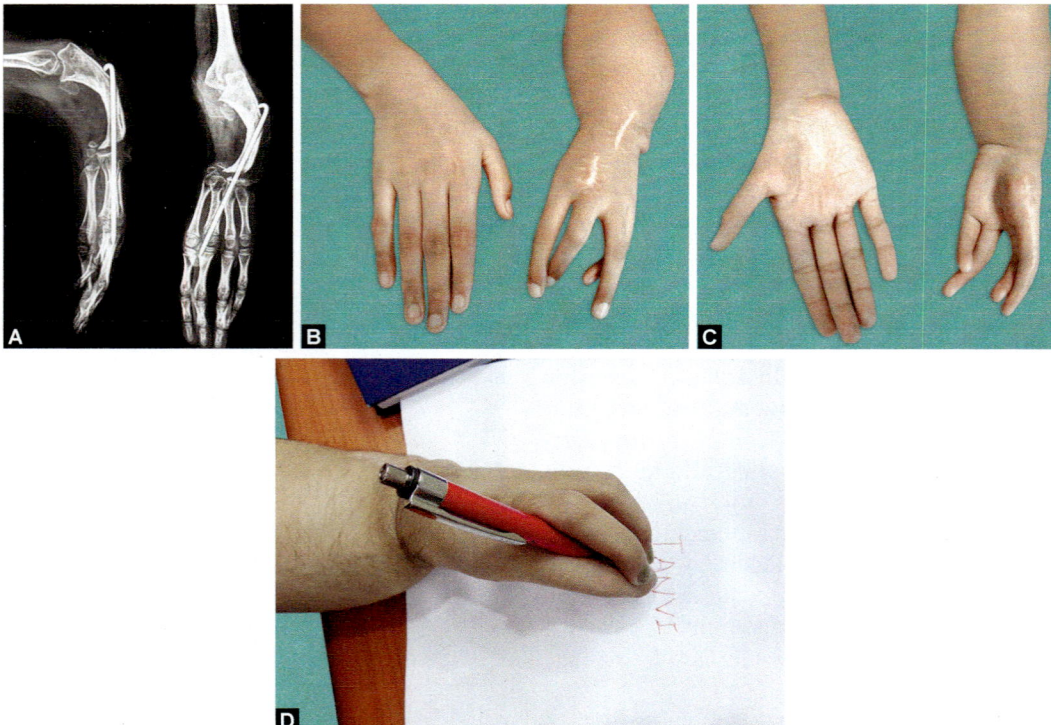

Figs. 13.6A to D: (A) X-rays of a child with congenital radial hemimelia: Treated by centralization of distal end of ulna. Note absence of radius and the first ray of the hand; (B and C) Follow-up shows some cosmetic improvement; (D) Patient now 18 years, attempting to write with left hand.

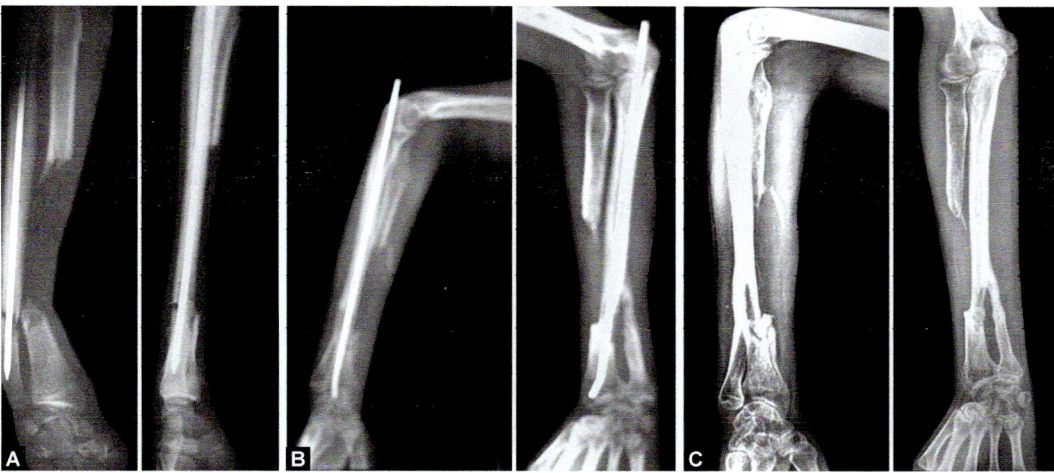

Figs. 13.7A to C: Follow-up of a case of (A) traumatic extrusion of a large segment of radius; (B) Single bone forearm was created by radialization of ulna. The ulna served as a pedicled bone graft; (C) 3-years postoperation appearance.

Pollicization of the most radial finger may improve some function. The forearm may need further corrective osteotomy of ulnar deformity prior to the skeletal maturity. Centralization of ulna for traumatic loss of radius can restore near full function **(Figs. 13.7A to C)**, unlike congenital absence of radius.

MYOSITIS OSSIFICANS (HETEROTOPIC OSSIFICATION)

It is a new bone formation in the periarticular muscles and soft tissues and has been observed around any joints (e.g., elbows, hips, knees), usually as a result of forceful passive manipulations and local massage. Involuntary spasmodic contraction of muscles in cases of severe head injuries or cord damage can also lead to myositis ossificans. Radiologically, heterotopic ossification passes through 3 phases of evolution: **stage of onset and progression** seen as fluffy radiolucent shadows around the joints, which increase in size for about 3 months: it is followed by the **stage of regression** as size of myositis decreases, the bone appears more solid and the margins are clearer, after about

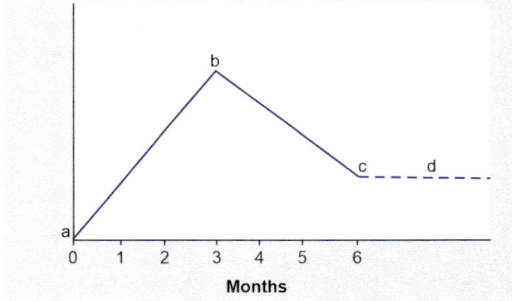

Fig. 13.8: Stages of myositis ossificans. (a) Onset often traumatic insult; (a)–(b) Stage of progression; (b)–(c) Stage of regression; (c)–(d) Stage of maturity, safe time for operative intervention.

6 months further decrease in the size does not take place, the bone margins are now clear and smooth, the bone texture has trabecular pattern and the myositis has reached the **stage of "maturity"**. Any operative intervention is justified only when the myositis has matured, surgery performed during the stages of "progression" or "regression" may further initiate the formation of more heterotopic ossification **(Fig. 13.8)**. Some surgeons have suggested for the use of radiation therapy and indomethacin prior to the operation if performed earlier than the stage of maturity.

SUGGESTED READINGS

1. Thorndike A Jr. Myositis ossificans traumatica. J Bone Joint Surg. 1940;22:315-23.
2. Douglas K, Cannada LK, Archer KR, Dean DB, Lee S, Obremskey W. Incidence and risk factors of heterotopic ossification following major elbow trauma. Orthopedics. 2012;35:815-22.

14 Wrist and Hand

For all practical purposes wrist and hand work as a single functional unit. When dealing with the problems of hand and wrist, both the upper limbs should be exposed for clinical examination. When dealing with subtle or less obvious defects or early stage of disease, it is wise to ask for X-rays of both sides in identical positions for comparison, [e.g., X-rays posteroanterior (PA) both wrists in maximum ulnar deviation]. A few common conditions encountered in clinical practice are described as follows.

WRIST DROP

This deformity is due to paralysis of extensors of the wrist and fingers due to pressure or damage to the radial nerve around the middle third of arm. The pressure on the nerve may be caused by the edge of a bed or chair while sleeping with hanging arm, or a pressure caused by the bodyweight while using the axillary crutches or by contusion of the nerve in fractures of humeral shaft or supracondylar fractures. A careless injection in the lower part of arm near the lateral part of spiral groove may result in a wrist drop. Perineural injections may cause a temporary paralysis, however, an intraneural injection damages a long segment of nerve. With suitable precautions radial nerve palsy is preventable. Most closed injuries would recover in 8–12 weeks by holding the wrist in 10–15 degrees of dorsiflexion and encouraging active exercises of fingers. If the nerve is cut due to an open injury or during internal fixation it should be repaired immediately. Nerve grafts may be needed if long segment is damaged. The results of radial nerve repair or grafting are usually gratifying because the nerve has essentially motor functions. Despite all efforts, if recovery does not occur within about 1 year, one should consider tendon transfers: pronator teres to extensor carpi radialis brevis, flexor carpi radialis to the long finger extensors, and palmaris longus to the abductor pollicis longus.

CLAW HAND

This deformity is caused by damage to the ulnar and median nerves above the wrist level. If both nerves are involved, it results in total claw hand, partial claw hand is due to involvement of ulnar or median nerve. Total claw hand also called "intrinsic minus hand"; because of the paralysis of intrinsic muscles of the hand, the fingers attain a position of extension at metacarpophalangeal joints and flexion of interphalangeal joints **(Fig. 14.1)**. In partial claw hand, 4th and 5th fingers would show the deformity in ulnar nerve palsy, and other fingers would exhibit deformity in median nerve involvement. Damage of the lower trunk of brachial plexus, leprosy involving the median and ulnar nerves and muscular dystrophy can also show the intrinsic minus deformity.

"Intrinsic plus" deformity presents as flexion at metacarpophalangeal joints and extension at interphalangeal joints. It is caused by the contracture of the intrinsic muscles of hand by rheumatoid inflammation, or contracture of intrinsic muscles, due to prior infection or ischemic changes (Volkmann's contracture).

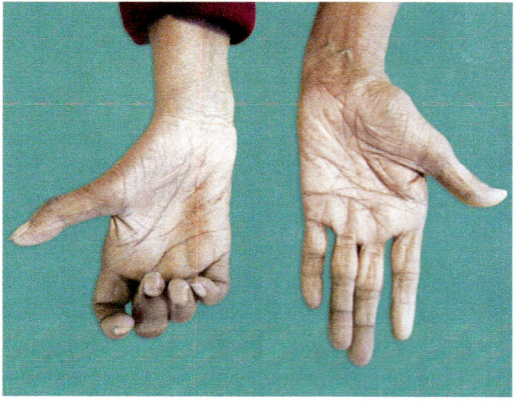

Fig. 14.1: Total intrinsic minus claw hand: Right hand on comparison with contralateral normal side shows the flattening of thenar and hypothenar eminences and extension at metacarpophalangeal joints with flexion of fingers.

Treatment

The appearance and function of the hand deformity can be improved by repeated active and assisted exercises. The correction of deformity achieved should be retained by corrective splints worn during night. In traumatic injuries above the wrist, the nerves must be repaired.

Repair of the damaged brachial plexus is a highly complex procedure with variable outcome. This falls within the preview of specialized centers. The function of intrinsic minus hand can be markedly improved by various tendon grafts as described earlier. The principles are the same for any paralytic condition.

CARPAL TUNNEL SYNDROME (SEE ALSO CHAPTER 10)

The carpal tunnel is a fibro-osseous tunnel formed by the palmar hollow of the articulated carpal bones that is roofed by the transverse carpal ligament. The tunnel contains all the flexor tendons supplying the fingers, median and ulnar nerves. Any space occupying lesion or swelling of the structures traversing the canal, cause pressure on the median nerve and rarely on ulnar nerve (passing through the Guyon's canal), deep to the pisohamate ligament.

The patient complains of pain, tingling and numbness in the thumb, index and middle fingers, the area of median nerve distribution. In long-standing cases, there would be wasting of thenar muscles. Usual causes of this syndrome are rheumatoid inflammation of the tendon sheaths contained within the tunnel, compound palmar ganglion (tubercular) or tenosynovitis of the flexor tendon sheath, traumatic dislocation or avascular necrosis of the lunate bone, malunited Colles fracture or distal radius osteochondral fractures, edema caused by hypothyroidism or pregnancy or renal disease. Symptoms are most disturbing at night. In the western population 6% of adults have been reported to have symptoms of carpal tunnel syndrome (CTS) once in their lifetime.

If there is a specific cause present, its treatment would relieve the symptoms. Conservative treatment like nonsteroidal anti-inflammatory drugs (NSAIDs), night splints, or a few injections of long-acting corticosteroids may provide relief. If symptoms are not relieved by nonoperative treatment **surgical division of the transverse carpal ligament** (flexor retinaculum) is warranted. The skin incision is made through one of the creases, with skin margins retracted open surgical division of whole length of transverse carpal ligament is performed. The ligament should be cut in line with the ring finger to prevent injury to the palmar cutaneous (sensory) and thenar motor branches of the median nerve taking origin from the radial border of the median nerve. At the distal end, the dissection need not go beyond the distal border of thumb (thumb held in extension), careful distraction at the distal end prevents damage to the vascular palmar arch. After hemostasis, suture only the skin and splint the wrist for 2–3 weeks. Endoscopic tunnel release is an alternative; however, the complication rates are higher in the hands of a general orthopedic surgeon.

Injection for Carpal Tunnel Syndrome

The point of entry is between the tendon of flexor carpi radialis and the tendon of palmaris longus. In case the palmaris longus is absent (about 10% of people) the needle should be inserted just medial to the tendon of flexor carpi radialis. The level of entry should be just proximal to the upper border of pisiform bone. The needle is inserted at an angle of almost 45 degrees pointing dorsally and distally. The carpal tunnel is a distensible space, the fluid should flow without much resistance. If problem is encountered during injection, tip of the needle is imbedded either in the flexor retinaculum or in any tendon. Correctly reposition the needle before you inject the fluid without resistance. In general the maximum number of injections should not exceed 3 with a minimum gap of 1 month between the injections.

CARPAL TUNNEL RELEASE

Open surgical division of the flexor retinaculum and transverse carpal ligament is safe and simple. Endoscopic carpal tunnel release is another alternative, however, it needs endoscopic expertise and the complication rate is higher. The skin incision is made through one of the palmar creases, ulnar to the thenar eminence. The distal end of the skin incision is upto the distal border of the thumb placed in extension. The proximal extent should not cross the flexion crease of the wrist, here the incision is continued ulnarwards in the wrist crease for about 2 cm and then curved proximally for another about 2 cm. Retract the skin flaps, cut the subcutaneous tissues, and the palmaris longus tendon is *retracted* radially, all further dissection is performed on the ulnar side of the retracted palmaris longus. Identify the upper border of the flexor retinaculum many a times by the presence of some fat. Insert a flat blunt dissector deep to the flexor retinaculum (transverse carpal ligament), from proximal to its distal border. At the distal end protect the superficial vascular palmar arch by retraction distally. Cut the entire length of the transverse carpal ligament in line with the ring finger. No deeper dissection should be done on the radial border of the median nerve, important motor branch from the median nerve generally arises from it radial border to supply the thenar muscles. Once the entire length of the median nerve deep to the transverse carpal ligament is visible no further dissection is required. If one encounters a tumor (lipoma, neurofibroma) or hypertrophied or granulomatous synovitis of the flexor tendon sheaths, it may need excision or debridement. About 2 cm of deep fascia is also released at the proximal end of the skin incision. At the end of surgery bleeding points are cauterized using bipolar coagulation, and the wound is closed by skin sutures only. Postoperatively a wrist splint may be used for about 2–3 weeks.

GANGLION

This is a cystic swelling most commonly observed on the dorsum of wrist usually fixed to the capsule of one of the carpal joints, less commonly one can occasionally find a ganglion on the anterior aspect of wrist or around the ankle. It consists of a synovial protrusion containing viscous jelly like (synovial fluids) material encased in a fibrous wall. The size varies between 1/2 to 1.5 cm. The patient may complain of the swelling and vague pain on movements. It is not a disabling condition and can be left alone. Manual compression of the ganglion while doing active exercise may resolve the mass, aspiration may help it to disappear. If the swelling is too big and disfiguring, it may be excised, however, it may recur after any attempted treatment, and the operative scar may be uglier than the ganglion (Figs. 14.2A and B).

DEFORMITIES IN WRIST AND HAND

Any pathology of osteoarticular system can be present in wrist and hands. Commoner affections are infections, inflammations, degenerative changes and tumorous conditions. In advanced rheumatoid arthritis,

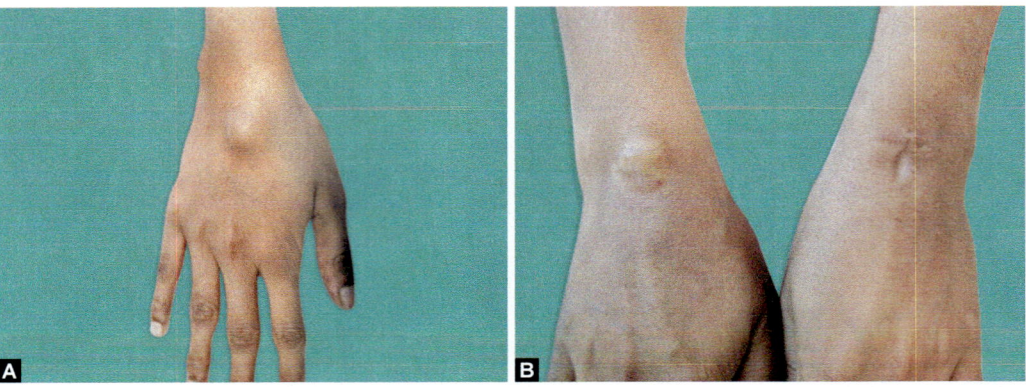

Figs. 14.2A and B: (A) A typical dorsal ganglion of the wrist; (B) Dorsal wrist ganglion, right nonoperated ganglion, left operated ganglion. Cosmetically the scar is more ugly than the ganglion.

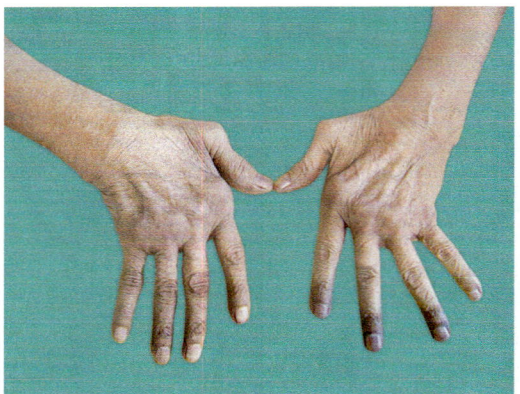

Fig. 14.3: An advanced case of rheumatoid arthritis of wrist and hands. Note radial deviation of carpus at wrist and ulnar drift at metacarpo-carpal joints.

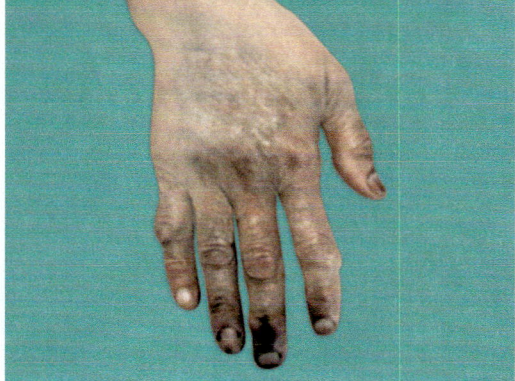

Fig. 14.4: Typical picture of osteoarthrosis involving distal interphalangeal joints. Note the prominent knobs on the dorsum of interphalangeal joints (Heberden's nodes).

the hand generally shows deformities with radial deviation at wrist, ulnar deviation at metacarpophalangeal joints and more involvement of proximal interphalangeal joints. In osteoarthrosis, frequent changes are present in first carpometacarpal joints and terminal interphalangeal joints (Figs. 14.3 and 14.4).

GROSS DEFORMITIES

Gross deformity around any joint can be corrected by Z-plasty of skin (or skin-grafting), excision of contracted deep fascia, lengthening of contracted tendons, capsulectomy (or arthrolysis), corrective osteotomies (or bone resection) and graduated correction of the clinical deformity. Prerequisites for such corrections are normal capillary circulation and sensations in hands (or feet). Corrective forces can be applied through change of plaster every 5–7 days or use of distracting external fixation (Figs. 14.5A and B).

CONSTRICTIVE TENOSYNOVITIS

De Quervain's Disease

De Quervain's disease is a chronic constrictive tenosynovitis affecting the abductor pollicis longus and extensor pollicis brevis

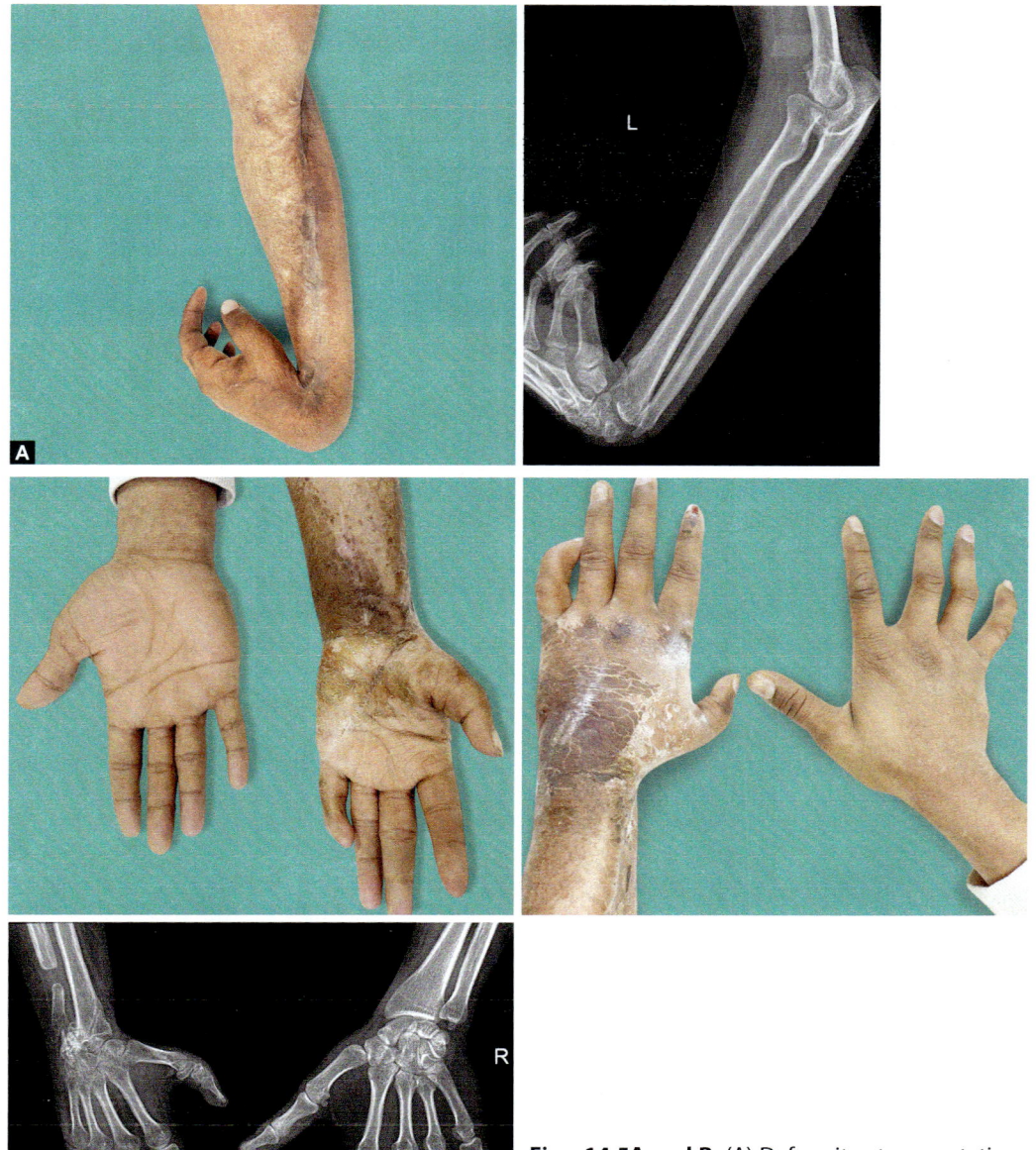

Figs. 14.5A and B: (A) Deformity at presentation; (B) Correction achieved.

tendons as these traverse in a groove over the lateral aspect of the lower end of radius. This results in obstruction in the free movements of thumb. The patient presents with diffuse pain over these tendons, there is tenderness on deep palpation, localized swelling is sometimes palpable. Active or passive extension and flexion of the thumb are painful, and in late cases, the movements are obstructed and on forceful movements, a palpable (or audible) snap may be present.

Treatment

In early stages, active exercises of the thumb and use of NSAIDs for about 2 weeks may relieve the condition, local ultrasonotherapy may help. In late stages, local injection of long-acting corticosteroids into the tendon sheath may relieve the stenosing effect. In cases refractory to these procedures, the stenosed tendon sheath should be surgically slit to relieve the symptoms. While operating prevent injury to the dorsal sensory branches of radial nerve.

Trigger Fingers

This is common in middle and ring fingers, there is stenosis or constriction of the flexor tendon sheath at the level of metacarpophalangeal joints with the development of a palpable nodule in the substance of the flexor tendon. The patient complains of difficulty and pain during flexion and extension of the finger. In later stages, after full flexion of the finger, the extension is not possible. On forceful extension, the finger extends suddenly with a palpable and audible snap. The principles of treatment are the same as for any stenosing tenosynovitis.

Congenital Trigger Thumb

It is a congenital constriction of the tendon sheath of the flexor pollicis longus at the level of metacarpophalangeal joint. The child keeps the thumb with flexion at the interphalangeal joint. Attempted extension releases the thumb into full extension with a click. A small nodule can be felt in the tendon at the level of metacarpophalangeal joint and the triggering can be palpated on passive flexion and extension of the distal phalanx.

Triggering often resolves by doing repetitive passive corrective exercises. If the condition persists beyond one year surgical division of the stenosed tendon sheath is required.

Dupuytren's Contracture

This is an uncommon condition in the Indian subcontinent **(Fig. 14.6)**. There is contracture of palmar fascia related to ring and little fingers. Generally, a male patient above the age of 40 years presents with gradually increasing flexion deformity of little and ring fingers at metacarpophalangeal joints. With advancing disease other fingers may also be involved. One can palpate cord like thickened palmar fascia, with nodules. The contracted fascia is adherent to the palmar skin and there may be formation of "pits" (small depressions) in the involved areas.

A high incidence is observed in epileptics, diabetics, smokers and those with liver cirrhosis. The condition may have familial aggregation. In some patients, both hands may be involved, and the condition may also be seen on the soles of feet. Clinical examination would reveal cords, nodules and pits in the plantar fascia.

Treatment

Treatment at early stages is active and passive exercises, control of comorbidities and local corticosteroids injections. In long established cases percutaneous focal multiple

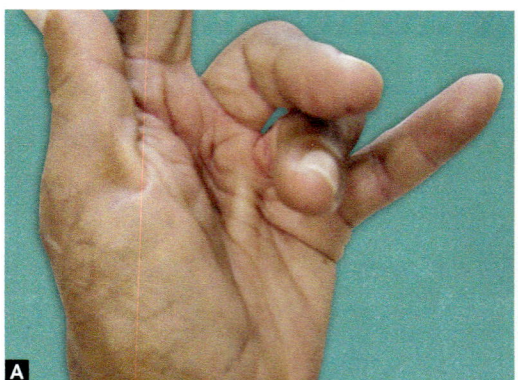
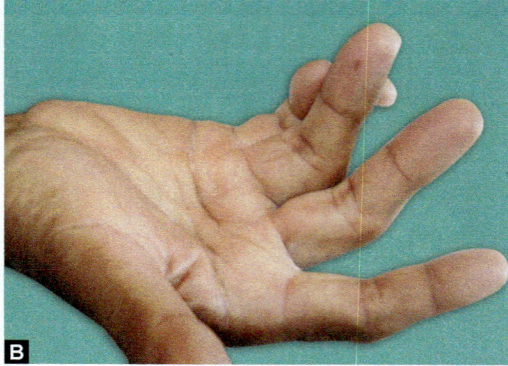

Figs. 14.6A and B: Dupuytren's contracture: It is a fibromatosis of palmar fascia. Cord like contractures are present in both hands of this patient leading to deformities of fingers (mostly fifth and fourth).

fasciotomies of the cord and contracted fascia is advised. If the contracture is more severe, the contracted cords are carefully removed by making Z-plasty skin incisions through various palmar creases. If skin closure is not possible, the palmar wound can be left open to heal within 10–15 days. After operation, corrective splint is applied till the healing of wound. Night splints should be continued for many months, corrective exercises are for lifetime to reduce the chance of recurrence.

Compound Palmar Ganglion

This expression is conventionally used to describe a subacute or chronic swelling of common flexor sheath of flexor group of muscles traversing deep to the carpal ligament (flexor retinaculum). The swelling is seen both proximal and distal to the carpal ligament, one is able to elicit cross fluctuation by pushing the fluid from one part to the other. The thickened flexor sheath contains fluid and sometimes fibrin particles. While eliciting cross-fluctuation, one may palpate creaking sensation. Most common causes are tuberculosis or rheumatoid inflammation. The patient presents because of swelling, local pain, tenderness and paresthesia due to median nerve compression. Start the treatment according to the pathology. Operative treatment may be required for confirmation of diagnosis and release of the median nerve. Subtotal excision of the inflamed synovial flexor sheath is performed followed by splintage for 2–3 weeks and medications according to the final diagnosis (Fig. 14.7).

KIENBÖCK'S DISEASE (SEE ALSO CHAPTER 5)

This is a form of avascular necrosis of lunate bone. Many causes have been discussed but none is convincingly proven. In the post-COVID era after 2020 many cases have been observed concomitantly associated with osteonecrosis of femoral head. Like osteonecrosis of any bone it may be classified as four stages:

1. X-rays normal, changes present in MRIs.
2. Lunate bones shows sclerosis in X-rays, height of bone is maintained.
3. X-rays show fragmentation and reduced height (collapse) of lunate.
4. Arthrosis of adjacent carpal bones plus changes at 3 above.

Nonoperative treatment like wrist splint, active exercises and NSAIDs may relieve the symptoms. If pain is disturbing and persists, X-rays show flattening and fragmentation, operative treatment is indicated. Many authors have tried vascular bundle implantation, core decompression with bone grafting, removal of lunate and its replacement with silicone prosthesis. With moderate facilities available the lunate can be removed, and the gap can be filled by a rounded ball made from the ipsilateral palmaris longus tendon. This autologous biological spacer has given good relief to the patients for long time.

SUDECK'S DYSTROPHY [CURRENTLY ADDRESSED AS COMPLEX REGIONAL PAIN SYNDROME (CRPS)], OR REFLEX PAIN SYNDROME (RPS)

In orthopedic field, it is generally precipitated by a trauma (many a times, a trivial injury)

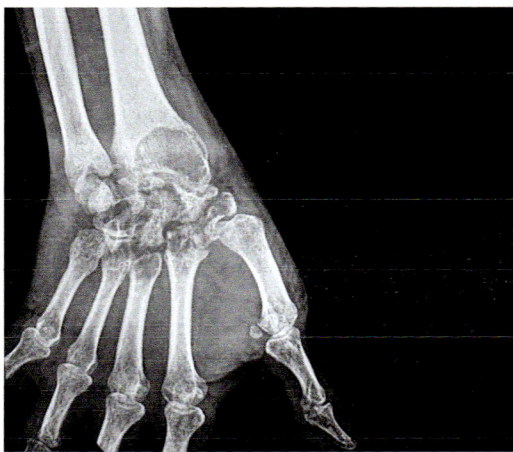

Fig. 14.7: Advanced tuberculous arthritis of wrist involving all carpal bones. Commonest bone for initial infection in the wrist is capitate. Distal end of radius has a lytic lesion. Note absence of reactive new bone formation.

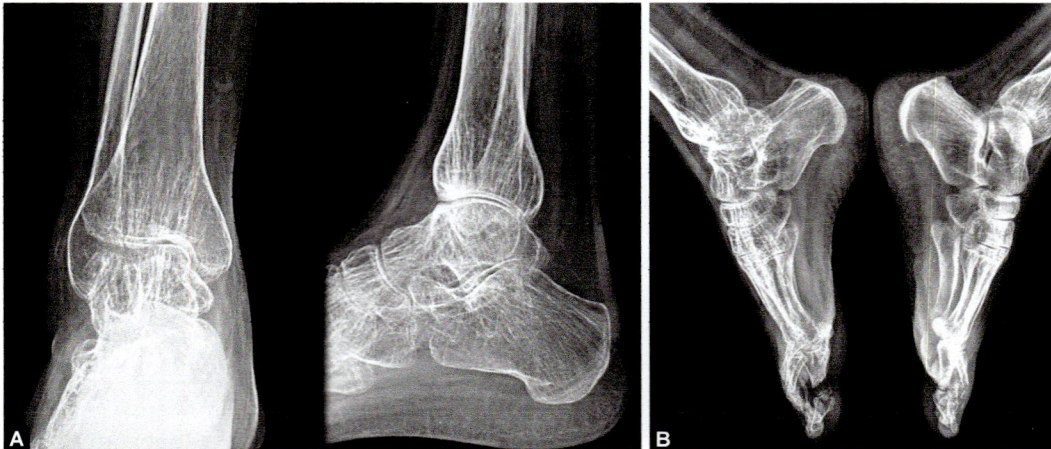

Figs. 14.8A and B: Complex regional pain syndrome (Sudeck's dystrophy) after an insignificant injury around the ankle the complaints of pain, swelling, warmth and tenderness persisted for many months, the X-rays show an unusual degree of osteoporosis: (A) The symptomatic (right) foot; (B) Lateral view of both feet for comparison with normal (left) foot.

like fractures around the wrist or around foot. The characteristic features are local swelling (hand or foot are most commonly involved), hypersensitive painful reaction to all types of stimuli (hot or cold wind), disproportionate loss of function and stiffness. The part is swollen, skin is stretched and shining with loss of wrinkles, the color may be cyanotic or have blotchy appearance and there may be local sweating. X-rays may show para-articular band like osteoporosis or it may be patchy or generalized demineralization **(Figs. 14.8A and B)**.

The exact cause and mechanism of this syndrome is not known, however, it is considered that many factors are involved such as abnormal cytokine release, neurogenic inflammation, enhanced cortical and sympathetic reaction to the noxious stimuli and emotionally hypersensitive personalities. Shoulder-hand syndrome is generally associated with Sudeck's like picture.

Treatment

Treatment should be started as soon as the diagnosis is made. Anti-inflammatory (NSAIDs) drugs, repetitive active exercise and elevation of the involved part is the most important modality of treatment. A short course of calcium channel blockers, amitriptyline, carbamazepine and gabapentin may help deal with emotional elements. Concomitant medical problems must be well-controlled. A short course of bisphosphanates and calcitonin may also help control local osteoporosis. Prolonged dedicated treatment is the mainstay for success. In nonresponders one may need to do sympathetic block at stellate ganglion or lumbar sympathetic chain, or regional nerve blocks. Transcutaneous nerve stimulation may help. Psychological treatment may be tried to dealt with emotional distress.

SUGGESTED READINGS

1. Sayegh ET, Strauch RJ. Open versus endoscopic carpal tunnel release. A meta-analysis of randomized controlled trials. Clin Orthop Relat Res. 2015;473:1120-32.
2. Tang CQY, Lai SWH, Tay SC. Long-term outcome of carpal tunnel release surgery in patients with severe carpal tunnel syndrome. Bone Joint J. 2017; 99-B:1348-53.

15 Back Pain and Spine

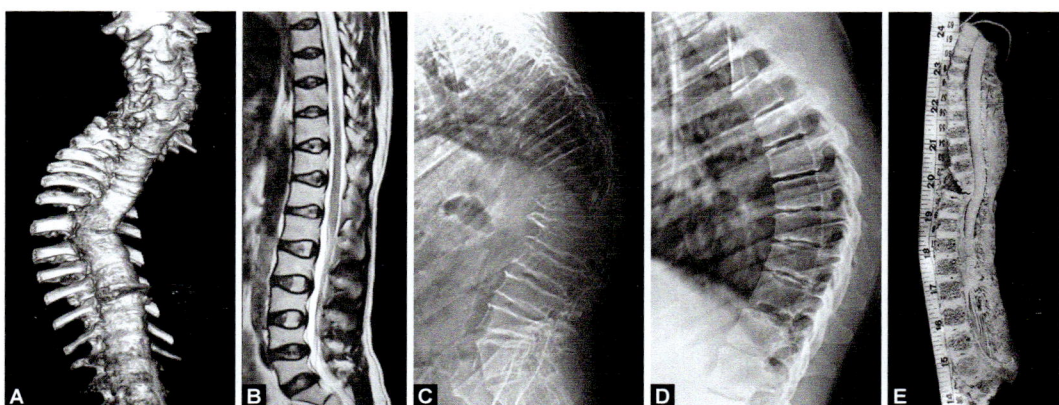

Typical images of common vertebral disorders. (A) 3D reconstruction of scoliosis = Lateral convexity + axial rotation + kyphosis. (B) Osteomalacia in a young person: Showing generalized biconcave vertebral bodies and biconvex discs. (C) Severe osteoporosis in an elderly person; note demineralized bones with compressed verterbal bodies and round kyphosis. (D) Scheuermann's disorder; mild vertebral anterior wedging, irregular disc shape round kyphosis. (E) Museum specimen: Mid-sagittal section of spine showing tuberculous destruction at lower dorsal spine. *Note*: Dural tube is not invaded by tuberculous pathology.
Courtesy: (Part E) Patna Medical College.

INTRODUCTION

Age-related changes in the vertebral column start around 40 years, however, most of the clinical symptoms present around the age of 50 years. The sequential changes that take place are desication of discs leading to decreased disc height, telescopy of vertebral bodies and infolding of ligamentum flavum. Degenerative changes lead to enthesopathy and formation of osteophytes and hypertrophy of ligaments. All images must be interpreted in relation to the clinical symptoms.

Low back pain (ache) is by far the most common spinal complaint in any general orthopedic consultation service. In majority of the cases, the cause or source of pain is "strain" or inflammation of myofascial structures and ligaments. The pain can originate from annulus fibrosus, vertebral periosteum, anterior and posterior longitudinal ligaments, supraspinous and interspinous ligaments and myofascial structures attached to various parts of the vertebral column. Rarely the symptoms of backache may be associated with viral infections and visceral disorders. As the source of pain in a particular patient is conjectural, there are many synonyms for low back pain such as lumbago, lumbosacral strain, sacroiliac strain and rheumatoid inflammation. A small number of these patients may at a later stage develop features of a prolapsed disc, ankylosing spondylitis and rheumatoid inflammatory disorder. Rarer conditions affecting the spine may give rise to backache primarily or secondarily. These less common conditions must be eliminated in every case. Careful clinical examination, appropriate investigations and periodic follow-up helps the clinicians to differentiate these conditions.

Age-related guidelines for "commoner" nontraumatic severe low back pain:
- **Age <20 years:** Spondylolysis or spondylolisthesis, infections, tumors (osseous or neural).
- **Age 20–40 years:** Prolapsed intervertebral disc, inflammatory disorders.
- **Age 40 years:** Osteoporosis, metastasis, myelomatosis.
- **Any age:** Infections, tumors, endocrinal, inflammatory disorders.

Of all the patients of backache, only 1–2% need operative interventions. However, because of many areas of uncertainty, the frequency of operative treatment varies widely in different parts of world. In the United States, the rate of surgical treatment is 5 times that of Great Britain. Appropriate surgical treatment may be considered for unrelieved patients having signs and symptoms disturbing his day-to-day activities.

There are only two indications for urgent operation on the spine; cauda equina syndrome, and an epidural abscess leading to neural deterioration.

Any other operation must be considered after elaborate investigations and sound preoperative planning.

For any patient with persistent back-ache standing X-rays are a standard requirement. The X-rays are able to show any abnormality in curvature, health of vertebral bodies and disc, destructive lesions like infection, trauma, osteoporosis, neoplastic lesions, paravertebral soft tissue collections, ossification of ligaments and disc spaces, kyphosis, scoliosis and loss of spinal curvatures. Lateral views in flexion and extension may reveal excessive intervertebral movements as in spondylolisthesis.

Broadly speaking, MRI images show T2- "water white" and T1- "water black". Fat looks white in both T1 and T2 images. Ligaments, desiccated discs, scarred tissue stay as black.

MRIs have provided the clinicians most helpful imaging modality now practically available in all countries. It is a "non-invasive" investigation, does not expose the patient to radiations. MRIs have practically done away with the need of myelography and discography. The scans can mostly reveal the biological status of the pathology (like active, healing, healed, deteriorating). It can provide information like dural tube compromise and intrinsic changes in the cord. However, we need to be aware that about 20% of asymptomatic persons above the age of 40 years may show significant abnormalities, therefore, all images must be interpreted in conjunction with the clinical picture.

Scheuermann's Disorder (Osteochondrosis of Vertebrae)

Scheuermann's disorder of spine presents as a round dorsal spine kyphosis in a juvenile. The deformity is considered a result of irregular growth of vertebral apophysis, the disc spaces are irregular and there is mild anterior wedging of vertebral bodies. Mostly presenting in dorsal spine, however, can occur upto lumbar vertebrae as well.

SCOLIOSIS (FIG. 15.1A)

Clinically, scoliosis appears to be a lateral curvature of the vertebral column. However, most of the scoliotic deformities are tri-planner [a combination of lateral convexity, posterior convexity (kyphosis)], and axial rotation of the vertebrae (the vertebral body rotates toward the convex side). There are a number of classifications of idiopathic scoliosis, the classification suggested by Scoliosis Research Society (SRS) is used currently. This (SRS) classification is based upon the chronological age at presentation of the deformity; *Infantile Scoliosis* (birth to 3 years), Juvenile Scoliosis (3–10 years), and Adolescent Scoliosis (10 years to skeletal

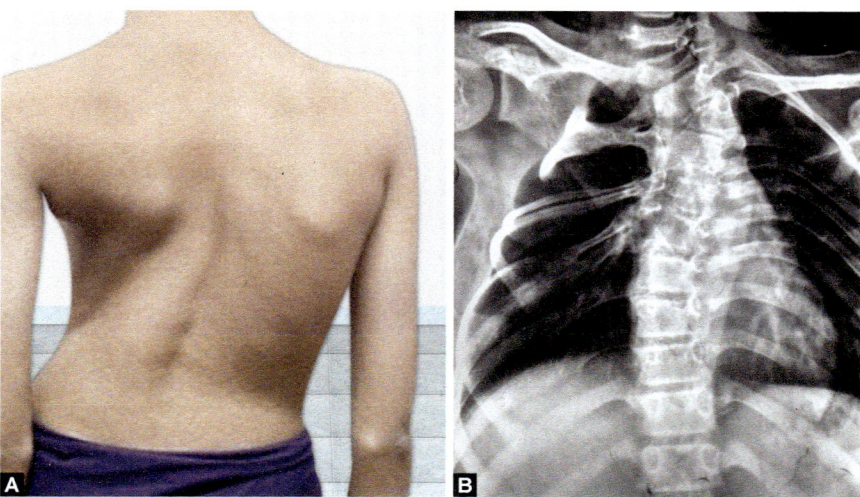

Figs. 15.1A and B: (A) Scoliosis in a young boy: Right dorsal scoliosis is generally idiopathic in nature; (B) Congenital right dorsal scoliosis: Incomplete formation of many vertebral bodies in the upper half of dorsal spine, also note fusion and incomplete formation of ribs on the right side.

maturity). Infantile and juvenile scoliosis are frequently associated with pulmonary complications. The SRS classification broadly serves as descriptive terms for communication and comparison. In general, scoliosis in young persons is painless, presence of pain suggests the possibility of spinal tumor. Right thoracic curve is most common in dorsal spine. In left-sided thoracic curve (unusual) presence of spinal tumor must be excluded by MRI studies. The scoliotic curvature may be idiopathic, structural, compensatory, congenital, neuropathic, or myopathic. Before any major operation for scoliosis, MRI of the spine is mandatory to exclude the presence of neural-defect (spinal dysraphism), tethering of cord or spinal tumors. For any major operation for scoliosis, the facilities for somatosensory and motor-evoked potential or for Stagnara wake up test must be available **(Figs. 15.1A and B)**.

For idiopathic scoliosis a simpler classification is being accepted now: "Early-onset" scoliosis (before puberty) and "late-onset" scoliosis (after puberty). About 4–6 monthly clinical examination and X-rays are used to assess the deterioration of deformity (progression of scoliosis). Younger age at presentation, deformity >30 degrees and incomplete (open) Risser's sign have more chance of deterioration.

For deformities <30 degrees, spinal exercises and spinal braces with "pads to push" the convexity toward normal alignment are used. Braces when used throughout the upright posture, at best help to minimize further deterioration.

Operative indications: Cosmetically unacceptable curves, deformity deteriorating beyond 30 degrees are indications for surgery.

The aim of planned surgery should be to halt the deterioration of deformity, restore near normal contours with instrumentations. This requires arthrodesis of entire primary curve using bone grafting.

Posterior surgery: It includes multiple pedicle screws connected to correcting rods. In case pedicles are too small sublaminar wires may be useful (with less cost to the patient). If deformity is too rigid resection of facet joints may be needed.

Anterior surgery: This is a transthoracic-transpleural approach, the discs at the deformity site are resected, screws are inserted in the vertebral bodies and fixed to the correcting rods to obtain correction of vertebral rotation and deformity. Transthoracic approach however, has more postoperative morbidity.

Rib-hump: Significant rib-hump deformity can be reduced by subperiosteal resection of 3–6 cm of 3–6 ribs near the attachment with transverse processes. The excised ribs can be used as autogenous bone-grafts for spinal arthrodesis.

Postoperative complication: Neurological compromise, pseudarthrosis at bone-grafting sites, implants debonding or dislodging from the bone insertion and metal-fatigue-fracture are observed in long-term follow-up.

Neural monitoring: During correction of any spine deformity (scoliosis and kyphosis) above the level of lumbar one vertebra, spinal cord can get damaged during the corrective procedure. All corrective procedures should be done under electrophysiological neural monitoring during operative correction and implant fixations. One should however, be aware of false-positive or false-negative responses in such monitoring.

If electrophysiological facility is not available, "Wake-up" test must be used to determine the safe extent of deformity correction and the placement of implants.

Semi-invasive techniques like elongation-derotation-flexion (EDF) have been tried using corrective plaster of Paris casts, growth or elongating rods or magnetically induced lengthening. Such procedures have a long learning curve, are at great cost, still being assessed for the practicability with moderate infrastructure facilities.

KYPHOSIS

Kyphosis clinically is a deformity of spine with convexity posteriorly. Flattening of lumbar lordosis and cervical lordosis is in reality a kyphotic deformity at an early stage. Kyphosis may be a round (regular) kyphosis commonly seen in Scheuermann's disorder, senile/osteoporotic kyphosis, ankylosing spondylitis. Angular kyphosis is generally associated with

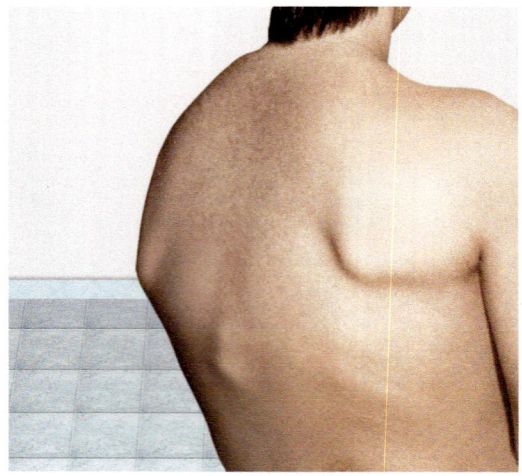

Fig. 15.2: Localized kyphotic deformity: Common causes in the Indian subcontinent are tuberculosis, trauma, osteoporosis or neoplasm.

trauma (vertebral fracture), tuberculosis, or tumorus conditions. Collapse of one or two vertebral bodies leads to a localized (knuckle) deformity, however, destruction of three or more vertebral bodies would create more obvious angular deformities (mild, moderate and severe) **(Fig. 15.2)**.

SPONDYLOLYSIS AND SPONDYLOLISTHESIS

In the erect posture, there is a tendency for the body of the fifth lumbar vertebra (carrying the weight of the trunk) to slide forward on the upper surface of the sacrum as the plane of the L5–S1 disc space slopes downwards anteriorly. The slipping (spondylolisthesis) occurs if there is a defect or weakness (spondylolysis) of the posterior articular facets. The commonest site for this defect is L5–S1, however, less commonly the defect and slipping may occur between L4 and L5 vertebrae. If listhesis is significant, one may clinically appreciate a "step-sign" at the back. Both these conditions may give rise to low back pain with radiation to buttocks and rarely distal to the knee joints. In mild cases, the symptoms may be controlled by spinal exercises and a corset support. Severe

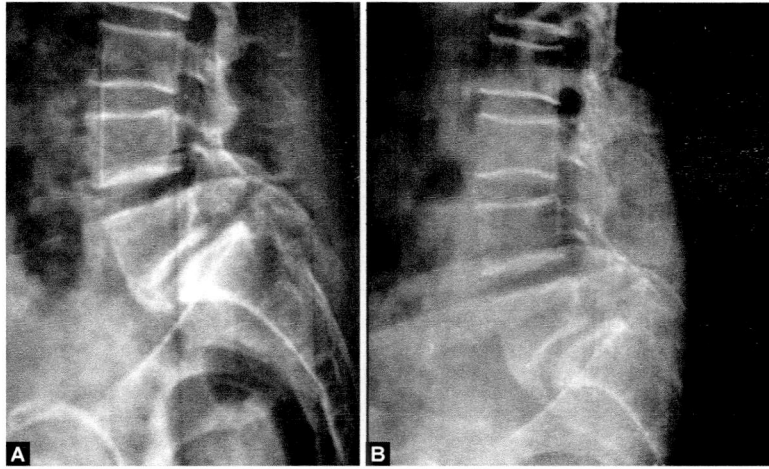

Figs. 15.3A and B: Classical appearance of spondylolisthesis L5 over S1: Upper border of S1 is dome-shaped in this case. The gap between (A) and (B) is 5 years; (B) Shows no instability, and there is development of an anterior buttress.

mechanical pain in the spine (axial pain) may need a localized spinal fusion. Gross spondylolisthesis with significant neurological disturbances may need decompression, discectomy, and a localized fusion **(Figs. 15.3A and B)**. If listhesis is >50% and is deteriorating on follow-up, in situ intertransverse fusion stabilizes the spine **(Figs. 15.3 and 15.14)**.

SPINA BIFIDA

It is a neural tube defect or spinal dysraphism which usually affects the lumbar or lumbosacral segments. In its mildest form, there is an incomplete closure of the lamina and nothing more. The severest form is associated with gross motor and sensory deficit and loss of bladder and bowel control. Clinical examination of the spine may reveal a midline dimple, a pigmented nevus, a tuft of hairs, a palpable fibrolipoma or myelomeningocele.

ANKYLOSING SPONDYLITIS AND RHEUMATOID SPONDYLITIS

Ankylosing spondylitis is more common in men during third and fourth decades. There is progressive ossification of the joints

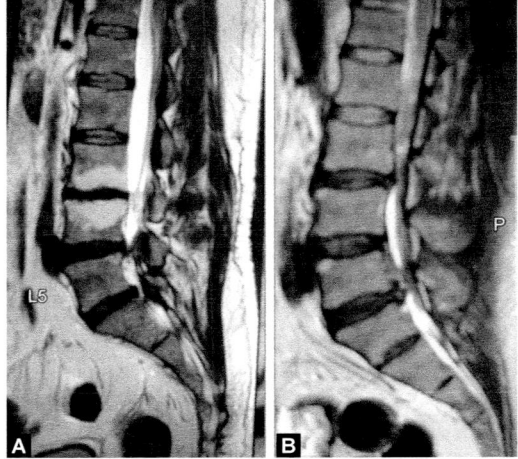

Figs. 15.4A and B: MRI images showing changes related to degenerative changes. (A) Lower disc spaces are dehydrated (black), paradiscal area between L3–L4 showing semilunar fat deposition in the bone; (B) Degenerative changes leading to secondary canal stenosis in another case.

of spine, generally starting from sacroiliac joints, proceeding to lumbar vertebrae, and costovertebral articulations. Low back pain with stiffness of spine and marked reduction in chest expansion are the presenting symptoms. Because of marked reduction of chest excursion and vital capacity, pulmonary tuberculosis is sometimes found as a complication in developing countries. The disease is progressive and generally leads to gross ankylosis of sacroiliac joints, spine (bamboo-spine) and costovertebral articulations. Involvement of rhizomelic joints (hips and shoulders) is not uncommon in advanced cases.

Rheumatoid spondylitis is generally associated with involvement of multiple peripheral joints. The management is that for generalized rheumatoid inflammatory disorder.

Osteoarthrosis (OA) of Spine

Primary osteoarthrosis of the spine is a common condition especially in the elderly. Generally, the symptoms of backache are mild. In majority, the changes are related to the degenerative process associated with aging. Normal age-related wear and tear processes get accelerated due to overweight, excessive use of the spine in heavy manual workers, previously healed disease like old fracture, prolonged intervertebral disc prolapse, healed infection of long-standing and diabetes **(Figs. 15.4A and B)**.

Radiologically, osteoarthrosis of spine is accompanied by disc degeneration (diminished disc space), anterior and posterior lipping (osteophytes) of vertebral bodies and facet joints. Sometimes lipping from adjacent vertebral bodies leads to abutment of the osteophytes giving an impression of kissing spines. Generalized osteophyte formation from posterior surface of vertebral bodies and facet joints may lead to secondary spinal canal stenosis. Generally, the symptoms are vague pains in the back and stiffness of the spine. The treatment is by weight reduction where applicable, spinal exercises to improve the musculature, and selective use of non-steroidal anti-inflammatory drugs. Short-wave-diathermy or ultrasonotherapy, and use of lumbosacral belt is generally helpful. Very rarely, a spinal fusion may be indicated in younger patients for disabling axial pain.

It is important to understand that a large number (20–30%) of older persons show degenerative changes in X-rays and MRI, and have no pain in the back. Thus in patients with nonspecific low back pain one is never certain about the cause and exact source of pain. Altered loading kinematics may exhibit degenerative changes in the paradiscal areas (in MRIs) like bone edema, fat replacement, fibrosis, sclerosis, generally in a "crescent-shaped" configuration; however, similar changes may be present in infective pathologies as well. All imaging findings must be correlated with clinical presentation prior to formulation of diagnosis and treatment plans.

Spinal Infections

Localized persistent pain, stiffness along with systemic features of infection may be caused by infections of the vertebral column. Any infective organism may lead to spinal infection. Hematogenous infections are generally caused by *Mycobacterium tuberculosis*, pyogenic microbes and enteric organism, like the involvement of any other bone. In tuberculous infection, the onset is often slow. **Pyogenic osteitis** is relatively uncommon, however, generally the onset is rapid: pain, stiffness and tenderness is more severe. Unlike tuberculosis, it may be accompanied by spikes of high fever. In acute stage, pyogenic organisms may be isolated from blood culture or from the diseased tissue obtained by needle biopsy or by operative exploration. Rarely pyogenic discitis may occur as a complication of operations on the vertebral column.

X-rays at the onset of infection may be normal. Earliest radiological features in tuberculous infection may be discernible when the infection has lasted for 3–4 months. In pyogenic infection, the X-rays may be positive by about 3–4 weeks. Earliest radiological picture in tuberculosis is narrowing (thinning) of the disc space with erosion (fuzziness) of the paradiscal borders of vertebral bodies, and localized osteoporosis. Exuberant new bone formation around the site of lesion favors the diagnosis of pyogenic infection.

Most of the cases of spinal infection would resolve with prolonged treatment with appropriate antibiotics, rest to the part, supportive therapy and spinal braces. Operative intervention is justified if there is doubt in the diagnosis, patient is refractory to the treatment being given or there are neurological complications. **Epidural abscess** though rare is a surgical emergency.

The patient generally presents with a short history of acute pain, impending neurological involvement with toxemia, fever, and elevated ESR and leukocytosis. X-rays may show bone erosion and MRI would show the epidural abscess collection. Treatment is by immediate decompression and antibiotics. Promptly start with "best guess" antibiotics, which may be changed as soon as the reports are available regarding the organisms and their sensitivity **(Figs. 15.5 to 15.7)**.

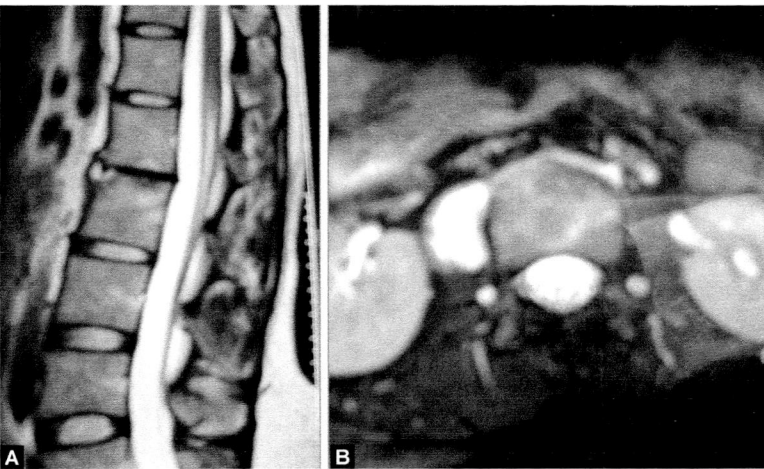

Figs. 15.5A and B: MRIs are the best investigation to diagnose infection at early stages of development. Note (A) A suspicious area between L1–L2; diminished disc space with paradiscal edema: The axial cut; (B) A paravertebral abscess collection on right side.

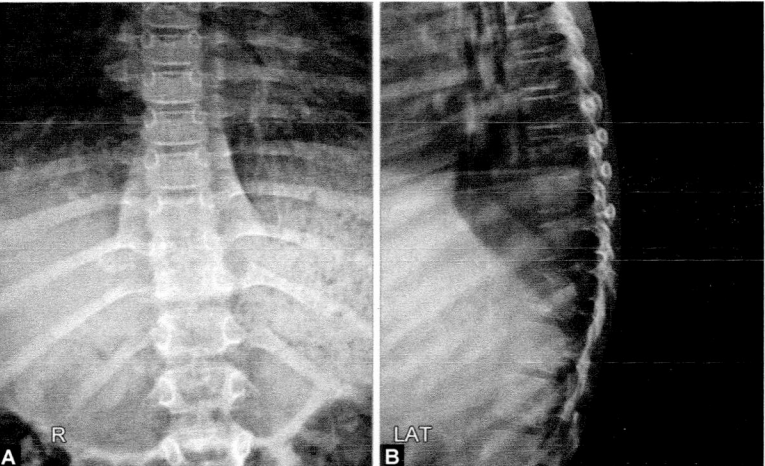

Figs. 15.6A and B: Classical radiological appearance of spinal tuberculosis. (A) Showing a triangular paravertebral abscess shadow; (B) Involvement of D9-D10-D11 vertebrae.

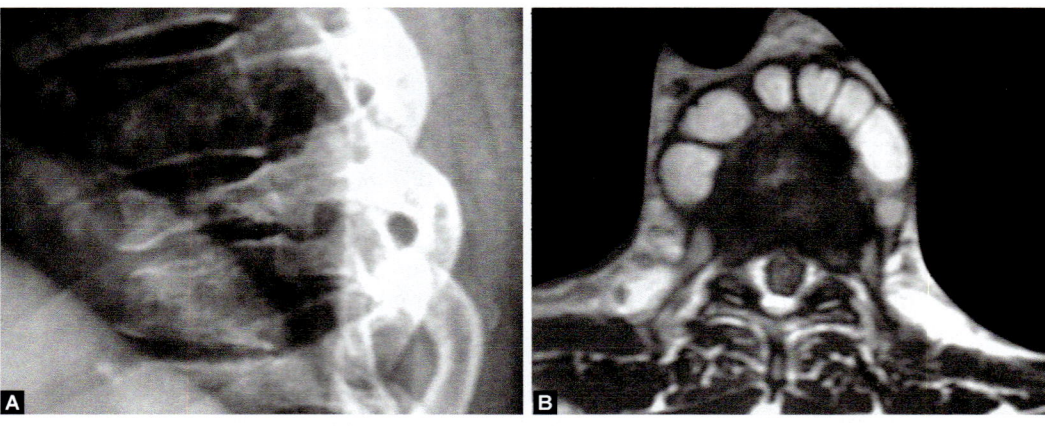

Figs. 15.7A and B: (A) X-ray: Vertebra plana in mid-dorsal spine; (B) The MRI shows a loculated cold abscess. Common causes of vertebrae plana in the Indian subcontinent in descending order are tuberculosis, osteoporosis, myeloma and mitotic deposits.

Lumbar Canal Stenosis

A decrease in the global diameter of the vertebral canal with or without narrowing of the nerve root canals may give rise to symptoms of vague backache and neurogenic symptoms in lower limbs. Most common variety of canal stenosis occurs in persons above the age of 60 years, and the cause is narrowing of the vertebral canal, secondary to age-related degenerative changes. Neurogenic claudication takes place in lower limbs related to walking and physical activities. There may be symptoms of temporary motor weakness, cramps, paresthesias (paresthesiae), and reduction of walking distance. Claudication distance is variable and sensory loss is segmental; impulse symptoms are usually present. The condition can be suspected on clinical grounds, however, at present an MRI is generally used for confirmation of the diagnosis and the extent and localization of stenosis. Rarely developemental canal stenosis and achondroplasia may produce neurogenic claudication in younger patients. Differentiation must be made from "vascular claudication" where the claudication distance is mostly constant, sensory loss is generally stocking type and peripheral arterial pulsations are weak or absent **(Table 15.1)**.

Many authors have suggested actual measurements of the vertebral canal. Boundaries of the canal are difficult to define in X-rays in the elderly because of degenerative changes. Accurate measurements can, however, be made on CT scans, anteroposterior diameter of <11 mm, and transverse diameter of <16 mm suggest canal stenosis. The round and ovoid shapes provide the greatest amount of space for the dural tube, whereas the trefoil shape has the smallest cross-sectional area and the highest incidence of neurogenic claudication.

Patients with lumbar canal stenosis that fail to respond to conservative treatment and have intractable symptoms are candidates for operative decompression. Despite many modifications and adjunct procedures, a standard laminectomy has been found to be most cost-effective and clinically rewarding procedure. The author has been performing a standard **laminectomy with spinoplasty** as a routine operation for symptomatic canal stenosis. Spinous processes along with supraspinous and interspinous ligaments are raised as a continuous "tongue-shaped flap" with base proximally. After adequate decompression the "flap" is replaced in position and sutured to paraspinal ligaments and muscles **(Figs. 15.8A to F)**.

CHAPTER 15: Back Pain and Spine

Table 15.1: Broad differentiating features of neurogenic claudication and vascular claudication.		
	Neurogenic claudication	**Vascular claudication**
Pain location	Back, buttocks, legs	Calf tightness and cramping
Radiation	Proximodistal	Distalo-proximal
Walking distance	Variable	Constant
Relief	Stooping (flexion) of spine, sitting, walking uphill	Rest to lower limbs
Lower limbs appearance	Normal healthy	Hair loss, toenail atrophy
Arterial pulsations	Normal	Diminished, dorsalis pedis ± posterior tibial
Note: In aged population lumbar canal stenosis and peripheral vascular disease can co-exist.		

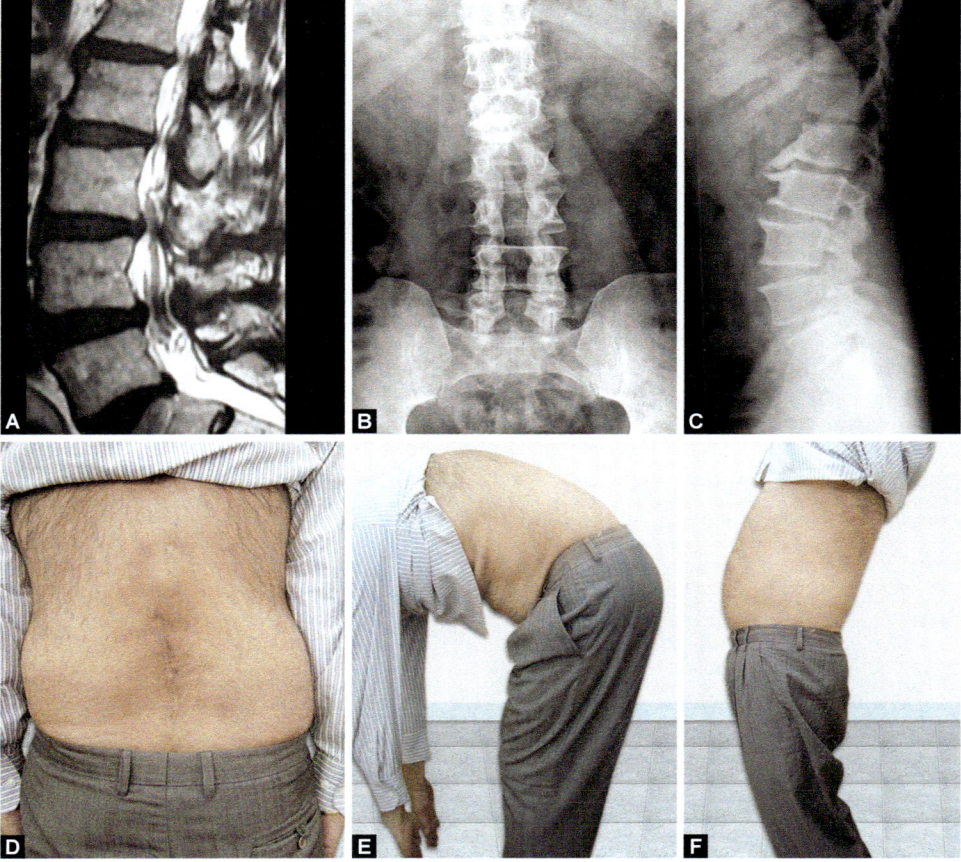

Figs. 15.8A to F: Developmental lumbar canal stenosis in a young man (26 years). (A) MRI showing stenosis from L2–L5; (B and C) 15 years follow-up X-rays of a standard laminectomy performed with retention of interspinous structures (spinoplasty); (D to F) Clinical function and relief of symptoms at 15 years of follow-up.

Neoplasms in the Lumbar Spine (Figs. 15.9A and B)

Tumors of the lumbar spine are rare causes of low backache. Hemangiomas are the commonest tumors of the vertebral column and most of these are asymptomatic. In anteroposterior and coronal images in X-rays and MRI hemangiomas may be suspected by corduroy appearance: prominent and coarse vertical trabeculae with surrounding osteoporosis. Axial cuts would generally exhibit an appearance of pinheads **(Figs. 15.10A and B)**. Extremely rarely vertebral hemangiomas may be associated with arteriovenous malformation and neural complications. The most common malignant tumors of the vertebral column are metastatic deposits. The commonest primary malignant tumor of the vertebrae is myeloma (arising from the marrow cells of the vertebrae). Myeloma and metastatic disease is particularly seen in the elderly, accompanied by pain and may be complicated by neural involvement. The diagnosis is made by X-rays and MRI, serological tests and tissue diagnosis. The treatment is dependent on the nature of the primary tumors. Local radiation, systemic chemotherapy, supportive treatment may help control of the tumor and give relief of pain. When neurological complication is present decompression should be undertaken unless the case is at terminal stages.

Lumbar Intervertebral Disc Prolapse

Lumbar disc prolapse produces back pain, loss of lumbar lordosis, restriction of

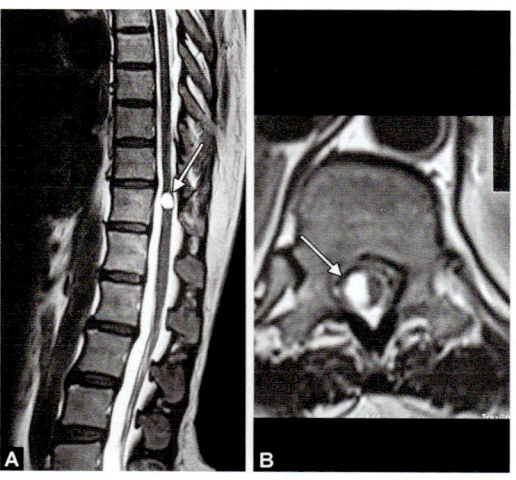

Figs. 15.9A and B: Schwannoma: Nerve sheath tumor situated intradural extramedullary.

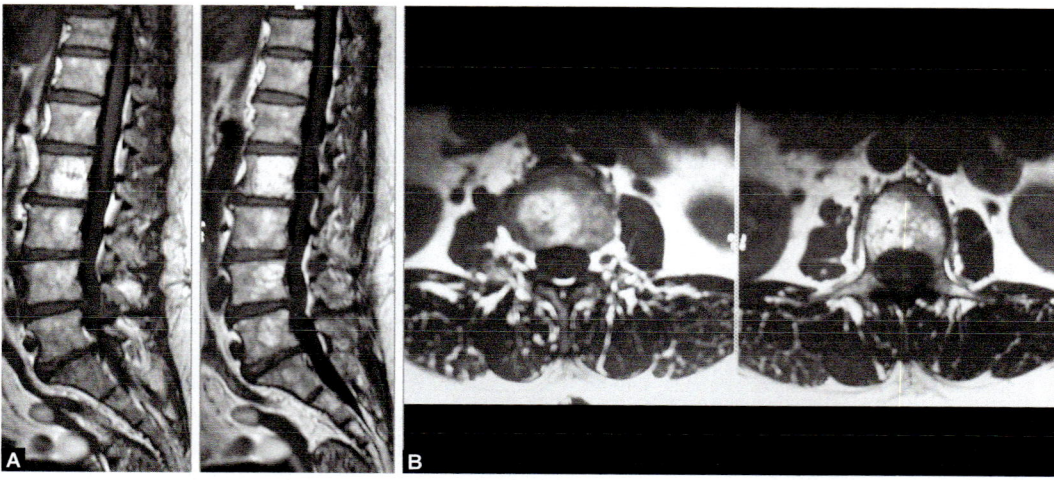

Figs. 15.10A and B: Vertebral body hemangioma: MRI scans showing multiple hemangiomas in the vertebral bodies of L2–L5. One can observe the "corduroy appearance" in the sagittal images and "pin-head appearance" in the axial cuts.

movements due to protective muscle spasm, sciatic scoliosis (list to one side) and radiation of pain in the lower limbs. If the prolapsed disc is in the "axila" of the exiting nerve root, the list is to the same side, if the disc is on the "shoulder" the list is to the opposite side. In a typical case, there is a history of "flexion stress" or weight lifting which leads to tears in the annulus fibrosis allowing the nucleus pulposus to herniate through. The protruding or extruding nucleus presses on the neighboring nerve roots giving rise to pain and paresthesiae in the sciatic distribution. In some cases, there may be muscle weakness, sensory impairment and diminution or absence of the ankle jerk. The common levels involved in decreasing order are L4–L5, L5–S1, L3–L4. Prolapse at higher levels may be associated with absent knee jerk. Neurological distribution is segmental in pattern and is dependent upon the level and extent of prolapse. In addition to back pain, impulse symptoms are common; increase of pain on coughing and sneezing. If there is a massive, sudden, and central prolapse, **cauda equina syndrome** is produced, leading to bladder and bowel sphincter disturbances, and neural deficit. This is one clinical situation where immediate operative exploration and decompression is indicated **(Figs. 15.11 and 15.12)**.

The intervertebral discs start undergoing desiccation (dehydration) around the age of 30 years. In the elderly, where the discs have already undergone degenerative changes, frank prolapse of nucleus pulposus is rare, however, there would be extensive posterior bulging of many discs compromising the space available for the nerves in the lumbar region. All cases of acute disc prolapse (except those with "cauda equina" syndrome) are first treated by conservative methods. Rest in recumbent position for 2–3 weeks, anti-inflammatory drugs, gentle exercises within the limits of pain and use of corset for toilet purposes would relieve the symptoms in most of the patients. Once acute symptoms are relieved, the patient is gradually allowed to resume his normal activities. To avoid recurrence, the patient must continue exercises for spine (to keep the mobility of spine and strength of muscles), keep a control on his weight, avoid lifting of heavy weights, and use corsets far strenuous work/activities **(Figs. 15.11A and B)**.

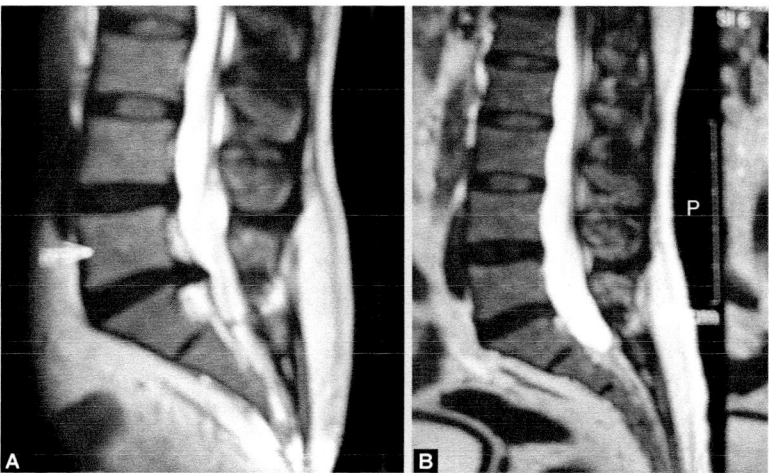

Figs. 15.11A and B: Resolution of lumbar disc herniation: First time, acute lumbar disc herniation in a young patient can undergo spontaneous resolution by conservative treatment: (A) At presensation the herniated L5–S1 disc; (B) Complete resolution after 3 months.

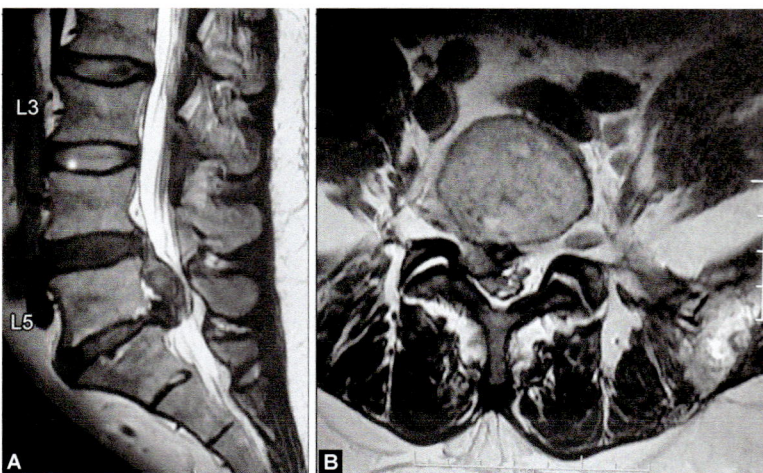

Figs. 15.12A and B: MRI images of a massive disc prolapse leading to cauda equina syndrome: Note (A) Caudal migration of the sequestrated disc from L4–L5 with concomitant disc prolapse at L5–S1; (B) Significant encroachment of the vertebral canal (spinal canal).

If there is no response in 2–3 weeks, or residual symptoms are disabling, or there is recurrence of symptoms, further investigations and operative intervention must be considered. MRIs of lumbar spine done in asymptomatic adults (above the age of 40 years) may show abnormalities in about 30%: prolapsed disc in 20% and spinal canal stenosis in 20%. One should consider these changes as a part of aging process, operative intervention must be considered only on clinical features correlating with investigative findings. Removal of the offending disc is the common procedure performed with moderate infrastructure facilities available. Minimally invasive techniques are being used in institutions with sophisticated infrastructure available. Whether operation is performed by conventional laminectomy or by more recent modifications with or without use of implants, the clinical outcome for the patient does not differ materially. It is rational for the surgeon to perform the procedure in which he has the most confidence. There is, however, no doubt that more extensive and complex procedures carry a higher complication rate. Like any orthopedic operation, the first operation on the spine gives the best result. One must do it very well, and adequately, avoid injuries to nerves, dural sac, minimize bleeding, rough handling of tissues and infections. Repeat operative procedures do not have a satisfactory success rate. As clinicians, let us not underestimate the emotional and financial stress on the family in case of repeat operations.

Spinal Decompression, Fusion, and Instrumentation

Conventional standard operations like laminectomy, posterior fusion and posterolateral fusion are successful, cost-effective, have least morbidity and can be performed with moderate infrastructure facilities **(Figs. 15.13 and 15.14)**.

Harrington rod fixation was first started in 1947 predominantly for spinal deformities caused by post-polio paralysis. The construct had long lever arms which had fixation only at upper and lower ends. Failure of the construct did occur.

Luque (2006) developed multisegmental fixation by using sublaminar wires. The wiring was further modified as wires traversing through the bases of spinous processes (Harri-Luque). Cotrel, Dubousset, Guillaumat (1988) evolved pedicle screws

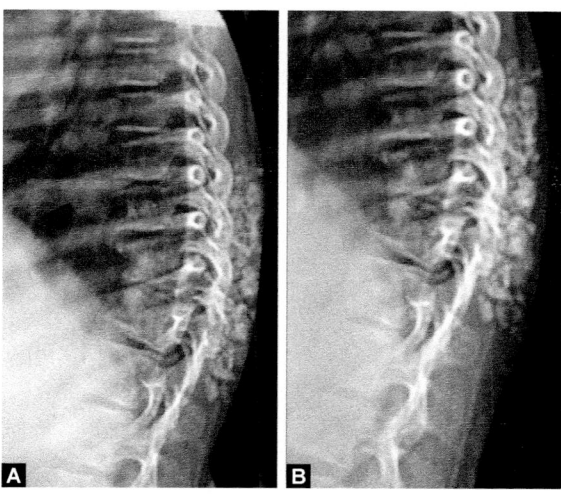

Figs. 15.13A and B: Deterioration of the kyphotic deformities of dorsal spine can be minimized by "convex fusion" between 6 to 10 years of age: Attempted posterior fusion for tuberculosis of D8–D11 in this case.

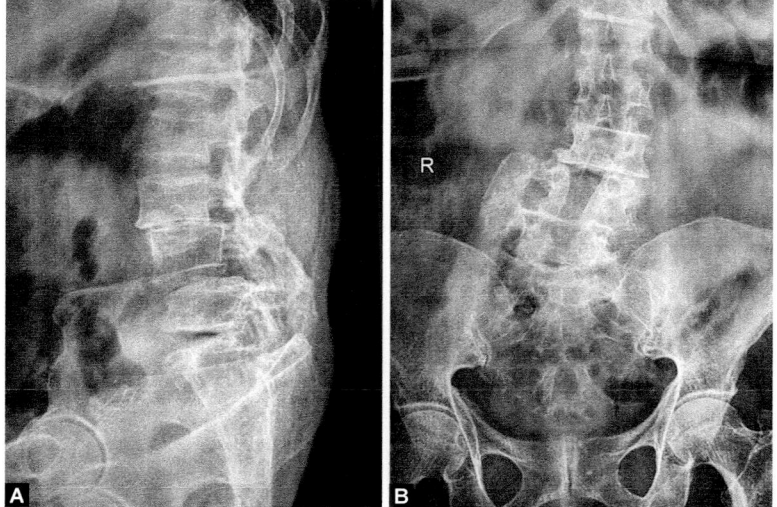

Figs. 15.14A and B: Symptomatic lumbar canal stenosis with concomitant anterolisthesis. (A) Decompressive laminectomy was performed; (B) L4–L5–S1 were stabilized by intertransverse fusion. The anterolisthesis here (L3/L4 and L4/L5) in addressed as step-ladder listhesis.

and hooks. At present there are dozens of hybrids and modifications. Internal fixation or stabilization are best suited for correction of spinal deformities or for stabilization of pan-vertebral destruction or gross instability. Extensive (multisegmental) spinal fusion in lumbar and cervical spine should be considered a drastic remedy. It is well known to lead to premature symptomatic degenerative changes or instability in the juxta-fusion segments in about 30% of patients followed for 10 years or more.

SUGGESTED READINGS

1. Lonstein JE, Carlson JM. The prediction of curve progression in untreated idiopathic scoliosis during growth. J Bone Joint Surg Am. 1984;66A:1061-71.
2. Grob D, Humke T, Dvorak J. Degenerative lumbar spinal stenosis. Decompression with and without arthrodesis. J Bone Joint Surg Am. 1995;77A:1036-41.
3. Fritzell P, Hagg O, Wessberg P, Nordwall A. Lumbar fusion versus nonsurgical treatment for chronic low back pain: A multicenter randomized controlled trial from Swedish Lumbar Spine Study Group. Spine (Phila Pa 1976). 2001;26:2521-32.
4. Van Tulder M, Koes B, Malmivaara A. Outcome of non-invasive treatment modalities on back pain: An evidence-based review. Eur Spine J. 2006:15:S64-S81.
5. Hedequist D, Emans J. Congenital scoliosis: A review and update. J Ped Orthop. 2007:27:106-16.
6. Todd NV. Spine: The surgical treatment of non-specific lowback pain. Bone Joint J. 2017:99B:1003-5.
7. Buchowski JM, Adogwa D. What is new in spine surgery. J Bone Joint Surg. 2019;101-A:1043-9.

CHAPTER 16

Hip

INTRODUCTION

The common presenting symptoms for which a patient presents in a hospital are "pain" in the hip region or pain referred to the knee, limitation of movements or "stiffness" and "limping". Information about the age at onset, duration of symptoms, mode of onset (sudden, insidious), previous trauma, fever, swelling and draining ulcers or sinuses, guide the clinicians to reach the diagnosis. Examination must follow the standard protocol of inspection (look), palpation (feel), measurements and movements. It is essential to remove clothings to the maximum socially permissible limits. Any step of examination which causes pain should be the last step.

WALKING AND STANDING

In a patient, who can walk, carefully watch the pattern of gait which may be antalgic gait (painful hip), stiff hip gait, unstable hip gait, or short limb gait. **In antalgic gait**, the patient leans the body over to the side of painful hip while bearing weight and takes a short stride (short step) to minimize the time the painful limb bears body weight. Unstable hip gait **(Trendelenburg gait)** is the outcome of weakness (paralysis) of hip abductors or inadequacy of the lever arm (femoral neck fracture, coxa vara, coxa breva), or misplacement of the fulcrum (dislocation or subluxation of the hip joint). The pelvis of the contralateral side will tilt downwards (dipping) on weight bearing during stance-phase or standing on the unstable hip. As an example while bearing weight on unstable left hip joint, the right-sided pelvis would tilt **downwards**.

Inspection (look) and feel: With the patient in recumbent position, visualize the position of limbs, pelvis and lumbar spine to detect the flexion deformity of hip (Thomas hip flexion test), tilting of pelvis as a result of fixed abduction, fixed adduction, and fixed flexion deformities. Be aware of pseudo hip flexion deformity due to iliopsoas abscess. Swelling, sinuses and scars around the hip would indicate an infective pathology. Palpation would help to detect any abnormality of tilting of pelvis, position and thickening of greater trochanter (infection or trauma or neoplasms), the relationship between various bony landmarks (through Bryant's triangle or Nelaton's line).

The greater trochanter is at a level higher than normal in many disorders of hip joint and femoral head and neck, causing shortening of the limb **(Figs. 16.1A to C)**.

MOVEMENTS

Active and passive movements of hip joints give very useful information regarding the pathology in the joint. Observe not only the range of motion but also the quality of movements, presence of pain and muscle spasm. With the patient in recumbent position, compare the range of passive movements of symptomatic and normal hip joint. Complete loss of movement is mostly due to bony ankylosis. Short fibrous ankylosis is due to fibrous healing of the hip pathology, hip has only a jog of movements. Fibrous ankylosis is generally due to healed status of tubercular arthritis and there is gross limitation of movements.

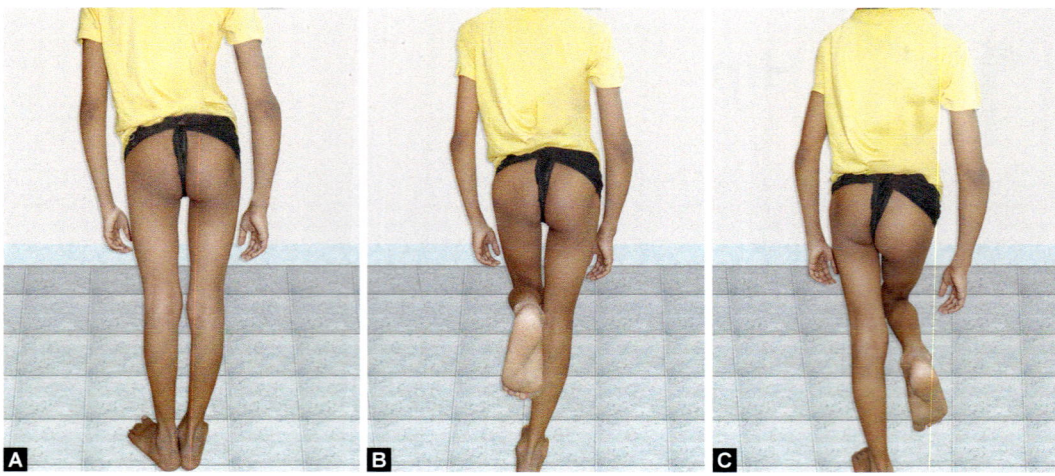

Figs. 16.1A to C: Trendelenburg test is a clinical sign to evaluate the competence of hip "abductor mechanism". Patient (A) standing on both feet showing identical gluteal folds. With single foot stance phase (standing) on normal side (right side), (B) the left side of pelvis is maintained in some elevation by contraction of right gluteal muscles. While standing on the (C) affected left foot (stance phase) the contralateral pelvis (right) drops because of disruption of abductor mechanism on the diseased side, left hip congenital dysplasia in this patient.

Telescoping Test

It is performed with the patient lying on the back and the hip and knee flexed to about 90 degrees. As an example for right hip dissease, the pelvis is steadied by the left hand with your thumb on the iliac crest. The flexed knee is held by the right hand, on pulling and pushing the femur vertically, in the presence of instability, one can feel the upper end of femur (trochanteric area) moving up and down. This abnormal movement is called telescopy. Commonly, this test is positive in cases of nonunion of fracture neck femur, healed septic arthritis of early childhood, congenital developmental dysplasia of hip or congenital absence of proximal femur **(Figs. 16.1A to C)**.

Measurements: Real length is measured, after "squaring" the pelvis in recumbent position of patient, adjust the position of both lower limbs in such a way as to arrange anterior superior iliac spine (ASIS) of both sides at identical levels. The measurements from ASIS to the medial malleolus will indicate the real shortening of the lower limbs. The shortening may be due to destruction or fracture of the upper end of femur or displacement of the femoral head or shortening in the femoral or tibial segments of the lower limbs. Apparent measurements are done from umbilicus or xiphisternum to the medial malleolus, the prerequisite for this measurement is placement of both lower limbs parallel to each other in the recumbent position. Adduction deformity of hip joint would result in upwards tilt of the ipsilateral pelvis (ASIS) creating apparent shortening of that limb. Abduction deformity of the hip joint would result in downwards tilt of the ipsilateral pelvis (ASIS) creating apparent lengthening of the limb. Let us take an example of a patient who has real shortening of 3 cm due to a destructive lesion of the hip joint. If this hip joint has abduction deformity the apparent shortening will be <3 cm; and in case the hip joint has adduction deformity the apparent shortening will be >3 cm.

If a real shortening has been detected, the next step is to localize the site of shortening by tests like Bryant's triangle or Nélaton's line. If the top of the greater trochanter is raised as compared to the opposite normal hip, the site of pathology is in the femoral head, neck, or the

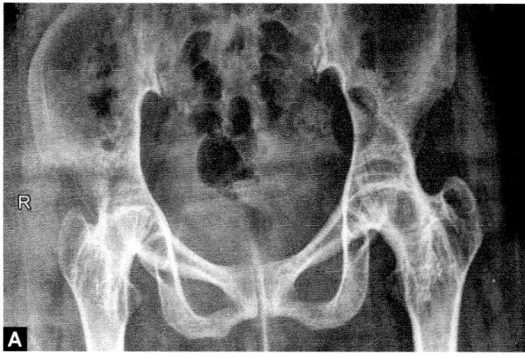
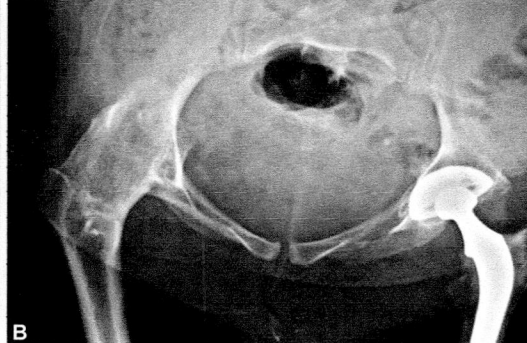

Figs. 16.2A and B: (A) Bilateral bony ankylosis of hips in a lady suffering from generalized rheumatoid arthritis. This is the patients for whom joint replacement at a younger age may be justified; (B) Bilateral bony ankylosis in another young lady; left hip joint has been replaced.

acetabulum (supratrochanteric shortening). If the greater trochanter is not elevated, the site of pathology is infratrochanteric. **Common hip disorders** would fall into one of the following broad clinical conditions:

- **Gross limitation of movements without much pain:** Suspect fusion due to septic arthritis in adults, ankylosing spondylitis, periarticular myositis ossificans **(Figs. 16.2 and 16.3)**.
- **Gross limitation of movements with acute pain:** Suspect septic arthritis, rheumatic arthritis, rheumatoid arthritis.
- **Gross limitation of movements with chronic pain:** Suspect tubercular arthritis, rheumatoid arthritis.
- **Moderate limitation of movements in the elderly or middle age:** Suspect osteoarthrosis secondary to old trauma, coxa vara, coxa plana (Perthes' disease), coxa profunda (protrusio-acetabuli), avascular necrosis of femoral head, primary osteoarthrosis.
- **Limitation of terminal movements only:** Suspect early cases of coxa vara, coxa plana (Perthes disease), coxa profunda, avascular necrosis of femoral head, infective lesions healed at early stage, early osteoarthrosis, juxta-articular lesions.
- **Presence of abnormal movements (telescoping hip joint):** Suspect developmental dysplasia of hip, sequel of suppurative arthritis of early childhood, (Tom-Smith hip), nonunion of femoral neck fracture, neuropathic hip (Charcot's joint).

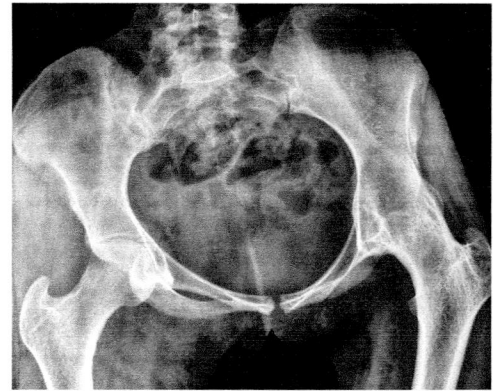

Fig. 16.3: With bony ankylosis of one hip joint, many patients can manage activities of daily living. 'Floor activities' are impossible. Disturbed kinematics lead to symptomatic premature degenerative changes in spine, ipsilateral knee and contralateral hip and knee.

After the clinical assessment, one should proceed for appropriate imaging and laboratory investigations. X-rays of pelvis with both hip joints should be an early investigation. Comparison of normal hip with the disease hip helps one to detect the abnormalities at an early stage. Some hip pathologies may be bilateral such as ankylosing spondylitis, rheumatoid arthritis, slipped capital femoral epiphysis, congenital coxa vara, rickets, osteomalacia, polyostotic skeletal dysplasia.

Protrusio acetabuli is best judged by comparison with contralateral normal hip by drawing ilioischial line. The cause may be rheumatoid disorder, infective lesions, developmental, traumatic or metabolic disorders or Paget's disease. Vertical shift of pelvis may be observed if there is concomitant destruction of sacroiliac joint and symphysis pubis caused by tuberculous infection or by trauma.

MRIs of hip joints and pelvis in general exhibit nonspecific findings like bone edema, soft tissue edema, fluid collection in soft tissues and in the joints. These findings are not suggestive of a specific pathology, however MRI does show the extent of the diseased (abnormal) area. MRIs are most helpful in the early diagnosis of avascular necrosis of femoral head.

Paget's Disease

Paget's disease is considered an unclassified metabolic disorder of bone. There is increased bone turnover and the new bone is laid in mosaic pattern. In early stages the patient, generally a middle age man, presents with pain, swelling and deformation (in weight bearing bones). X-rays show thickened and sclerotic bone with coarse trabeculations. Histology reveals a mosaic pattern. Electron microscopy has exhibited inclusion bodies in osteoclasts, suggesting virus as possible causative factor. Untreated or uncontrolled patients may develop a pathological fracture or a malignant change. Commoner bones involved are pelvis, femur, skull, tibia and spine. Bisphosphonates and calcitonin have been found to suppress the disease process; the author has observed many patients whose disease remained static, suppressed or had partial resolution during an observation of 15–25 years **(Figs. 16.4A to C)**. Surgical treatment may be needed for complications.

Coxa vara: Normally, the femoral neck and shaft angle is considered to be 125 degrees. The reduction of this angle is called coxa vara. Many conditions can lead to this deformity; a few less uncommon are Perthes disease, rickets, chondro-osteodystrophy, slipped capital femoral epiphysis, fibrous dysplasia, malunited femoral neck fracture and cretinism. There is restriction of movements of abduction and internal rotation depending upon the degree of varus deformity. Uniaxial movements of flexion and extension are retained for a long time. Many of these hips develop symptomatic early degenerative osteoarthrosis in the fourth and fifth decade of life. Because the greater trochanter is at a higher level, the length of the lever arm is reduced, the efficiency of hip abductors becomes inadequate. The patients walk with Trendelenburg gait and there is limitation of terminal degrees of hip abduction and internal rotation.

Congenital coxa vara: It is the result of a congenital defect in the femoral neck. X-ray may reveal an inverted V-shaped cartilaginous defect in the femoral neck **(Fig. 16.5)**.

PERTHES DISEASE (LEGG–CALVÉ–PERTHES DISEASE)

It is a vaguely painful disorder of childhood characterized by avascular necrosis of femoral head. It is an uncommon condition, usually between the age of 4–10 years, the incidence is approximately one in 10,000, and boys are affected 5 times as often as girls. Bilateral hip involvement is generally associated with generalized osteochondraldysplasia. Affected children may have slightly retarded growth.

The child presents with a history of periodic attacks of limping and pain. The local symptoms of muscle spasm, and limitation of movements (especially abduction and internal rotation) would clear up with bed rest and use of NSAIDs for about 2 weeks not unlike "transient synovitis". In later stages, there may be no local symptoms of muscle spasm and synovial irritation, however, the child walks with a limp, there is only selective restriction of hip movements, there may be true supratrochanteric shortening by about 2 cm, and on palpation the greater trochanter may be thickened and elevated.

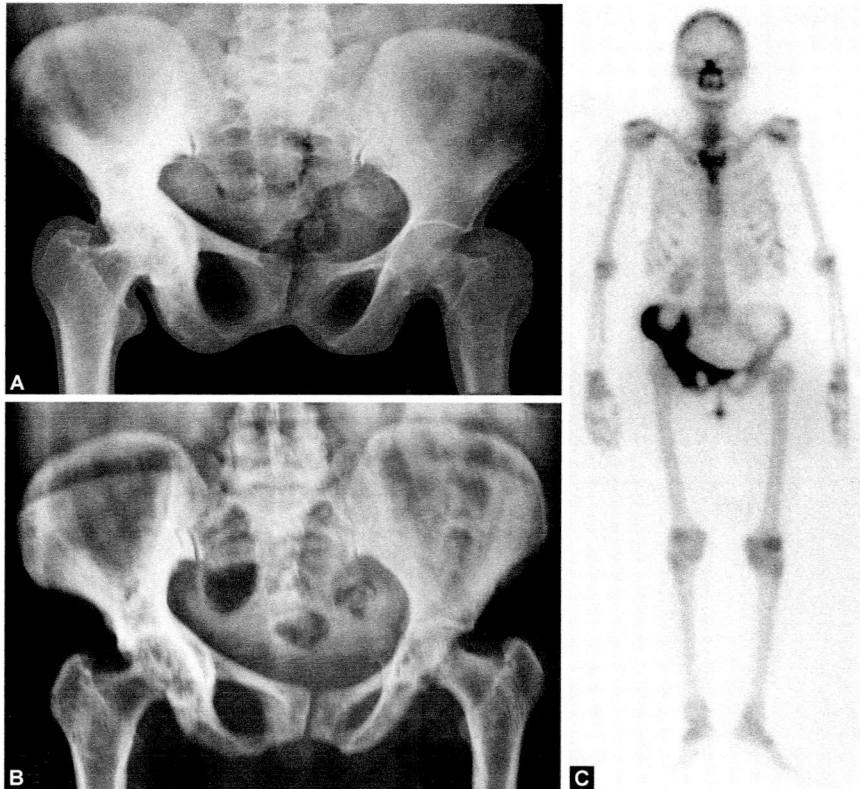

Figs. 16.4A to C: Paget's disease: (A) X-ray of pelvis showing irregular thickening in the right half of pelvis due to Paget's disease; (B) Isotope bone scan shows the hyperactivity of the involved bone; (C) Follow-up after 3 years of intermittent treatment with bisphosphonates shows some degree of resolution.

CLASSIFICATION OF PERTHES DISEASE

There are a number of radiological classifications of Perthes disease. Elizabethtown classification is based upon the radiological appearance corresponding to the natural history of disease. It was classified as stage I, II, III and IV. Benjamin Joseph (2015) further subdivided first three stages into a and b, as follows:

Stage Ia: Sclerosis of the epiphysis with normal height.

Stage Ib: In addition to stage Ia, there is decrease in the height of the epiphysis.

Stage IIa: The abnormal epiphysis as above, begins to fragment with one or two vertical fissures.

Stage IIb: There is advanced multiple fragmentation without any new bone formation lateral to the epiphysis.

Stage IIIa: Reparative new bone (porous) forms to cover (replace) the necrosed bone by about one-third of the epiphysis.

Stage IIIb: The newly formed bone now evolves normal texture and covers more than one-third of the epiphysis.

Stage IV: Reossification or repair is complete. The shape of the femoral head may be normal or deformed.

Despite the large number of classifications there are however exceptions to the orderly pattern of evolution of the disease. Following phases of the biological reaction and repair of the avascular femoral epiphysis

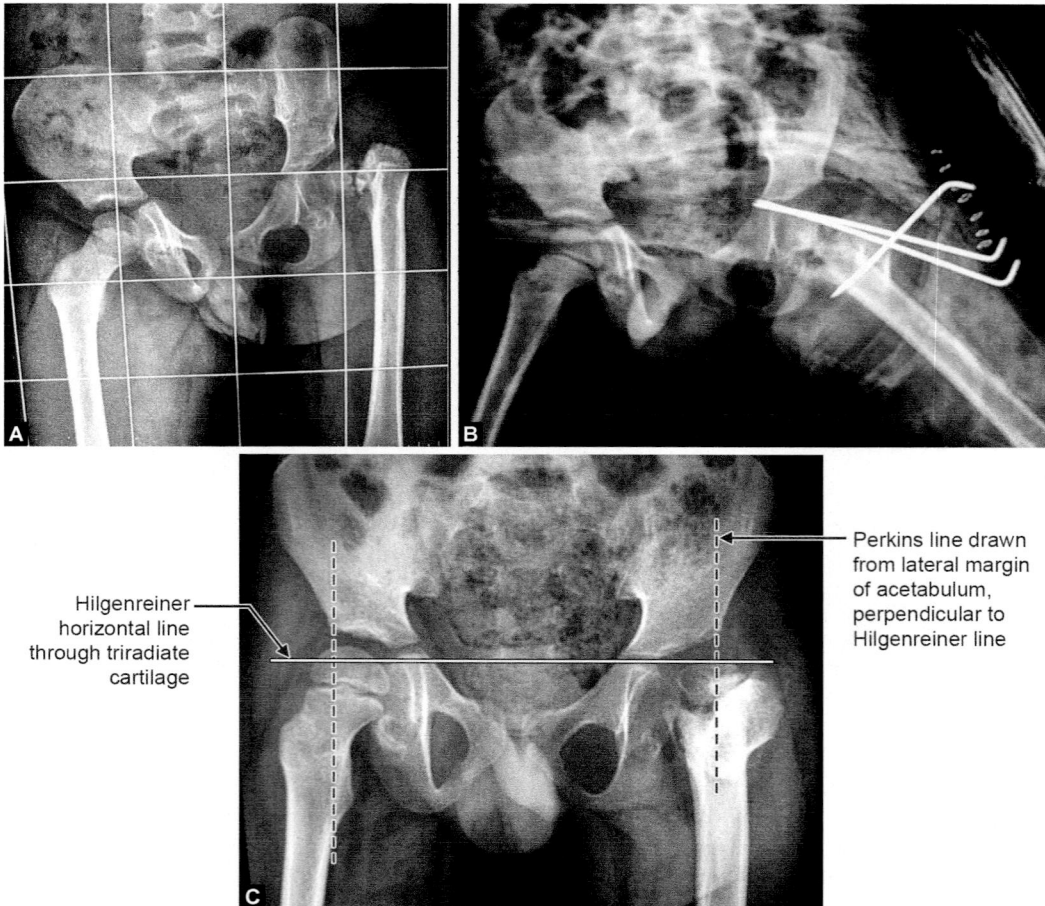

Figs. 16.5A to C: Follow-up X-rays of a case of congenital coxa vara: (A) At presentation; (B) soon after upper femoral osteotomy; (C) 2 years after osteotomy, note the improvement in the configuration of femoral head and neck. Hilgenreiner's horizontal line and Perkin's vertical line form a quadrant, the femoral head should lie in the inner lower quadrant.

may be related to the radiological stages of Elizabethtown and Joseph's classification.

Stage of synovitis (1–3 weeks): There is synovial effusion and synovial thickening as a reaction by the living tissues surrounding the avascular femoral epiphysis. X-rays may show thickening of synovium.

Stage of avascular necrosis (1–12 months): Avascular necrosis may affect either a part of epiphysis or the whole of it. There is hyperemic reaction in the living tissues (bone in metaphyseal region) and X-rays show dense epiphysis (Stage I).

Stage of vascular invasion and fragmentation (1–3 years): The intense vascular response from the tissues (ligamentum teres, retinacular capsule, metaphysis) surrounding the necrosed bone invades the avascular bone for its replacement and repair. The X-rays would reveal fragmentation of the necrosed epiphysis (Stage II).

Stage of healing (2–3 years): The necrosed bone gets replaced by new bone (Stage III). If contained at appropriate time the head maintains its sphericity (Stage IV), if loaded prematurely the head gets compressed and

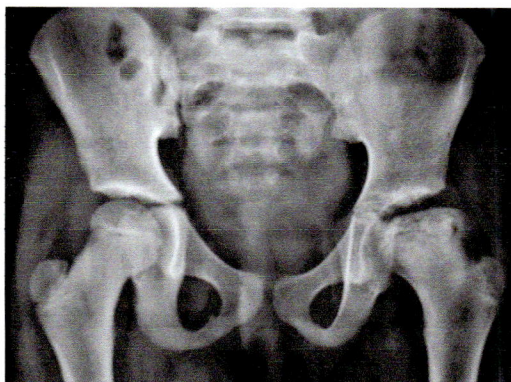

Fig. 16.6: A neglected case of Perthes disease in left hip, note coxa magna, spheroidal femoral head and flattening of the weight-bearing area.

flattened (coxa plana), if left uncontained the head may show a depression (hinge-abduction defect), the head size may be increased (coxa magna) and get deformed (mushrooming) **(Fig. 16.6)**.

X-rays on comparison with the contra-lateral normal side would show changes: in **early stages** like widening of the joint space and increased density of the capital femoral epiphysis. **In later stages,** there is a vascular response for revascularization of the avascular femoral head. This results in fragmentation of the femoral head and flattening of its contour. Reactive hyperemia in the adjacent metaphyseal area may be seen as an osteoporotic area. **With further delay,** there is broadening and flattening of the femoral head (mushrooming), and broadening (coxa magna) and shortening (coxa breva) of the femoral neck. After the age of 20 years, evidence of secondary osteoarthrosis starts becoming evident.

Treatment

If diagnosed at an early stage, the femoral head is well contained in the acetabulum, nonweight-bearing exercises are encouraged, the disease may heal within 12–18 months with near normal hip joints. Many classifications have been described with the hope of prognostication and planning of treatment. Catterall's classification is based upon the amount of head that is "avascular". Herring's lateral pillar classification is more popular at this stage. In the anteroposterior X-ray, the femoral head is divided into 3 segments by 2 vertical lines on each side of the avascular segments. The height of the lateral pillar (the prime weight bearing area) determines the Herring's grouping. Group A has normal height of the lateral vertical pillar (best prognosis), group B has reduction of vertical height up to 50% and in group C the height has reduced by >50% (worst prognosis). Based upon the observations of many workers, a concept has evolved about the "head at-risk" radiological signs. These signs, if present, the preferred approach is to achieve head containment by operative means.

Head at-risk signs are:
1. Progressive uncovering of femoral head.
2. Calcification in the cartilage lateral to the ossific nucleus.
3. Radiolucent area at the lateral edge of the bony epiphysis.
4. Severe metaphyseal osteoporosis.
5. Avascularity of more than half of the epiphysis.
6. Hinge-abduction defect as seen in X-rays or in the MRIs. Now addressed as Femoroacetabular Impingement (FAI).
7. Age of the patient >7 years.

Femoral head containment or coverage of the weight bearing (anterolateral) part of femoral head by acetabulum can be achieved by 2 methods:
1. **Upper femoral varus—derotation osteotomy;** proximal fragment is abducted and internally rotated (15–20 degrees) to hold the femoral head deep in the acetabulum. Varus derotation osteotomy is indicated if the preoperative X-rays in abduction and internal rotation of hip show good containment of femoral head in the acetabulum. The correction obtained is fixed with a suitable angle-plate. Best results are obtained in patients aged 6–8 years.

2. **Innominate osteotomy:** Salter's redirectional osteotomy for patients younger than 6 years, and displacement Chiari's shelf osteotomy for those above 6 years of age. In Salter's, the distal fragment of pelvis is tilted (anterolaterally) to cover the femoral head. In Chiari's, the proximal fragment is shifted as a shelf to cover the anterolateral part of the femoral head. Innominate osteotomies are best held in corrected position with 2 or 3 K-wires.

SLIPPED CAPITAL FEMORAL EPIPHYSIS (ADOLESCENT COXA VARA)

In slipped capital femoral epiphysis (SCFE), there is a slipping of femoral head epiphysis downwards and posteriorly. Exact etiology is not known, a mild trauma precipitating the slipping has often been suspected. The disease is bilateral in about 30%, most of the patients are boys between 10 years and 15 years of age, many of them are obese with suspicion of subtle endocrine disorders.

Generally the patient is brought to the hospital for moderate pain in hip joint and pain during walking. The pain is worse on walking and is relieved by rest. On examination, the leg lies in external rotation and there is supratrochanteric shortening by about 2 cm. There may be limitation of terminal range of abduction (in extended position as well as in flexed position) and internal rotation. On complete flexion of the hip, the knee gets directed toward ipsilateral axilla.

X-ray of the pelvis with both hips shows slipping down of the femoral head epiphysis, the lateral view (clinically best revealed in X-ray of pelvis in maximum "frog position" of both hips) would show the posterior slip. Another clinically practical method is to X-ray of the pelvis with both hips is maximum frog-position. A line drawn along the superior border of the femoral neck should normally intersect the femoral head epiphysis, when slipping has occurred the slipped epiphysis would be just flush with the line or well below it. The presence of the element of posterior slip may be seen in the lateral view as a double density in the metaphyseal area because of the superimposed shadow of the slipped epiphysis. **Radiological grading** has been suggested according to the percentage of slipping **(Fig. 16.5)**.
1. **Mild**—displacement less than one-third of the femoral neck width.
2. **Moderate**—the displacement between one-third and a half.
3. **Severe**—the displacement is greater than half of the femoral neck width.

Treatment

The basic principle is to very gently reduce the slip to as close to the normal alignment as possible and fix the femoral head in position with one or two Moore's pins or sliding screws, under C-arm control. "Perfect reduction and perfect fixation" is easier said than achieved. The safer technique is to accept the "reduction" one is able to achieve by gentle manipulations. Fix the reduction by inserting one or two threaded pins; insert the pins on the anterior part of femoral neck and direct them posteromedially to have purchase on the slipped epiphysis. During follow-up, once the physeal plate has fused gradual bone remodeling would minimize the deformity and the disability. If after one or 2 years of the fusion of physis, there is a noticeable limitation of function, a corrective osteotomy would help improve deformity and function. The osteotomy is best performed just proximal to the lesser trochanter. The proximal fragment is repositioned into valgus, internal rotation and flexion. Osteotomy is fixed with suitable blade-plate and screws after wedge resection of bone at the site of osteotomy, most of the deformities are corrected to achieve a functional hip joint for many years.

Complications

1. The patient and attendants must be well-informed that in about 30% of patients the slipping occurs in the other hip as well,

sometimes even while the patient is in bed for the treatment of presenting SCFE. The asymptomatic hip should be kept under observation throughout the period of growth and at the earliest signs of slipping the epiphysis should be pinned.
2. Forceful manipulative reduction may damage the posterior retinacular vessels leading to avascular necrosis of the femoral head.
3. In some cases, necrosis of the articular cartilage may lead to chondrolysis and joint stiffness.
4. Inadequately treated patient may result in coxa vara, and early onset osteoarthrosis.

Pyogenic Infection and Tuberculosis (*See* also Chapter 2)

The common age for pyogenic infection is during early childhood. The hip joint may be involved directly by hematogenous spread from a distant focus or osteomyelitis of femur may spread directly into the joint. If the infection is not controlled at an early stage the femoral head and acetabular socket undergo rapid destruction.

Hip joint gets involved by tuberculosis is nearly 15–20% of cases of skeletal tuberculosis. As mentioned in Chapter 2 tuberculous infection passes through different stages of disease; synovitis, early arthritis, established arthritis, arthritis with subluxation or dislocation. With currently available diagnostic facilities (MRIs, bacteriological, histological, serological) it is possible to make diagnosis at stage of synovitis and early arthritis and achieve a fairly mobile and painless hip by multidrug antitubercular therapy **(Figs. 16.7A to E)**.

Patients presenting late or diagnosed at an advanced stage would end up with shortening, gross limitation of movements and deformities, generally with flexion and adduction. X-rays may show destruction of femoral head and acetabulum with wandering acetabulum (or protrusio acetabulum in some cases) **(Fig. 16.8)**.

Correction of deformities may be achieved by traction, some useful range of motion may be retained or regained by active assisted exercises when the pain has subsided under the influence of multidrug therapy. If diagnosis is not clear or the disease does not subside, arthrotomy and debridement is justified. If disease has healed with fibrous ankylosis with retention of some joint space, arthrolysis may help gain a useful range of motion. If healed status was achieved in an adult with bony ankylosis or gross deformity, Girdlestone's excisional arthroplasty is an acceptable option. In middle age or older patients with disease healed for >2 years total hip replacement under cover of multidrug therapy is now feasible and a viable option. Arthrodesis of hip joint should now be considered as historical.

OSTEOTOMIES OF PROXIMAL FEMUR

Prerequisites for upper femoral osteotomy: These operations are useful for active persons younger than 50 years with reasonable good range of hip movements (at least 60 degrees of flexion). Preoperatively do an anteroposterior X-ray of pelvis with both hips in standing positions, X-rays of pelvis with both hips in maximum abduction and maximum adduction. A "false lateral" view in standing position is very useful; stand with knee and foot pointing straight forward to the beam, and tilt the pelvis forward by 25 degrees. Careful examination of these X-rays suggests which type of upper femoral osteotomy is indicated and likely to benefit the patient. One may then perform an abduction (valgus) osteotomy, adduction (varus) osteotomy without or with addition of internal or external rotation of the proximal fragment. For good results, the patient should be active and <50 years of age. The range of hip flexion should be 60 degrees or more. If valgus osteotomy is planned, ensure that patient has 20–30 degrees of adduction range beyond his fixed adduction deformity. Having achieved the desired correction of

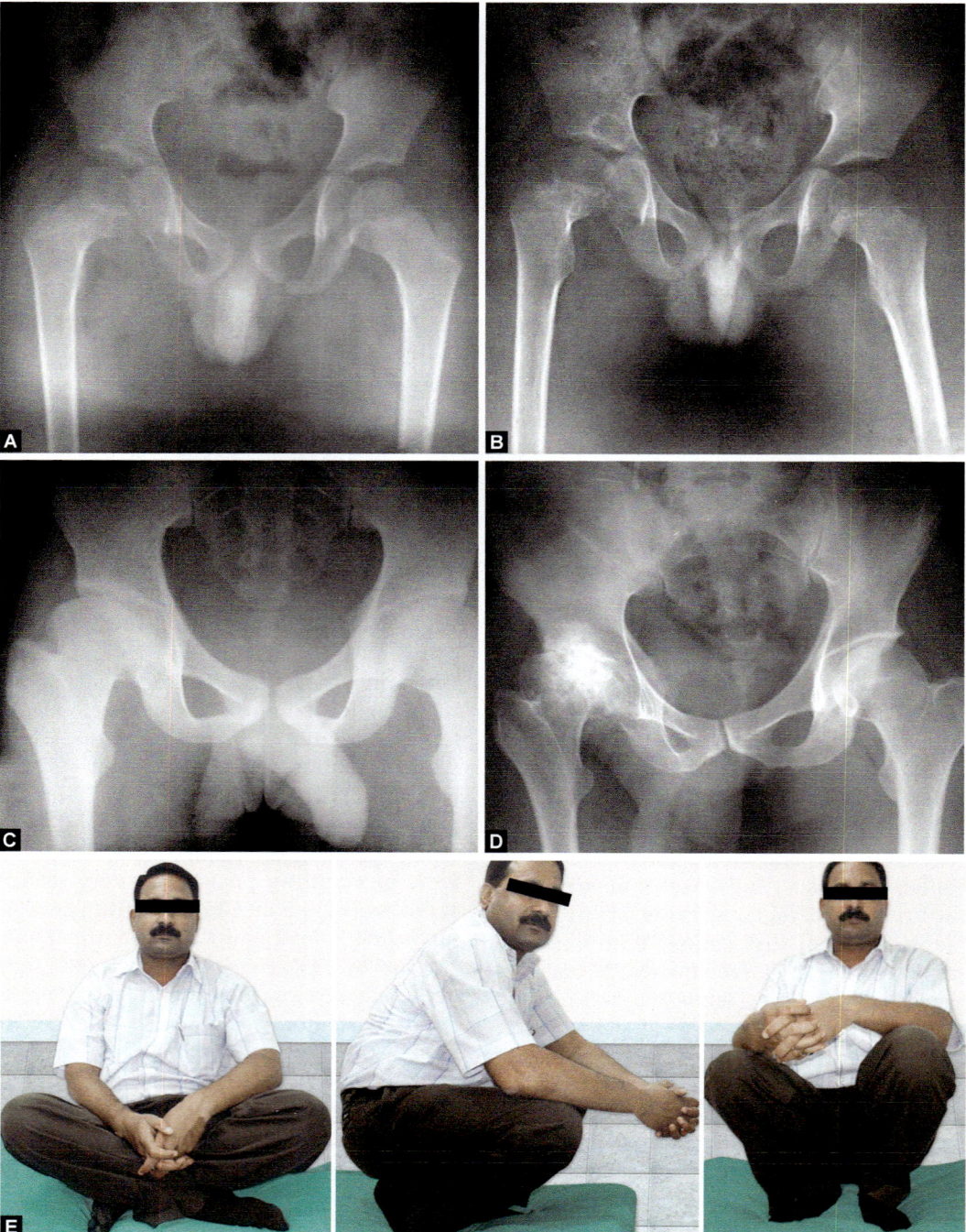

Figs. 16.7A to E: Follow-up of a treated case of tuberculosis of right hip joint: (A) At presentation; (B) After one year treatment healed status; (C) Developed coxa magna; (D) Degenerative changes; (E) Clinical function >45 years after the diagnosis.

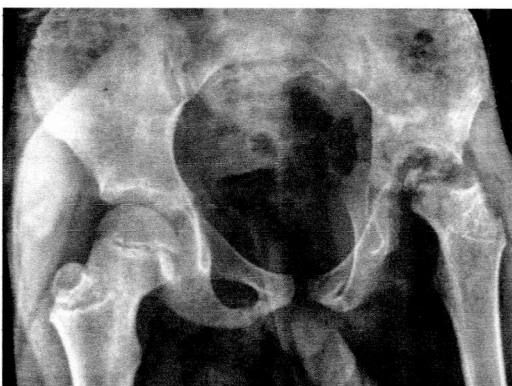

Fig. 16.8: X-ray shows advanced tuberculous arthritis of left hip stage IV: Note gross destruction of articular margins, upward migration of femoral head, empty lower half of acetabulum, break in the Shenton's line (arc) and adduction deformity.

hip joint in adults, almost rigid fixation is desired usually by a blade-plate fixation of the osteotomy site. In children, semi-rigid implants are acceptable because one can supplement with postoperative hip-spica. In adults, there are difficulties in nursing if the patient is in a hip-spica, in such cases (after blade-plate fixation) postoperatively give a derotation plaster-cast or an orthosis to minimize rotational stress at the site of osteotomy. Encourage soon after surgery, in bed exercises for hip and knee for 10 minutes six-times a day. Permit ambulation 4–6 weeks after the operation using a walker; toe-touch walking for 3–4 weeks, forefoot touch walking for 3–4 weeks, and then permit walking with one elbow crutch in contralateral hand for another 4–6 weeks. When X-rays at the end of 4–6 months show adequate union in an adult, permit unprotected loading and walking. In children 6–8 weeks after the osteotomy, one may remove the plaster-cast and encourage walking with a walker.

Osteotomy of proximal femur is one of the oldest operation performed by our ancestors. Currently with the availability of good results after replacement arthroplasty, the indications for such operations are rare after the age of 60 years. However, proximal femoral osteotomy is a very useful operation between the age of 6 years and 50 years for many conditions of the hip joint. This is an important biological option available to obtain a better function with less pain and to delay the indication of joint replacement **(Figs. 16.9A to C)**. A few useful osteotomies are outlined below:

A. **To improve the angle of ankylosis:** A hip joint fused or ankylosed due to any disease in unacceptable position can be brought to the best functional position. Though currently fusion of a hip joint is not considered a good option, however, the patient may present to you with grossly destroyed joint going into fusion. Aim at obtaining a fused joint in neutral position between abduction and adduction, add 5–30 degrees of hip flexion, 5 degrees in children, add 1 degree for each year; however, maximum flexion advised is 30 degrees. In children below the age of 11 years, a rare indication (for a totally destroyed hip joint), about 10 degrees of abduction is advised because with growth some degree of adduction deformity is added during the process of healing. Aim at 5 degrees of external rotation at hip joint for any age **(Figs. 16.10A to C)**.

B. **To improve arc of movements:** If a hip joint has partial ankylosis with some degrees (30–40 degrees) of a useful arc in flexion-extension range, upper femoral osteotomy can bring the range of motion to the best functional arc, say from 10 degrees of flexion to 40 degrees of flexion; 30–40 degrees of range of hip in the functional arc (flexion-extension) facilitates traveling in public transport.

C. **To improve weight-bearing area:** To bring healthier part of femoral head to the weight-bearing (loading) area of acetabulum (the sourcil in normal hips). The best indications are for certain cases of osteonecrosis of femoral head, and for certain cases of symptomatic hips due to early primary or secondary osteoarthrosis. Indications for varus osteotomy

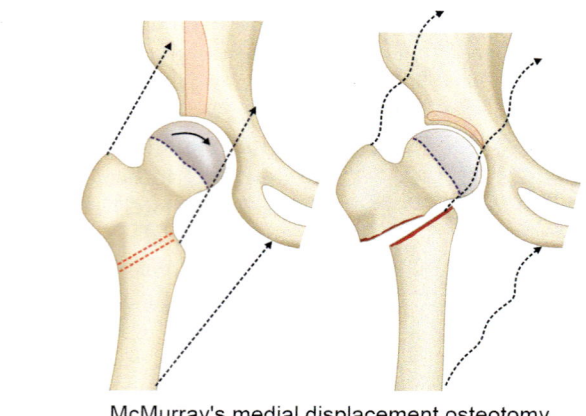

McMurray's medial displacement osteotomy used for osteoarthrosis and neglected femoral neck fractures

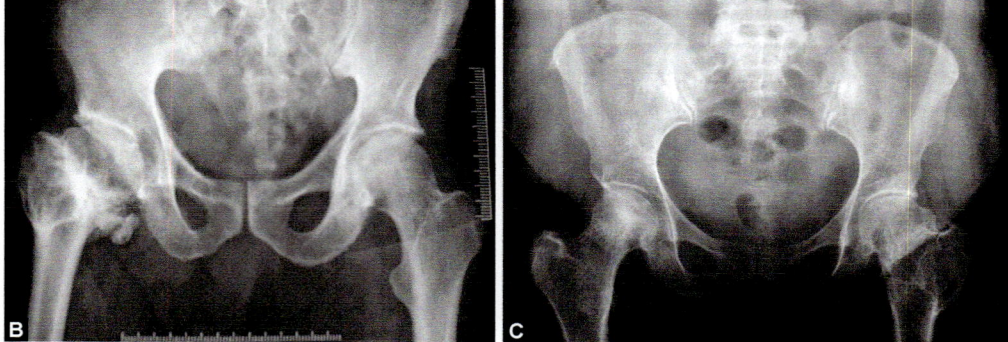

Figs. 16.9A to C: An outline of McMurray's osteotomy (A); More than 20 years of follow-up of two patients (B and C) showing united femoral neck fracture and retained joint space (B) right and (C) left hip.

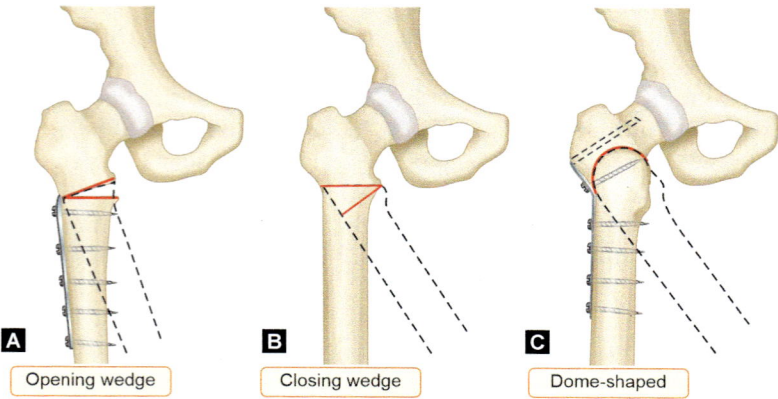

Opening wedge   Closing wedge   Dome-shaped

Fixed adduction deformity of hip can be corrected by any one of these osteotomies

Figs. 16.10A to C: An outline of upper femoral osteotomy. (A) Opening wedge would require bone grafting to fill up the gap; (B) Closing wedge; and (C) Dome osteotomy; do not create a gap.

or valgus osteotomy would be determined by assessment of the "best position". If the healthiest segment of femoral head comes under the sourcil in abduction X-rays, one opts for varus osteotomy. If adduction X-rays bring the healthiest part of femoral head under the sourcil, then valgus osteotomy is indicated. By such operations, the movements are preserved, pain becomes less and the patient can continue for many years and delay the necessity for replacement procedures to a more mature age.

D. **To improve femoral head coverage (in developmental dysplasia of hip and in Perthes' disease):** Upper femoral osteotomy may be used as one of the options to improve the femoral head coverage. It is intended that proximal femoral varus osteotomy without or with internal rotation to undo excessive anteversion (undo no more than 15–30 degrees of anteversion by doing internal rotation) would thus place the femoral head deepest in the acetabulum. The acetabular development over the well contained femoral head encourages the remodeling of a deeper acetabulum. The acetabular development is best up to the age of 5 years, however no significant development of acetabulum takes place after 8 years of age. Some surgeons prefer proximal femoral varus osteotomy to provide a cover to the femoral head "at-risk" in Perthes' disease. Most of the advanced cases of Perthes' disease would heal with coxa magna with resultant uncovered femoral head. When the femoral head is large and uncovered due to Perthes disease, or associated with developmental hip dysplasia or as a result of old healed (infective) disease during growing age (coxa magna as a consequence of prolonged hyperemic state), the author prefers to prepare a supra-acetabular shelf to provide adequate coverage to the femoral head. For long-term useful hip function, at least 60% of femoral head should have coverage.

Although upper femoral osteotomy has been reported to be successful in the treatment of Perthes' disease and in developmental dysplasia of hip joint; at present, there is a tendency to use it less often than in the past. Most of the correction achieved by femoral osteotomy during childhood, resolves within 3 years of the operation.

E. **Proximal femoral osteotomy as a pelvic support procedure:** It is a useful procedure when the proximal part of femoral head is grossly destroyed by infection, or as a consequence of excisional arthroplasty, or developmental proximal femoral deficiency. Such "joints" are fairly mobile, however these are unstable and have pain on loading. An upper femoral osteotomy (like Schanz) or pelvic support osteotomy helps decrease limp and instability, preserves existing mobility and decreases pain to some extent. The osteotomy is performed almost at the level of ischial tuberosity, the upper fragment of femur is parallel to the outer surface of pelvis, the angle desired at the site of osteotomy is 30–40 degree with convexity to medial side, almost centering at ischial tuberosity **(Figs. 16.5, 16.11 and 16.12)**.

F. **Osteotomy to reconstruct femoral head:** In young adolescents (age 7–12 years) when the femoral head and neck have been grossly destroyed or iatrogenically removed, following 2 operations are described for the sake of completion of the possible use of proximal femoral osteotomies. Trochanteric arthroplasty has been described by Dal Monte et al. and by Colona. In first stage, greater trochanter is placed into the acetabulum, hip abductors are shifted distally on the femur and the limb is held in abduction in a plaster-cast. About one month later, an upper femoral varus osteotomy is performed, fixed with implants to create an angle of about 135 degrees between the proximal and distal femoral fragments with convexity laterally.

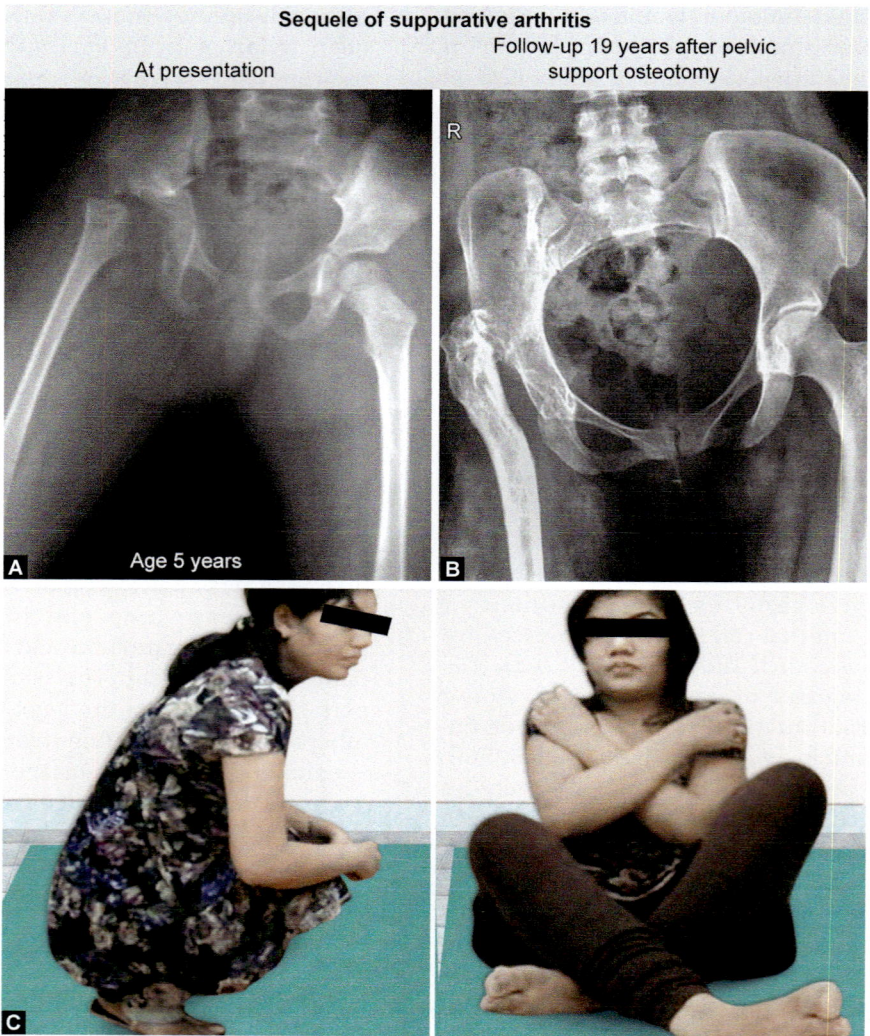

Figs. 16.11A to C: A pelvic support upper femoral osteotomy. (A) Gross destruction of right hip is a sequel of suppurative arthritis; (B) 20 years after the osteotomy; (C) Clinical function >25 years after the osteotomy.

In **Harmon's reconstructive procedure** (Y-osteotomy of upper femur), a new femoral head and neck is fashioned by bifurcation of the upper end of femur. The osteotomy is held open by bonegrafts and the fashioned out femoral head (the medial half of upper end of femur) is placed in the acetabulum, held in position with stout Kirschner's wires. The limb is held in plaster spica for 6–8 weeks, followed by gradual rehabilitation and weight-bearing. The author has no experience of the Colona's procedure, however Harmon's procedure performed in 3 young children aged 8–9 years reshaped a femoral head and gave a useful joint as observed for about 5 years.

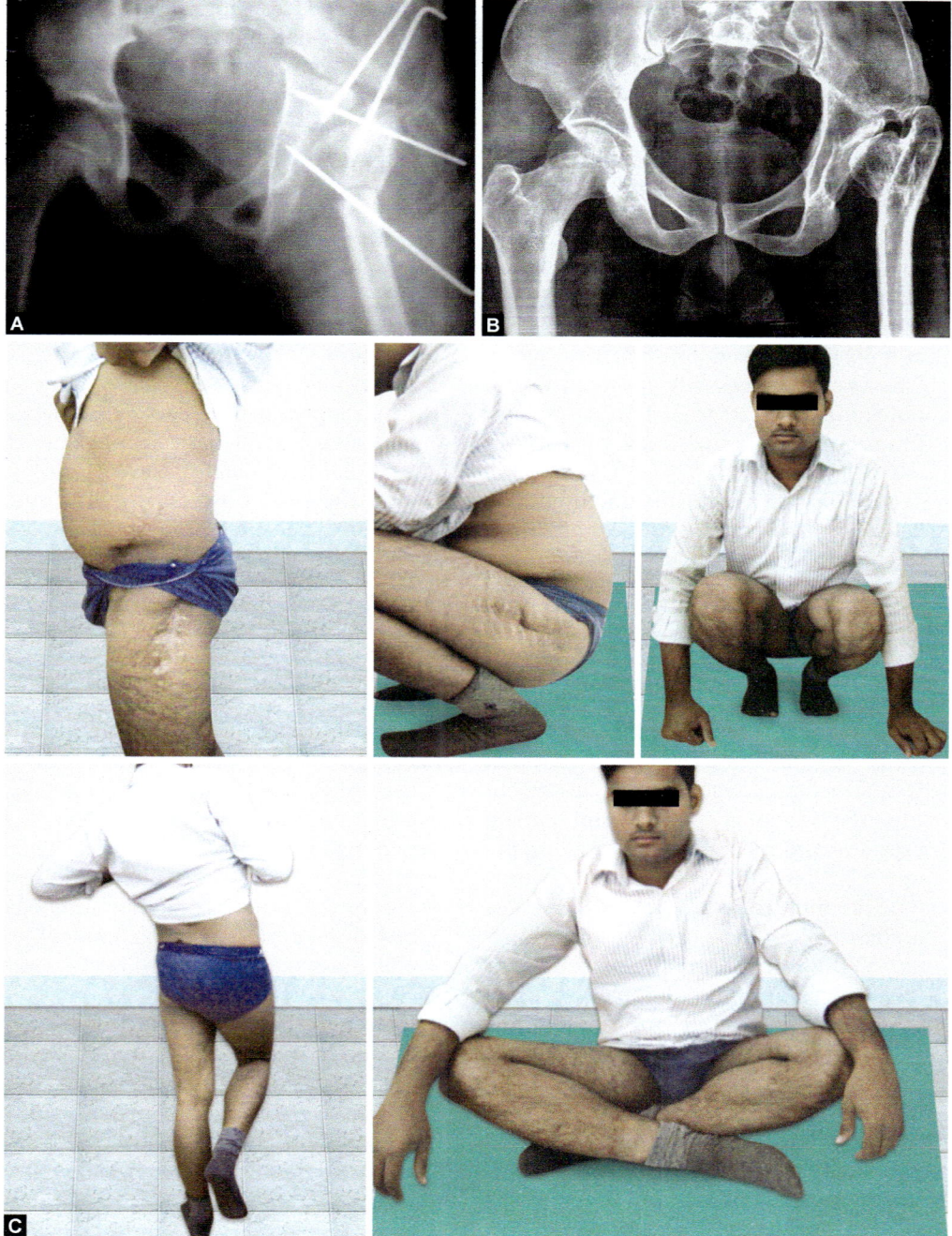

Figs. 16.12A to C: A young boy about 8 years presented with an unstable left hip joint (A). Note marked coxa breva and flattened acetabulum. Pelvic support osteotomy and innominate osteotomy were performed; follow-up after 20 years; (B) X-ray shows the remodeling of femoral and innominate osteotomies and retention of "joint space". The clinical pictures (C) show the scars of previous operations and the function obtained.

G. **McMurray's upper femoral osteotomy:** It was originally devised for treatment of osteoarthrosis of hip joint. An oblique inter trochanteric osteotomy is performed above the level of lesser trochanter running from the base of greater trochanter medially and about 20-30 degrees upwards almost parallel to the inferior border of the femoral neck. In addition to the original indication of McMurray's osteotomy for osteoarthrosis of hip, many surgeons (including the author) in the developing half of the world have used it successfully for treatment of old (older than 3 weeks), intracapsular fracture neck femur with or without avascular necrosis.

On a hip spica table, the fractured limb is fixed in neutral position with adequate traction to bring down the overlapping at the fracture site. Expose the lateral surface of femur centering at the base of greater trochanter by a mid-lateral 10-15 cm incision cutting through skin, fascia, and vastus lateralis. Expose the bone subperiosteally, insert long narrow bone levers skirting along the upper border of lesser trochanter. Osteotomy is carried out from the base of greater trochanter going upwards and medially skirting along the upper border of lesser trochanter. It is wise to make the first cut of bone in the most medial part of the proposed osteotomy line at the calcar femorale, to minimize the chances of comminution (shattering) of bone. Now complete the osteotomy starting from the base of greater trochanter proceeding upwards and medially. The distal fragment is displaced medially using a broad osteotome as a "shoe-horn". This places the part of raw surface of distal fragment medially under the femoral head extracapsularly, and the lateral part stays in contact with the trochanteric fragment. The distal fragment may be displaced medially by 50-75%. Give an abduction of 25-35 degrees at the site of osteotomy, and hold the limb in one and a half hip spica. The spica is changed to neutral position after about 4 weeks when stitches are removed, the abducted limb is brought to neutral position and a new plaster is applied for another 2 months. After the change of plaster, the patient is encouraged to start weight bearing with the plaster on and with the help of a walker. Some adults may not be comfortable in one and a half hip spica. One can manage to hold the osteotomy site by a single hip spica if you transfix the intermediate fragment (trochanteric fragment) to the femoral head by inserting 2 stout Kirschner wires, and while applying plaster keep the ipsilateral knee flexed at 30 degrees of flexion. With availability of fixation devices, one may hold the site of osteotomy by a double angled blade-plate, one must, however, ensure good apposition at the osteotomy site at the time of implant fixation. If done carefully, osteotomy site unites in every case, fracture unites in all the recent (Stage I) cases of nonunions, and in some of the late (Stage II) non-unions. In very late cases (Stage III and IV—Sandhu 2005), though fracture does not unite; however, the united osteotomy offers a very useful and long-lasting arm-chair effect for the patient to walk well. Hundreds of such operations have been followed up by the author and other orthopedic surgeons in our country. Most of the patients achieved a painless, stable and mobile hip joint for 10-20 years **(Fig. 16.13)**.

H. **Upper femoral angular osteotomy:** Upper femoral osteotomy is best performed below the greater trochanter and above the lesser trochanter. If the upper end of femur has markedly shifted upwards, and the femoral head is placed higher than the upper lip of acetabulum, it is wise to pull it down by pre-osteotomy skeletal traction (for 10-15 days) and release of origin of adductor tendons from the pubic bone, and release of iliopsoas from its insertion at the lesser trochanter. If the femoral head is fixed or ankylosed in the abnormal position, it

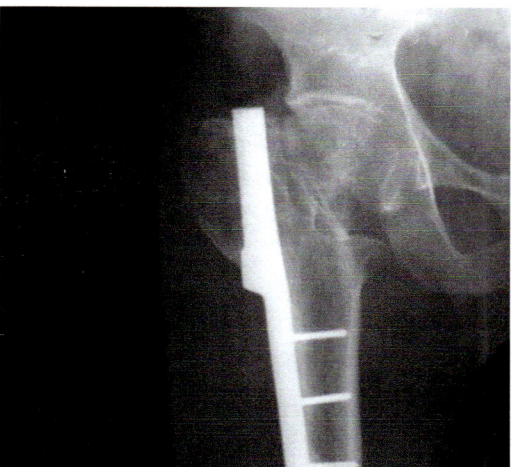

Fig. 16.13: McMurray osteotomy for un-united or neglected femoral neck fracture in young patients is still a good option. This is an X-ray of the osteotomy (with a plate fixation) 20 years after the operation. The patient has nearly full function.

Table 16.1: Results of excision-arthroplasty of hip done for deep infections in adults (follow-up >6 years).

	Percentage
Control of infection	95
Standing un-supported on operated limb	67
Ability in climbing stairs	70
Walking unaided/with one stick	90
Squatting	90
Sitting cross-legged	70
Significant relief of pain	80
Average shortening	4 cm

may be wise to excise the femoral head or perform the femoral neck osteotomy leaving the femoral head in situ. Excision of a (long-standing) fixed femoral head is accompanied by excessive bleeding, it is wise to leave it in situ; now you can gradually pull down the upper femur by skeletal traction. After 10–15 days of traction, one can now perform a pelvic support osteotomy (Schanz or Pauwels like) centering the angle of osteotomy almost at the level of ischeal tuberosity. The osteotomy may be fixed with an angled plate. If fixation is not adequate, supplement it with a plaster spica for 4–6 weeks. Nonloading ambulation may be permitted with a walker after 6–12 weeks, the walker may be replaced by an elbow crutch in the contralateral hand for 6–12 months till the consolidation of osteotomy, and maturation of the post-operative fibrous response around the "hip joint".

Upper femoral angular osteotomy in children is best performed above the age of 6 years. If osteotomy is performed at a younger age, despite fixation with angled plate remodeling due to the growth of upper end of femur may negate the correction obtained at operation.

Girdleston's like excisional arthroplasty is an acceptable procedure for grossly destroyed (ankylosed and painful) hip joint with poor functions. It is a useful salvage procedure for deep infections of hip joint due to tuberculosis, pyogenic infection, or iatrogenic uncontrolled deep infection after hip joint replacement procedures **(Table 16.1)**. Consider the option of this procedure only after completion of the growth of upper end of femur. Upper tibial pin traction (2–3 months) and concomitant exercises for the hip joint minimize the shortening, and possibly help development of fibro-cartilage at the site of pseudarthrosis. If performed for infective pathologies, gross post-excision instability is rare; however, if required, the stability can be improved by adding a pelvic support osteotomy **(Figs. 16.14, and 16.15)**.

INNOMINATE OSTEOTOMIES

Innominate osteotomies and shelf operations have been used since 1900. The description in literature started appearing around 1950s (Chiari 1953, Salter 1961, Pemberton 1965). Steel (1973) and many others modified these procedures. Main

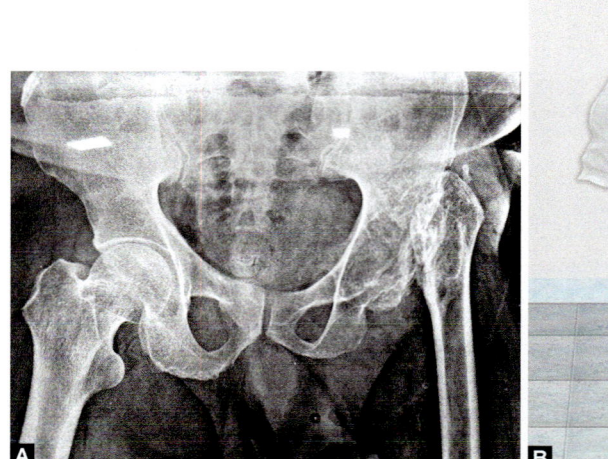
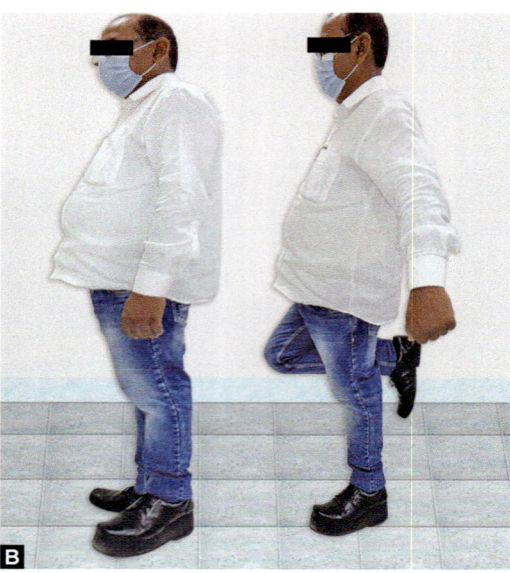

Figs. 16.14A and B: Fusion of HIP and Knee are now for Historical Records. However, for persisting hip infections, (A) Girdlestone—Excisional arthroplasty is still a biological and viable option. (B) Clinical function 40 years Post-operative, patient with stance-phase on operated (Left) side.

indications of innominate osteotomies have been for coverage of femoral head, to provide stability and to minimize redislocation of a dysplastic hip. Most of the dysplastic hips reaching the medical facility after the walking age, patients who present to you after a failed/unsuccessful previous operation, patients who are found to have unstable reduction on the operating table, and patients suffering from arthrogryposis-multiplex congenita are suitable for concomitant innominate osteotomy at the time of operative reduction of the hips. The stress to the child and family of multiple hip operations in childhood should not be underestimated. The surgeon should both reduce the hip and stabilize the hip to minimize the chances of redislocation and another surgery. In children younger than 6 years, it is best to reshape and orientate the acetabulum so that articular cartilage of the acetabulum covers the femoral head. The potential of remodeling of the acetabular cavity becomes almost negligible after age of 6 years. For flattened acetabulum, enlarged femoral head (coxa magna), irreversible subluxation, medial displacement Chiari osteotomy, or a shelf operation are rational options. Intuitively, it seems better to cover the femoral head with articular cartilage than to rely upon the joint capsule between the supporting shelf superiorly and the femoral head, in medial displacement Chiari's osteotomy and other shelf operations. However, even normally acetabular cartilage covers just about 60% of the femoral head. A significant part of femoral head articular cartilage articulates with joint capsule. When a supra-acetabular shelf is created, the undersurface of the shelf supports the capsule, which by function and weight-bearing is likely to undergo metaplasia to fibrocartilage (Hiranuma, 1992). The raw under-surface of the supra-acetabular shelf would undergo remodeling induced by function and loading of the joint.

After any innominate osteotomy or supra-acetabular shelf procedure, the hip should be held in moderate flexion, abduction, and internal rotation for 6–8 weeks. If one is using the procedure after complete transiliac osteotomy, preoperative shortening, if

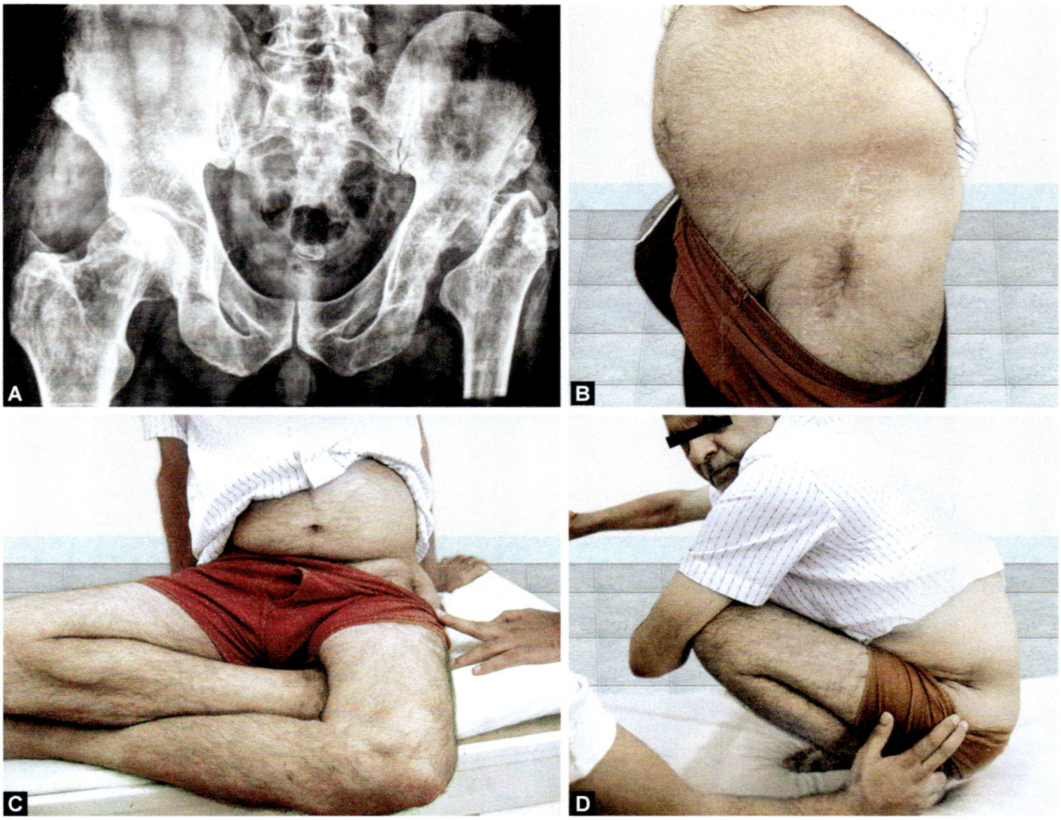

Figs. 16.15A to D: Follow-up case of Girdlestone's excisional arthroplasty for a grossly infected and ankylosed left hip; (A) X-rays of the pseudarthrosis functioning for >20 years; (B) In standing patient, one can see scars of multiple operations; (C and D) Clinical functions.

present, can be to some extent compensated by inserting a suitable sized bone graft (about 2–3 cm) at the osteotomy site. If the iliac bone is hypoplastic and there is not much of width of bone mass available at osteotomy site, one can insert a bone graft at the osteotomy site projecting laterally, anteriorly and posteriorly as a shelf providing a cover to the femoral head **(Figs. 16.16 to 16.19).**

In Salter's osteotomy, the distal pelvic fragment (acetabular fragment) is rotated anterolaterally. Its direction may be helped by gentle downward traction using a towel clip through the distal fragment or by pulling the acetabular segment with a small bone hook. Aim is to cover the femoral head

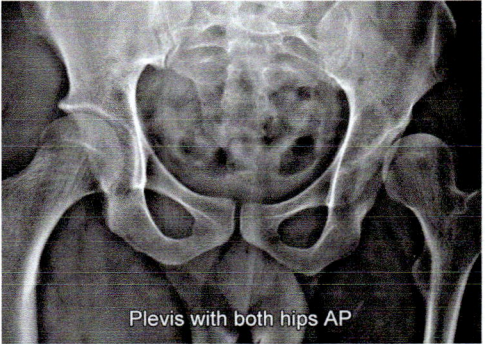

Fig. 16.16: Neglected congenital dislocation of left hip. The acetabulum is flattened. Patient has been walking up to her adulthood with limping but no pain.

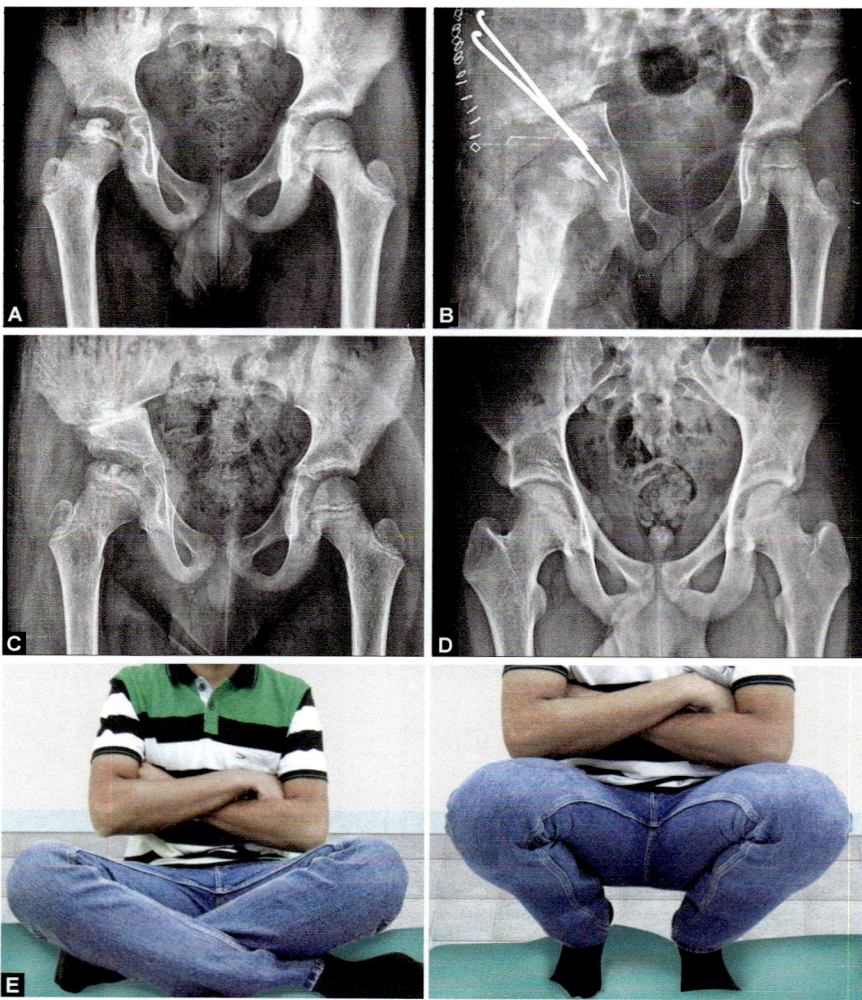

Figs. 16.17A to E: Legg–Calvé–Perthes disease: (A) X-ray shows fragmentation of the central part and uncovering of the femoral head. Following an innominate osteotomy (B); (C) The femoral head is much better "contained"; at maturity; (D) The femoral head is almost normal; (E) Shows the clinical function as at 22 years.

anterolaterally. The triangular wedge-shaped gap thus created between the 2 fragments (of osteotomy) is filled with a wedge-shaped bone graft obtained from the iliac bone. The graft and osteotomy are held secure in desired position by inserting 2 Kirschner's wires from the iliac crest. The wires are bent at right angle, cut short, slightly projecting from (pround of) the iliac crest **(Figs. 16.20A to D)**.

In Chiari's osteotomy, the acetabular fragment is displaced medially hinging at the symphysis pubis, and some degree of lateral shift of upper fragment takes place hinging at the sacroiliac joint **(Figs. 16.20A to D)**.

In Steel's triple osteotomy, the complete cuts made at transiliac site, superior and inferior pubic rami, permit the acetabular segment to be tilted/reinclined in the desired direction pivoting at the ischial tuberosity

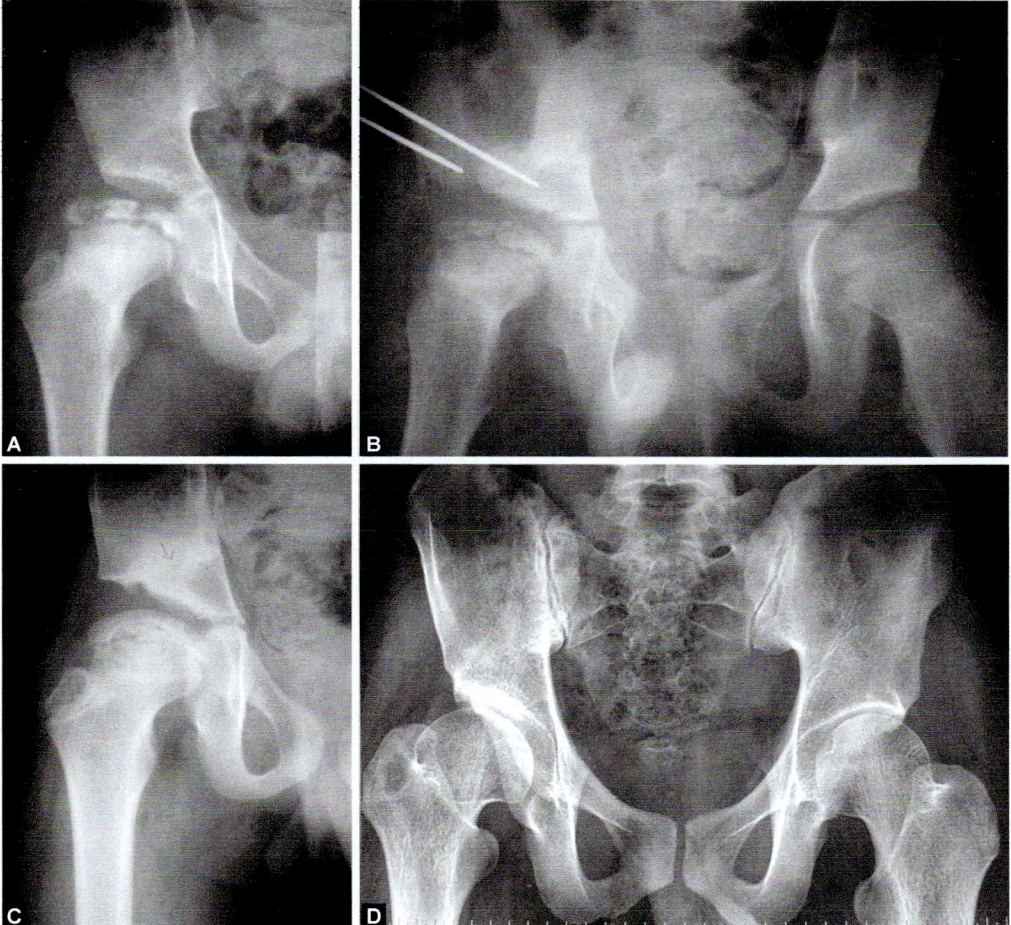

Figs. 16.18A to D: Legg–Calvé–Perthes disease in a boy (A) involving the whole of right femoral head, uncovered femoral head with possible hinge-abduction defect making corrective displacement difficult [Femoroacetabular impingement (FAI)]. (B) Because of coxa magna, the head was covered by innominate osteotomy, the follow-up (C) shows the remodeling and the appearance (D) at maturity. Note some degree of coxa magna and coxa breva with nearly full function at 22 years of age.

and sacrotuberous ligament. All osteotomies must be held in the best desired position using suitable bone grafts and 2 or more Kirschner's wires.

Transilial osteotomies are easy to master by general orthopedic surgeons; however, multilevel osteotomies are complicated and difficult to perform. Staheli popularized a supra-acetabular shelf procedure like tectoplasty, and a canopy procedure was described by Japanese orthopedic surgeons. These are like supra-acetabular shelf augmentation procedures.

Operative Procedure for Innominate Osteotomy (Transiliac Osteotomy)

If facilities are available, use a translucent table and make C-arm available in case of necessity. Earlier descriptions advised either splitting of iliac apophysis into medial and lateral halves or separation of cartilaginous

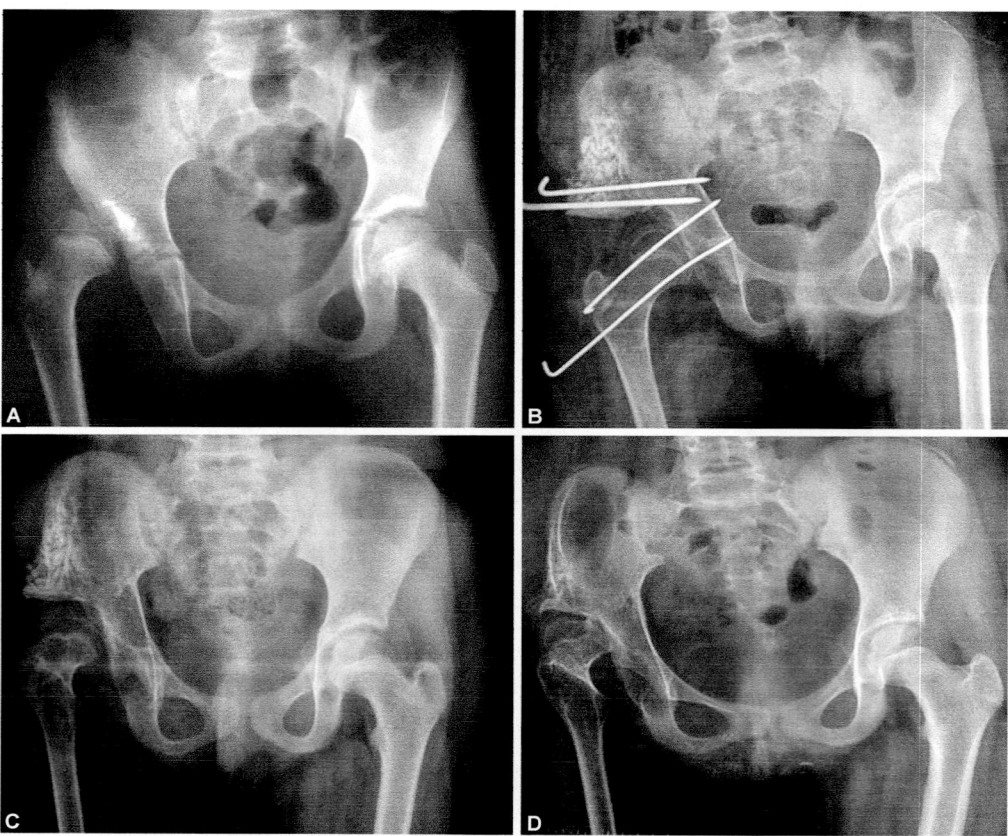

Figs. 16.19A to D: Follow-up of developmental dysplasia of right hip after (A) failed prior operations. As there was no acetabulum and the pelvic bones were hypoplastic (B) tectoplasty was performed using bone bank. (C and D) Follow-up X-rays show adequate coverage for the femoral head and adequate articulating "joint space" (note hypoplastic right pelvic bones and femur).

apophysis from the underlying bone. We, however, do not disturb the iliac apophysis and the muscles attached to it. Make the standard iliofemoral (Smith-Petersen) skin incision on the lateral border of iliac crest and curve it distally inferior to the anterosuperior iliac spine by 2–3 cm. Strip the muscles and periosteum from the lateral surface of iliac bone anteriorly up to anteroinferior iliac spine, inferiorly up to the superior lip of acetabulum and its capsular attachments, posteriorly up to greater sciatic notch. In neglected dislocation, the superior capsule is usually firmly adherent to the side wall of the ilium and this needs to be mobilized uptil the superior margin of true acetabulum. Pack the space between the reflected muscles and the outer surface of iliac bone. Strip the iliacus muscle and periosteum from the medial surface of the iliac bone extending from anteroinferior iliac spine to the greater sciatic notch. One should now be able to insert a smooth curved narrow dissector (as a retractor) skirting along the medial surface of iliac bone to become visible subperiosteally at the greater sciatic notch. Pack the area between the iliacus muscle and the bone. As a rule, it is not essential to cut the origin of sartorius from the anterosuperior iliac spine **(Figs. 16.20A to D)**.

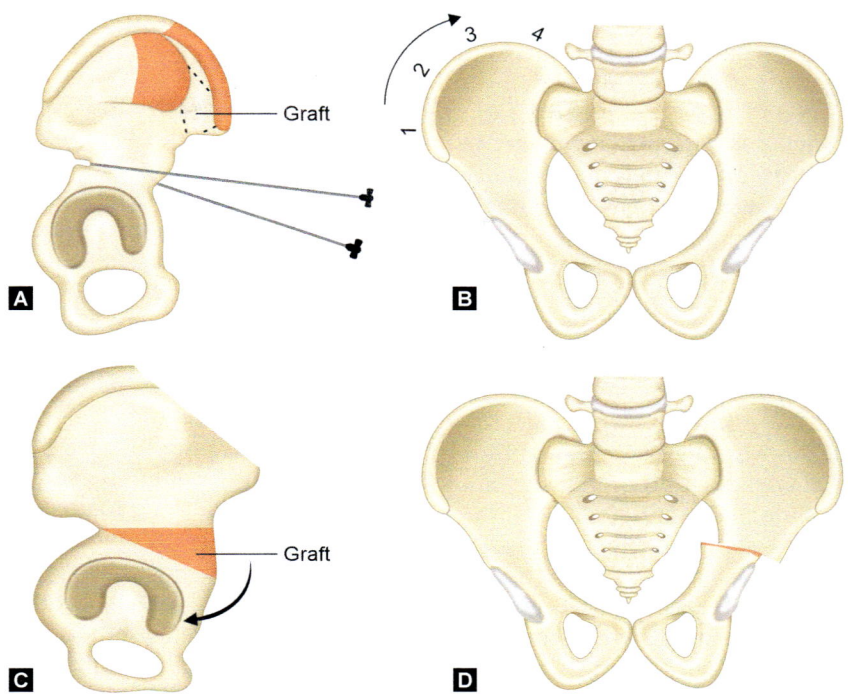

Figs. 16.20A to D: An outline of the innominate osteotomy. (A) A supra-acetabular cut is made from most anterior part of greater sciatic notch to the anterior inferior iliac spine; (B) Risser's sign is expressed in 5 stages: 0—not visible, 1—in anterior ¼, 2—upto middle, 3—posterior to mid-point, 4—complete, 5—fused; (C) Distal fragment is redirected with the help of bone grafts in Salter's procedures; (D) Distal fragment is shifted medially in Chiari's osteotomy.

Steps for difficult cases: Through a separate small incision, do adductor tenotomy if these are tight. In long standing cases of dislocated hips, identify the insertion of iliopsoas tendon on the lesser trochanter, use a right-angled curved artery forceps or a small bone hook to lift the tendon at the site of insertion, cut it complete nearest to the insertion. Stripping of the iliofemoral muscles, release of tight adductors and iliopsoas insertion enables the surgeon to bring down (descend) the femoral head into the deepest part of acetabulum. Hold the femoral head in the best (fit) possible position, about 30-40 degrees of abduction and about 10-20 degrees of internal rotation, 20-30 degrees of flexion and fix it with 2 Kirschner's wires. Insert a right angled curved artery forceps skirting along the medial surface of iliac bone and protruding through the greater sciatic notch. Hold a Gigli saw with the curved forceps and negotiate the saw through the greater sciatic notch onto the medial surface of iliac bone presenting at antero-inferior iliac spine. Use the saw to cut the waist of the iliac bone from the most anterior part of the sciatic notch to the anteroinferior iliac spine or slightly distal to it. The osteotomy cut is aimed at either horizontal (for Salter's), or 10-15 degrees of up-slope medially (for Chiari's) abutting the capsular attachments. The cut on the inner table should be slightly higher than the cut on the outer table, the up-slope medially (10-15 degrees) minimizes the redisplacement of the fragments after obtaining the desired position. With too much of medial up-slope, the osteotomy line is likely to enter into the sacroiliac joint, making corrective displacement difficult. In small children, this operation does not provide a generously wide access. In bigger children, one may try to do the osteotomy cut with convexity upwards parallel to the acetabulum. Osteotomy is held in desired position by insertion of 2 Kirschner's wires. Postoperation hip spica is required for 6–8 weeks. Kirschner's wires may be removed around 4–6 weeks after the innominate osteotomy to be followed by another plaster. About 6–8 weeks after the osteotomy, the hip spica is replaced by an abduction plaster with broomstick to hold the hips at 80 degrees of angle between the two thighs for 4–6 weeks more. As the hips and knees are now left free, mobility of hip joints is encouraged. About 8–12 weeks after the osteotomy, the patients are encouraged, ambulation with weight-bearing.

The ideal age for Salter's osteotomy is in children younger than 6 years of age, the Chiari's osteotomy is ideal for children >6 years of age. If indicated in adults, the innominate osteotomy can be performed up to the age of 50 years. The Chiari's medial displacement osteotomy is very useful operation for neglected congenital subluxations, untreated or inadequately treated congenital hip dysplasias, failed previous operations, hypoplastic acetabulum, coxa magna in Perthes disease, paralytic or spastic hip subluxations/dislocations, sequele of childhood hip infections or primary acetabular dysplasia.

PEMBERTON'S (1965) ACETABULOPLASTY

This is applicable where the femoral head is located in a wider and flattened acetabular socket. The triradiate cartilage must be open for this procedure to be accomplished, therefore its greatest use is between the ages of 4 and 11 years. The external surface of the iliac bone is exposed in the standard fashion. Two or 3 curved narrow osteotomes are used to cut the outer cortex of iliac bone starting about 1 cm proximal to the level of acetabulum. The outer cortex is cut in a convex manner parallel to the acetabular margin anteriorly, superiorly and posteriorly. The bone is cut curving medially just short of the location of triradiate cartilage. Two or 3 curved osteotomes inserted at the site of osteotomy are used to lever down the upper part of acetabulum to provide a closer coverage to the deeply seated femoral head. The levered down acetabular wall is held in position by inserting (packing) suitable size of bone grafts in the gap created between the levered down outer wall and the intact inner table of iliac bone. The desired position may be secured by using Kirschner wires.

Dega's pelvic osteotomy: Dega pelvic osteotomy is almost similar to the Pemberton's except that the curvilinear osteotomy is about 2 cm above and parallel to the acetabular margin. Once complete the outer table of iliac bone above the acetabulum is levered down over the femoral head capsule, and held in position by compact bone grafts. This is suitable for patients aged 3–11 years.

SUGGESTED READINGS

1. Salter RB. Innominate osteotomy in the treatment of congenital dislocation and subluxation of the hip. J Bone Joint Surg Am. 1961;43B:518-639.
2. Pemberton PA. Pericapsular osteotomy of the ilium for treatment of congenital subluxation and dislocation of the hip. J Bone Joint Surg Am. 1965;47A:65-86.
3. Salter RB. Role of innominate osteotomy in the treatment of congenital dislocation and subluxation of the hip in the older child. J Bone Joint Surg Am. 1966;45A:1413-39.
4. Tuli SM, Mukherjee SK. Excision arthoplasty for tuberculous and pyogenic arthritis of the hip. J Bone Joint Surg. 1981;63B:29-32.

5. Catterall A. Legg-Calvé-Perthes syndrome. Clin Orthop Relat Res. 1981;158:41-52.
6. De Waal, Malefijt MC, Hodgland T, Nielsen HK. Chiari osteotomy in the treatment of congenital dislocation and subluxation of the hip. J Bone Joint Surg. 1982;64-A:996-1004.
7. Graham S, Westin GW, Dawson E, Oppenheim WL. The Chiari osteotomy-A review of 58 cases. Clin Orthop Relat Res. 1986;208:249-58.
8. Hadjipavlou AG, Gaitanis IN, Kontakis GM. Paget's disease of the bone and its management. J Bone Joint Surg. 2002;84B:160-9.
9. Herring JA, Kim HT, Browne R. Legg-Calvé-Perthes disease. Part II: Prospective multicenter study of the effect of treatment on outcome. J Bone Joint Surg Am. 2004;86A:2121-34.
10. Kocher MS, Mandiga R, Zurakowski D, Barnewolt C, Kasser JR. Validation of a clinical prediction rule for the differentiation between septic arthritis and transient synovitis of the hip in children. J Bone Joint Surg Am. 2004:86A:1629-35.
11. Sharma H, De Leeuw J, Rowley DI. Girdlestone resection arthroplasty following failed surgical procedures. Int Orthop. 2005;26:92-5.
12. Choi H, Yoo WJ, Cho TJ, Chung CY. Operative reconstruction for septic arthritis of the hip. Orthop Clin North Am. 2006;37:173-83.
13. Ganz R, Horowitz K, Leunig M. Algorithm for femoral and periacetabular osteotomies in complex hip deformities. Clin Orthop Relat Res. 2010;468: 3168-80.
14. Cordero-Ampuero J. Girdlestone procedures: when and why. Hip Int. 2012;22(suppl 8):S36-39.
15. Joseph B, Management of Perthes' disease. Indian J Orthop. 2015;49:10-6.
16. Loder RT. Slipped capital femoral epiphysis: a spectrum of surgical care and changes over time. J Child Orthop. 2017;11:154-9.
17. Talbot C, Adam J, Paton R. Late presentation of developmental dysplasia of the hip: a 15-year observational study. Bone Joint J. 2017;99B:1250-5.

CHAPTER 17
Knee and Leg

INTRODUCTION

Most of the patients presenting with knee problems would consult the orthopedist for pain, swelling, stiffness, instability, locking, limping and loss of function, inability to squat, and kneel or sit cross-legged. The first clinical examination must be done by suitable exposure of both lower limbs. A comparison with contralateral normal limb is essential. The first X-ray should be a standing X-ray of both knees for comparison of normal with abnormal. Lateral view is done as a routine, skyline tangential views should be asked for when one suspects maltracking patella.

If clinically one suspects an internal derangement of knee, one may ask for MRIs. MRIs provide reliable diagnoses for meniscal tears, cruciate ligament injuries, osteochondral lesions and osteonecrosis. For most of the synovial pathologies, the MRI findings generally remain nonspecific **(Figs. 17.1 and 17.2)**. Rheumatoid inflammation, tuberculosis, pyogenic infection, post-traumatic effusions and villonodular synovitis would essentially show thickening of synovium and collection of fluid. Any pathology of osteoarticular system can be present at the knee joint **(Figs. 17.3 and 17.4)**, it is, however, important to remember that pain in the knee region may be a pain radiating from a hip pathology. Arthroscopy in the specialized hands is currently used for certain operative procedures with more precision.

Age and common knee pathologies: while most disorder can occur at any age, however,

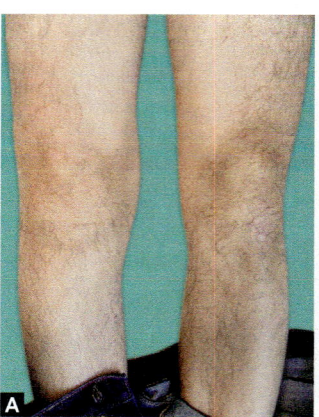 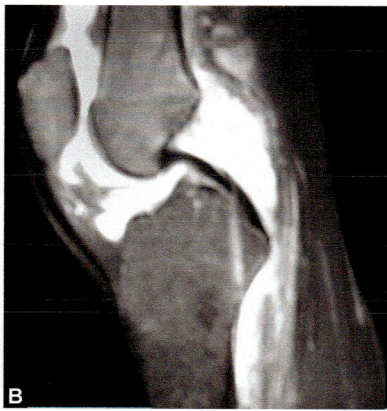 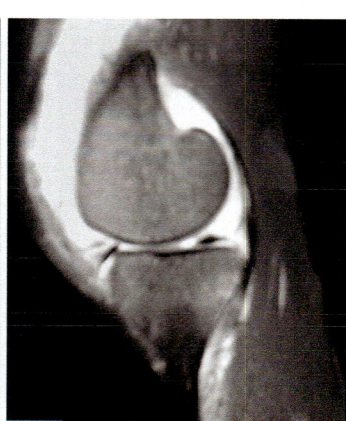

Figs. 17.1A and B: Comparison of both knees. (A) A diffuse swelling of the right knee; (B) MRIs generally show nonspecific synovial fluid collection, multiple images may give information regarding mechanical damage to osteochondral structures, ligaments and semilunar cartilages.

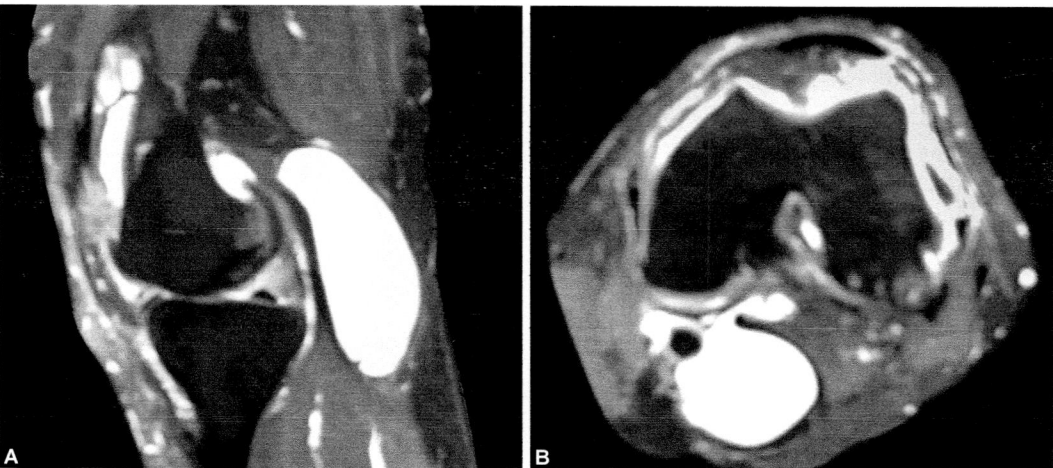

Figs. 17.2A and B: Synovial effusion: Synovial effusion due to "any pathology" would exhibit presence of fluid within the joint: (A) Suprapatellar pouch and popliteal cyst; (B) Many recesses around the joint.

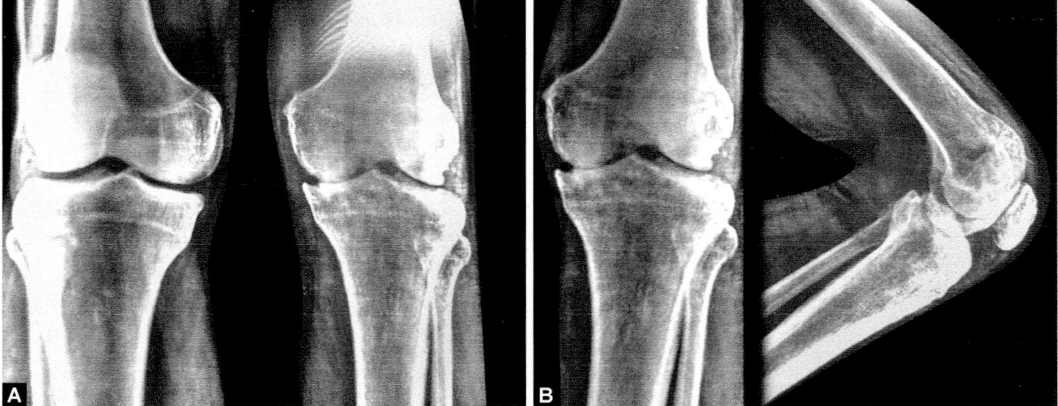

Figs. 17.3A and B: Knee is the third common site for tuberculous infection: (A) Note diminished joint space (left knee) and eroded articular margins. Antitubercular drugs and functional treatment (B) healed the disease with retention of motion from 0 to 90 degrees.

certain conditions present more commonly during specific age periods. Congenital disorders would present before 15 years of age. Conditions like chondromalacia patellae, instability of patellae, osteochondritis would present during adolescence. Young active adults especially those engaged in sports are common victims of ligament and meniscal injuries. Patients with primary or secondary osteoarthrosis generally present above the middle age.

DEFORMITIES OF THE KNEE

At birth children have varus angulation at the knee joints, around 3 years it starts resolving to the adult angles, generally by 8th year 5–7 degrees of valgus is achieved.

By the end of growth period, the knees usually (normally) show, 5–7 degrees of valgus. Moderate deviations from this may be considered "abnormal", however, many of such persons have no symptoms. A few common deformities are described as follows.

Genu Valgum (Knock Knees)

This is an outwards deviation of the legs at the knee joints. Mostly it is an acquired deformity and is generally bilateral in metabolic disorders (rickets). Unilateral deformity is due to premature arrest of the lateral half of distal femoral physis as a sequel to trauma or infection. Continued growth of the medial femoral condyle in the presence of suppressed growth of the lateral condyle would result in the progressive genu valgum deformity. The degree of genu valgum is measured by the distance between the medial malleoli (intermalleolar distance) when the child stands with medial surface of knee touching each other. In unilateral cases, the measurement is done from the midline to the medial malleolus. Excessive genu valgum is often associated with secondary (adaptive) flat feet. In some cases of genu valgum, the patella may show lateral subluxation on flexion of the knee. Intermalleolar distance by >10 cm, or >5 cm when measured from the midline in a unilateral deformity, is generally labeled as "genu valgum". Depending upon the height of patient if the intermalleolar distance is >13 cm, the deformity will require operative correction. There are many techniques to perform distal femoral osteotomy (DFO) like closing medial wedge, opening lateral wedge or dome shaped osteotomy with convexity toward the knee. Like high tibial osteotomy there are number of fixation devices employed postoperatively, multiple Kirschner's wires, staples, blade-plates and external fixators, with or without cast immobilization.

Treatment

In younger children, where the deformity is moderate, 1/4 inch raise on medial side of heel like flat feet shoes may correct the deformity with growth by the age of 6 years. Active rickets or metabolic disorders must be controlled by suitable measures. In severe deformity, supracondylar corrective osteotomy of distal femur is warranted. As a general principal corrective osteotomy must be performed near the skeletal maturity. If, however, a corrective osteotomy is indicated at a younger age, the family must be well-informed that a second operation may be needed near the skeletal maturity. A few degrees of overcorrection is advised depending upon the future growth potential of the bone.

Genu Varum (Bow Legs)

This is inward deformity of leg at the knee. Bilateral deformity is usually the result of rickets or metabolic disorders. Many children may show concomitant bowing of tibia with convexity to the lateral side. With the child standing, heels touching and knees looking forward, the distance between the knee joints up to 6 cm is considered normal. If the distance is >6 cm the deformity is addressed as genu varum. Unilateral varus deformity (like genu valgum) may be caused by damage to the medial half of upper tibial physis. During growing age, varus deformities are corrected by upper tibial osteotomies.

Earlier than 6 years of age, many deformities of knee and tibia may resolve on their own by remodeling and use of suitable orthosis. Stapling of the growing segment of physis or hemiepiphysiodesis, (on the convex side of deformity) can achieve the correction during growing period, however, both these procedures require careful timing and more precision. Distal femoral corrective osteotomy for genu valgum and proximal tibial osteotomy for genu varum are more simple and practical in the hands of a general orthopedic surgeon. As a rule corrective osteotomy is not advised before 6 years of age, the ideal age is a few years prior to the maturity of bone. Most of the deformities seen in adults or middle-aged persons are considered a sequel to the childhood deformities. These have remained painless for many years. Corrective osteotomy in adults is indicated for severe pain in the joints and difficulty in walking **(Fig. 17.4)**.

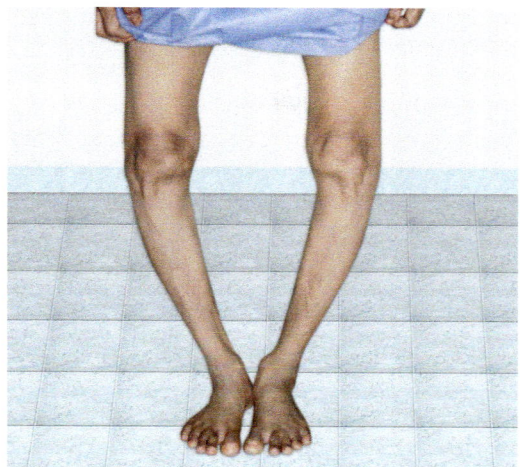

Fig. 17.4: Gross genu varum: This patient had near normal range of motion, if the range of motion is >100 degrees, high tibial osteotomy is a good option. If the range is <90 degrees, knee replacement, would be a better option.

Genu Recurvatum

This is a hyperextension deformity of knee (with convexity backward). Common causes are congenital weakness or contracture of quadriceps, or weakness due to poliomyelitis (rarely seen now), quadriceps fibrosis due to osteomyelitis or infection in thigh. The patient complains of inability to flex the knee joint. In some cases, genu recurvatum (with or without anterior subluxation of tibia) may be a part of arthrogryposis multiplex congenita.

Treatment

In paralytic condition, the range of motion is improved by active assisted exercises and protection of the paralyzed muscles by suitable orthosis till the return of power in the quadriceps. Early cases of quadriceps fibrosis may also improve by exercises and instillation of corticosteroids in the local fibrous cords. In gross fibrosis, the contracture may be released by selective division of the band-like contractures or by inverted V-Y-plasty. Contractures due to arthrogryposis do not give satisfactory outcome. In gross paralysis of quadriceps, hyperextension may be controlled by fixing the patella on the tibial plateau to act as a bone block.

Recurrent Dislocation of Patella (Maltracking Patella)

This condition is characterized by repeated lateral subluxation or dislocation of patella. The patient generally presents in childhood, girls are affected more commonly than boys and, in some, the condition may be bilateral. If patella dislocates every time with flexion of knee, it is labeled as "habitual dislocation" of patella, an occasional dislocating patella is addressed as "recurrent dislocation", rarely the patella may remain permanently dislocated on the lateral side (congenital dislocated patella). Currently recognized, predisposing factors are often present: (1) Generalized ligamentous instability; (2) Underdevelopment of lateral femoral condyle; (3) Fibrosis or contracture of lateral part of quadriceps; (4) Laterally placed insertion of ligamentum patellae or tibial tubercle; (5) Maldevelopment of patella (too high and or too small); (6) Valgus deformity of knee **(Figs. 17.5 and 17.6)**.

Treatment

For milder symptoms, muscle strengthening exercises are helpful, nonoperative treatment would suffice as with growth the patellar mechanism tends to get stabilized. For repeated and distressing episodes in children up to the age of 15 years operative intervention is justified. Try correction of predisposing factors, release the lateral side of quadriceps expansion by a longitudinal incision parallel to the patella, do double breasting of medial side of quadriceps expansion by suturing it to the medial border of patella, shift the lateral half of ligamentum patella more medially and distally, before closing check that patella moves in its normal track when the knee is flexed about 80 degrees. Postoperative apply a plaster-cast holding the knee at about 60 degrees of flexion for about 6 weeks. The plaster is then removed, active exercises are started

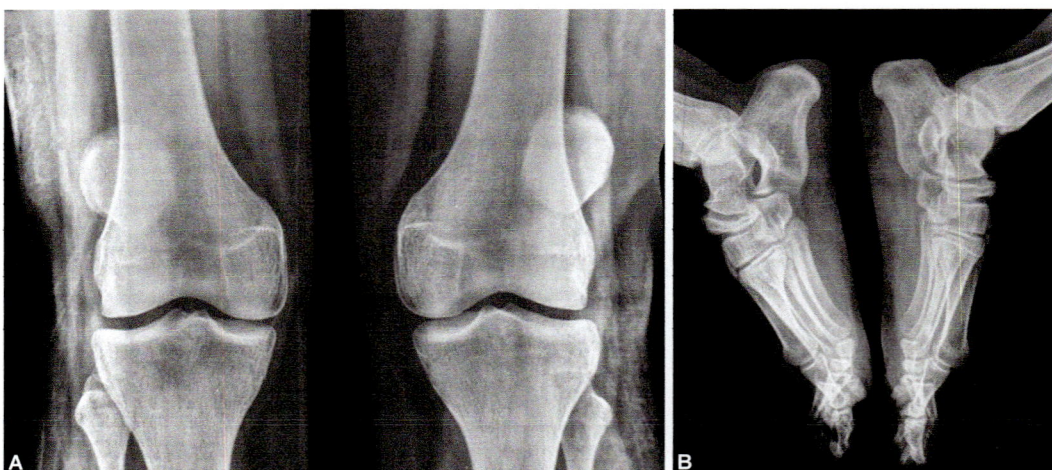

Figs. 17.5A and B: Maltracking patellae. (A) Both knees: The patient also had congenital; (B) Vertical talus on both feet operated during childhood, note the flattening of the navicular bones and talar heads.

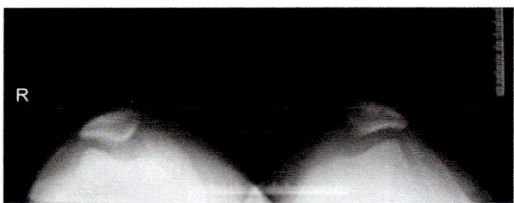

Fig. 17.6: Maltracking patellae in both knees as seen in skyline view X-rays, in another patient.

and loading is permitted 12 weeks, after the operation. The author has been able to get favorable outcome by this procedure in most of the children younger than 15 years.

Patients who do not get satisfactory outcome after realignment procedures or who get painful patellofemoral arthrosis or who present for problems as adults would benefit by patellectomy with concomitant medial transfer of the lateral half of ligamentum patellae (infrapatellar medial realignment).

Tibia Varum due to Blount's Disease

This is a progressive bow-leg deformity due to congenital defects in the posteromedial part of upper tibial physis. The deformity is worse and progressive as compared to the physiological bowing of legs. The tibia also shows internal torsion. Most of these children are overweight. The deformity is bilateral in 80% of cases. X-rays show flattening and fragmentation of proximal tibial epiphysis, hypoplasia of the medial half of the physis and a beak-shaped appearance of the superomedial corner of tibial metaphysis (**Figs. 17.7A and B**).

Treatment

Spontaneous resolution of deformity seldom occurs. Once one is sure of the progressive deformity, corrective osteotomy should be performed to correct the varus and torsional components. There is a wisdom to elevate the medial side by inserting a wedge of bone. The graft may be obtained from distal fibula which may reduce the risk of postoperative compartment syndrome. Overcorrection should be done because some degrees of recurrence is inevitable with many years of growth. The family must be counseled before the corrective operations that the child may need another corrective procedure near the skeletal maturity.

Popliteal Bursa (Semimembranosus Bursitis)

A chronic inflammatory swelling of bursal sheaths may present a patient with a cystic,

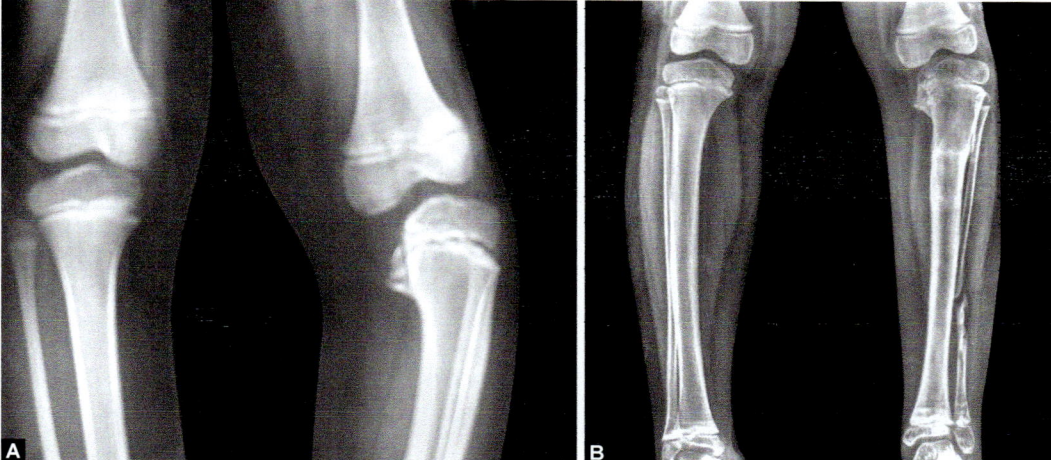

Figs. 17.7A and B: X-rays of a child showing tibia varum deformity in (A) Left leg: Note defective (retarded) physeal area in superomedial corner and angulation of the tibia; (B) Two years after the corrective osteotomy with bone grafting (from fibula).

fluctuant and transilluminant swelling in the popliteal fossa. The commonest bursa that is involved is the semimembranosus bursa situated between the insertion of semimembranosus tendon and the origin of medial head of gastrocnemius. There is moderate bulge at the back of knee with slight discomfort on the movements of knee. Occasionally, the bursal sheath in the popliteal fossa may communicate with the synovial cavity of knee. In such a situation, any effusion and inflammation of the knee joint would be associated with a swelling in the popliteal bursa (*See* **Figs. 17.1 and 17.2**).

Midline cysts generally communicate with the knee joint. Tubercular infection, rheumatoid disorder and osteoarthritis may be the pathology in such cases. Treatment of the causative pathology would diminish the popliteal bulge. If aspiration is performed, the material must be submitted for laboratory investigations.

If the swelling causes appreciable discomfort or the bulge is not acceptable cosmetically surgical excision of the bursa is considered. However, recurrence after excision is also known. A less aggressive approach may be tried by aspiration of the viscous fluid, instillation of local steroids, and a compression bandage for a few days.

Knee Synovial Chondromatosis

This is a rare condition that may develop in any joint. The commonest location is the knee joint. The cells of the synovial membrane undergo metaplastic changes to cartilage cells, which break free to float in the synovial cavity. The cartilaginous loose bodies proliferate, get ossified, become osteocartilaginous and then become visible in the X-rays (**Figs. 17.8A and B**).

Rarely an isolated loose body may be the result of a chip of bone or osteophyte or a piece from osteochondritis dissecans. The usual complaints of articular loose bodies are mechanical symptoms like sudden locking or feeling of loose body popping in and out of the knee joint. The treatment is to remove the loose bodies and remove the abnormal synovial membrane by arthroscopic technique or conventional arthrotomy.

Grossly Destroyed Joints

The usual causes in the Indian-subcontinent are neglected tuberculous or pyogenic arthritis, post-traumatic infections, gross osteoarticular fractures or rheumatoid arthritis. Earlier such patients were treated by arthrodesis following Charnley's principles. Arthrodesis of any major joint, however, leads to symptomatic early degenerative changes in the neighboring joints. Currently, total knee arthroplasty (TKA) also referred to as total knee replacement (TKR) is considered a rational option once the infection has remained healed for 2 years or more **(Fig. 17.9)**. Any operation for healed articular tuberculosis must be done under cover (umbrella) of antitubercular drugs for 4–6 months **(Figs. 17.10A and B)**.

Arthrodesis of hip or knee is now rarely advised because of the availability of arthroplasty procedures. When arthrodesis is being considered the patient should be given the experience of "trial fusion" by encouraging the patient to walk with a hip spica (like hip fusion) or walk with an above knee plaster cast (like knee fusion). This helps the patient to understand what would be the function and limitations after arthrodesis.

HIGH TIBIAL OSTEOTOMY (HTO)

Under a common diagnosis of "osteoarthrosis of knee joints" there are two groups of patients, one best suited for HTO and the other best suited for TKR. It is just natural that there would be a small gray area in between. The patients best suited for HTO are:
- Predominantly medial compartment degeneration
  - At least 100 degrees of flexion-extension range of motion
  - Varus deformity not >20 degrees, fixed flexion deformity not >10 degrees

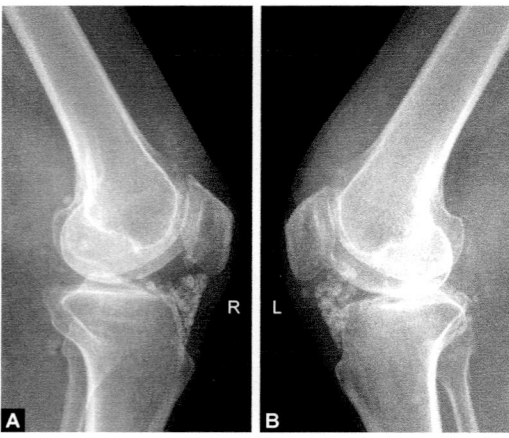

Figs. 17.8A and B: X-rays of knee joints. (A) Right knee and (B) left knee of a patient showing synovial chondromatosis present in both knees.

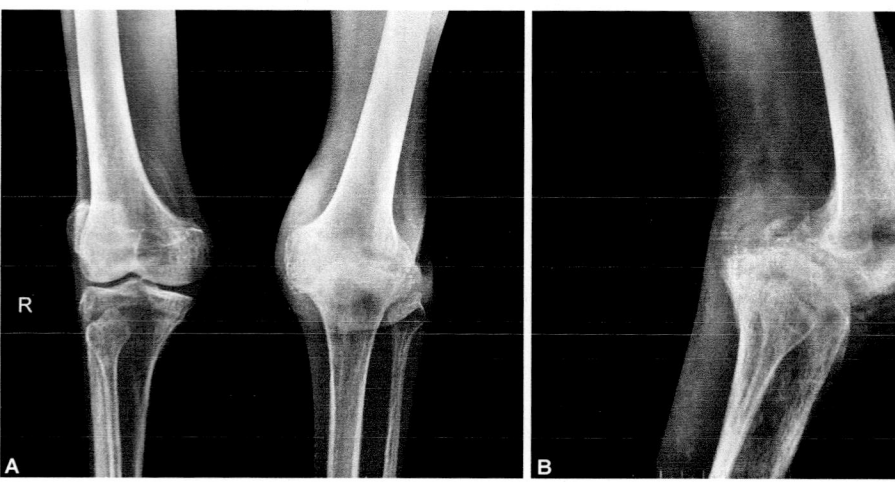

Figs. 17.9A and B: Grossly destroyed left knee joint; Note fixed flexion deformity, posterior and lateral subluxation (triple deformity); when arthrodesis was the standard procedure for such patients. Currently joint replacement is appropriate when infection is healed for more than 2 years.

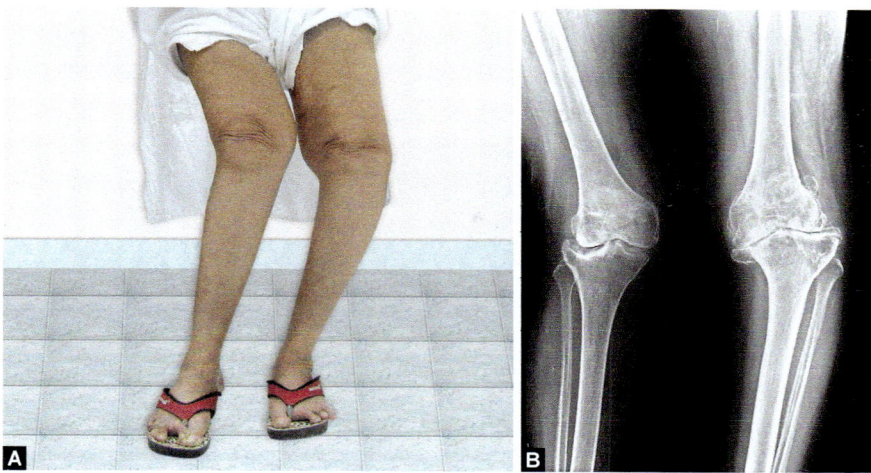

Figs. 17.10A and B: Classical Wind Swept deformity both lower limbs; One can observe valgus in right and varus in left knee; the commonest cause of such deformity is polyarticular rheumatoid arthritis. One can observe deformities of toes of both feet.

- Lateral subluxation (displacement) of tibia not >1 cm
- Weight of the patient within normal limits.

If a patient has to kneel, squat, sit cross-legged, work at farm for livelihood, or he wishes to run, dance and play sports, options of HTO should be seriously considered. If a person is not keen for joint replacement, HTO can be extended to correct a varus deformity of >20 degrees. Correction of such a gross deformity does improve the kinematics of ambulation for a few years, without losing any function at the knee joints.

There are many varieties of osteotomy described and practiced by various authors. The basics, however, are that the line of osteotomy must be proximal to the level of tibial tuberosity. One may use a lateral closing wedge osteotomy, medial open wedge osteotomy, or a dome-shaped osteotomy with convexity toward the joint line. What does HTO aim to do **(Figs. 17.11 and 17.12)**:

- Corrects the varus deformity and over corrects to 7–10 degrees of valgus. Improves the limb alignment for better walking
- In valgus position at knee, the medial compartment (the painful degenrated compartment) gets unloaded. Lateral healthier compartment bears the weight
- Both above would retarded the degeneration process in the joint
- Pain is reduced, movements are maintained and the necessity for replacement is delayed
- A juxta-articular osteotomy hopefully reduces the intraosseous tension and probably increases the blood supply of the osteotomized bones
- After HTO, the patient retains a natural joint (though repaired) which permits higher degree and freedom of activities without the concern of potential wear of arthroplasty components
- Proprioception is retained.

In early cases of genu varum deformity one can try outside (lateral) wedge raise in the heels or as shoe-inserts. While walking, outside raise of the heels almost creats a valgus effect on the upper end of tibia shifting the stress of loading to the lateral compartment (less involved) of knee joint. If patient gets comfort, such a modification can be used for long time.

Best results of HTO are obtained in active patients <50 years of age, having normal

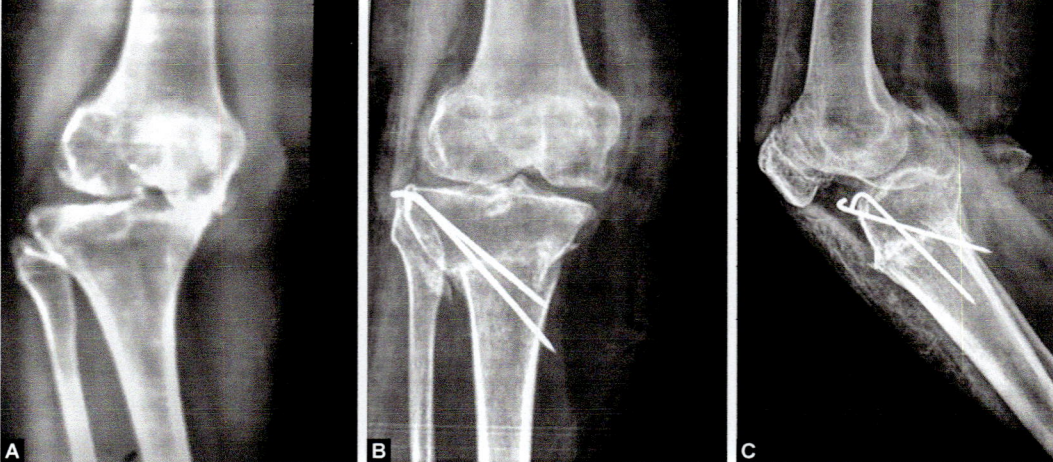

Figs. 17.11A to C: Genu varum (A) with gross reduction of medial joint space; (B and C) X-rays 2 years after high tibial osteotomy show the correction of the deformity and appearance of medial joint space. Note the lateral ledge from the proximal fragment and anteriorly positioned tibial tuberosity.

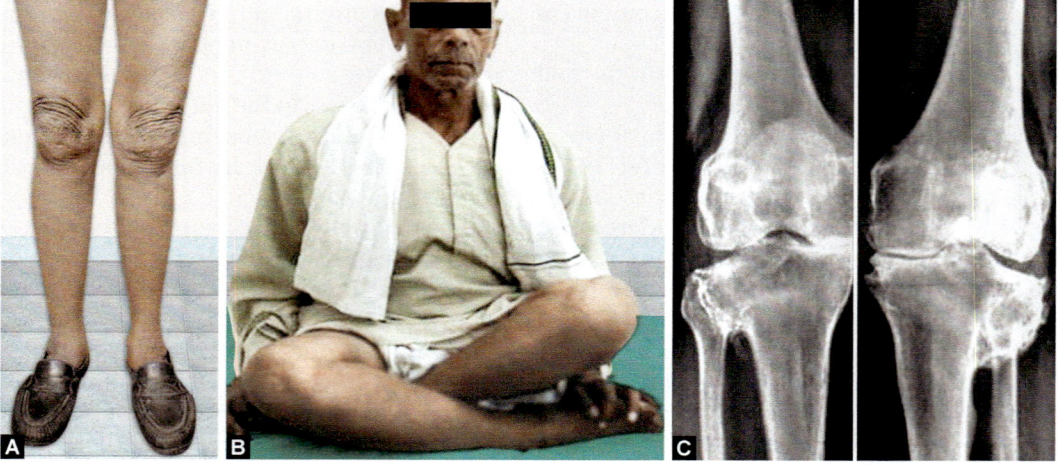

Figs. 17.12A to C: Clinical appearance, function and X-rays of a 70-year-old patient: High tibial osteotomy of both knees follow-up for 12 years (right) and 10 years (left).

weight, fixed flexion deformity at knee <15 degrees, varus deformity <20 degree, and postoperation valgus achieved and maintained was between 8 and 10 degrees.

Significant relief of pain, improvement in walking pattern, preservation of preoperative range of motion, and no restrictions to floor activities are the advantages of this procedure. If performed for correct indications results are satisfactory in >80% at 5 years, about 60% at 10 years and 50% when followed up for >10 years. The author has observed many patients with satisfactory outcome at 15 years after the operation.

There are many techniques of doing high tibial valgus osteotomy. We have been using slight modification of techniques used by Coventry, Slocum and Koshino.

OPERATIVE TECHNIQUES

Keep the knee joint flexed at 90 degrees throughout the operative procedure. Make a curved incision starting from lateral femoral epicondyle touching the upper end of fibula and coming up to the lateral border of tibial tubercle. Lift all the attachments of iliotibial band, lateral head of biceps femoris and lateral collateral ligament from the upper end of fibula, and the origin of tibialis anterior from the upper part of lateral surface of tibia as one continuous flap.

Identify superior tibiofibular articulation, cut about 1 cm of head of fibula and excise the articular surfaces of the tibiofibular joint. While stripping the muscles from the upper part of tibia, insert a pad subperiosteally behind the upper fourth of tibia to protect the major vessels and nerves.

Insert one stout K-wire through the knee joint from lateral to medial side. This represents the level of articular surface of upper end of tibia. The proximal cut of the wedge is made parallel to this K-wire about 1–1.5 cm distal to the joint line by gentle cutting using multiple drill holes and small osteotomes. The distal cut is made in an oblique fashion (starting about 2.5–3.5 cm distal to the first cut) from lateral to medial side upwards to meet the first cut on the medial side. The intervening wedge-shaped bone can be removed, osteotomy completed with gentle pressure to obtain the desired corrected position of about 8–10 degrees of valgus, about 5 degrees of external rotation and about 5 mm of anteriorly positioned tibial tubercle (distal fragment).

Over the years we have been using a modified lateral closing wedge osteotomy as follows: (1) The proximal cut made parallel to the joint line osteotomizes only the anterior half of the tibia; (2) The distal osteotomy cuts the whole width of tibia proximal to the tibial tubercle to meet the proximal cut on the medial aspect of tibia; (3) A third cut is a vertical osteotomy through the middle of lateral surface of the exposed tibia connecting the first and second cuts; (4) Remove the wedge-shaped bone (composed of the anterior half of tibia) between the 3 osteotomy cuts deep to the ligamentum patellae; (5) Complete the osteotomy by gentle force; (6) Enucleate a few mm of cancellous bone from the lateral ledge of the proximal fragment and the anterior surface of its posterior ledge; (7) A small ledge (5–8 mm) of cortical bone of proximal fragment is thus created laterally and posteriorly; (8) The distal fragment (after the completion of osteotomy) is gently telescoped to fit in the proximal fragment within the lateral and posterior ledges; (9) The distal fragment of tibia is now held in the best corrected position (8–10 degrees of valgus, 5 degrees of external rotation and about 5 mm of anterior transposition of the distal fragment) and transfixed with 2 or 3 stout K-wires; (10) All the bone collected from the excision of superior tibiofibular joint, wedge of bone from anterior tibia and enucleated cancellous bone is packed around the osteotomy site. The limb is supported in a plaster cast after the wound closure.

Osteotomy generally unites by 3–4 months when plaster is removed, knee exercises are started and normal loading is encouraged.

Alternative techniques: Recently there has been a surge for correcting the deformity by medial opening wedge osteotomy of tibia. This is because of development of strong fixation devices. This, however, involves extended operative procedures, necessity of bone grafts and more elaborate fixation devices, it may have more complications and failures thus making it less attractive in places with moderate infrastructure facilities **(Figs. 17.13 and 17.14)**.

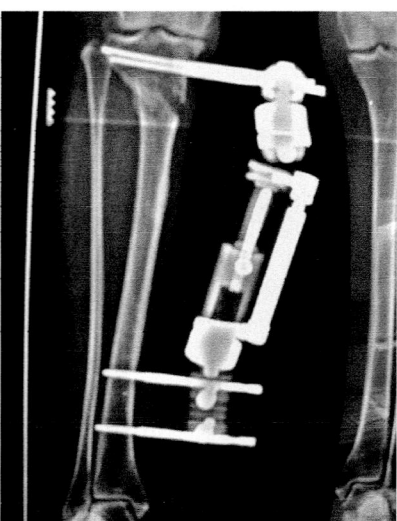

Fig. 17.13: Medial open-wedge high tibial osteotomy: External fixation device is used here to achieve the desired correction.

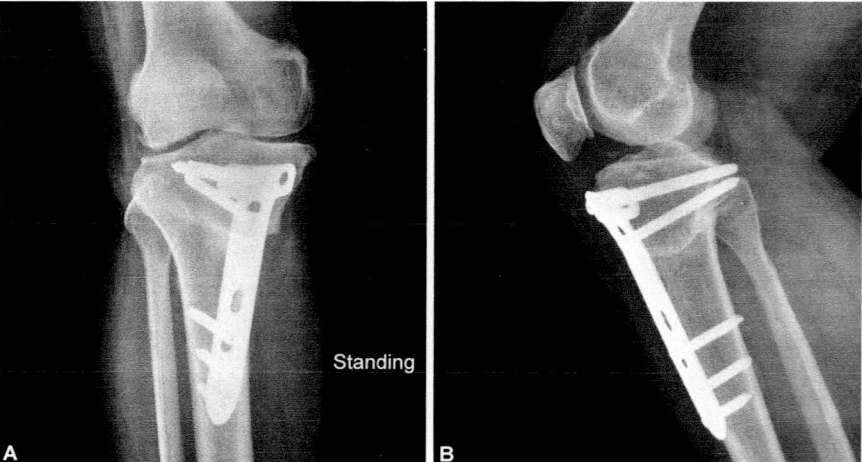

Figs. 17.14A and B: Medial open-wedge high tibial osteotomy: Blade-plate fixation is used here to achieve the desired correction.

SUGGESTED READINGS

1. Coventry MB. Upper tibial osteotomy. Clin Orthop Relat Res. 1983;182:46-52.
2. Illizarov GA. Clinical application of the tension-stress effects for limb lengthening. Clin Orthop Relat Res. 1990;250:8-26.
3. Virolainen P, Aro HT. High tibial osteotomy for the treatment of osteoarthritis of the knee: A review of the literature and meta-analysis of follow-up studies. Arch Orthop Trauma Surg. 2004;124(4): 258-61.

4. Brinkman JM, Lobenhoffer P, Agneskirchner JD, Staublic AE, Wymenga AB, Heerwaarden RJ. Osteotomies around the knee: Patient selection, stability of fixation and bone healing in high tibial osteotomies. J Bone Joint Surg. 2008;90B:1548-57.
5. Sabharwal S. Blount disease. J Bone Joint Surg. 2009;91A:1758-76.
6. Portner O. High tibial vagus osteotomy: closing, opening or combined? Patellar height as a determining factor. Clin Orthop Relat Res. 2014; 472:3432-40.
7. Thorlund JB, Juhl CB, Roos EM, Lohmander LS. Arthroscopic surgery for degenerative knee: systemic review and meta-analysis of benefits and harms. BMJ. 2015;350:h2747.
8. Mc Clelland D, Barlow D, Moores TS, Wynn-Jones C, Griffiths D, Ogrodnik PJ, et al. Medium- and long-term results of high tibial osteotomy using Graches external fixator and gait analysis for dynamic correction in varus osteoarthritis of the knee. Bone Joint J. 2016;98B:601-7.
9. Nerhus TK, Ekeland A, Solberg G, Olsen BH, Madsen JE, Heir S. No difference in time-dependent improvement in functional outcome following closing wedge versus opening wedge high tibial osteotomy: a randomised controlled trial with two-year follow-up. Bone Joint J. 2017;99B: 1157-66.

CHAPTER 18

Ankle and Foot

ANKLE

For all clinical purposes, the ankle and foot work as a single functional unit. Any pathology of osteoarticular system can present in an ankle and foot. Besides a traumatic condition, common affections for which a patient would seek an orthopedic advice are osteoarthrosis (as a sequel of old fracture or osteonecrosis of talus), neurovascular complications associated with diabetes and peripheral vascular disease, rheumatoid disorder, infective lesions and Charcot's neuroarthropathy. After clinical examination of other extremities, ask for X-rays of both ankles in anteroposterior and lateral projections in identical position.

Stress fracture (fatigue fracture): Rarely some patients may present with pain in the distal part of leg or foot without any history of trauma. The pain may be result of a "stress fracture" in newly recruited soldiers, nurses or ballet dancers. Usual fracture line is present in the distal fourth of tibia or in metatarsal bones (commonest second metatarsal). Plain X-rays may show a transverse defect with localized subperiosteal reaction about 2–3 weeks after the fracture. In difficult presentations radio scintigraphy (Tc-99m bone scan) would show increased up-take at a very early stage.

Standard treatment for specific conditions and comorbidities is essential. Once the primary condition has healed, active exercises, suitable orthosis, or boots and anti-inflammatory drugs would make the patient comfortable for normal activities. Rarely removal of impinging osteophytes on the anterior lip of distal tibia or from the neck of talus and loose bodies may require removal for disabling mechanical symptoms. When the pain is very severe arthrodesis of ankle may be considered. Postoperatively (after arthrodesis), there is no difficulty in using normal shoes; running may be difficult and ladies who wish to wear heels of varying height may not be comfortable. Ankle joint replacement at present is not as successful as those for hip and knee. Attempted arthrodesis of ankle for Charcot's condition as a rule fails **(Figs. 18.1 and 18.2)**.

FOOT

A significant number of people in the Indian subcontinent have been walking bare feet. This has a mixed blessing—the feet are more exposed to injury and infection and on the other hand the Indian feet have retained suppleness of the joints, and the intrinsic muscle power for better grip on the ground during walking. Some of the common disorders are described as follows:

Diabetic Foot

Diabetes mellitus is a very common disorder, affecting nearly 15% of people in the Indian subcontinent. Most of the patients presenting with foot complications have a long standing disease and belong to lower socioeconomic group. The predisposing factors are peripheral vascular disease, peripheral neuropathy, poor immunity and osteoporosis caused by poorly controlled diabetes. Nearly 30% patients of diabetes show clinical evidence of neuropathy and peripheral vascular disease.

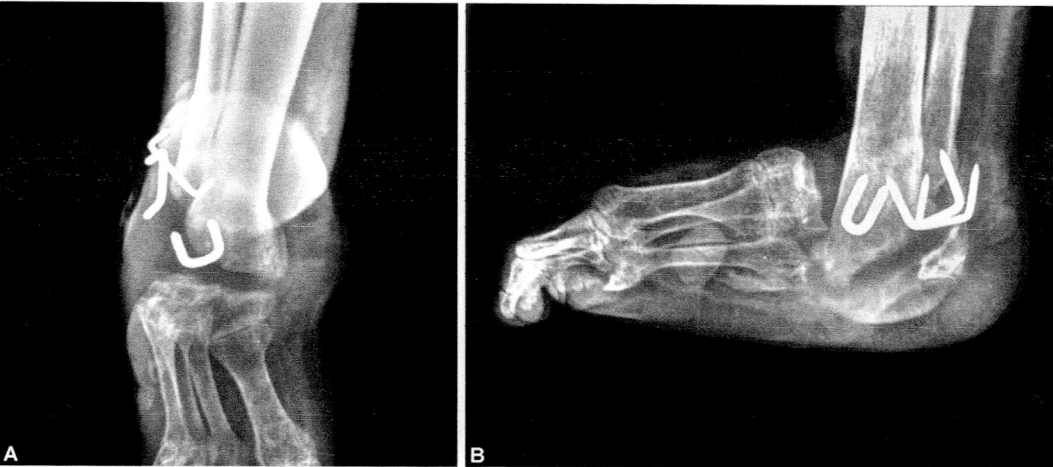

Figs. 18.1A and B: Charcot's arthropathy: Gross erosion and disruption of the joints of ankle and foot. X-rays show the failure of an attempted arthrodesis, the usual feature of an attempted fusion.

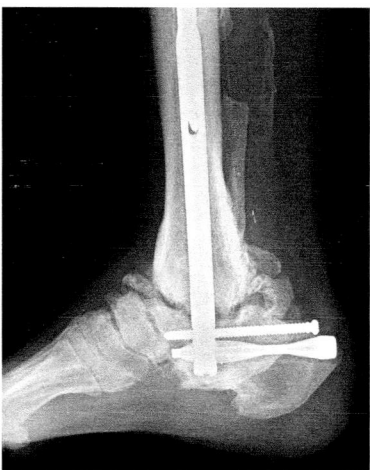

Fig. 18.2: Another patient of Charcot's arthropathy of ankle joint showing failure of attempted pantalar fusion.

Diabetic feet may develop Charcot's joint (neuroarthropathy) which may have pain in initial stages, however gradually the bones and articular surfaces undergo destruction, disorganization, panarticular debris, and collapse with gross abnormal painless movements of ankle and foot. Neuroarthropathic changes are caused by repetitive micro-trauma in feet with impaired sensations (insensate feet) and pathological neurovascular changes. The incidence of Charcot's neuropathic feet is increasing with rising incidence of diabetes.

The patients may present with swelling of foot and ankle, claudication on walking and ulceration on the sole of the feet and toes. The feet are colder than the uninvolved parts, dorsalis pedis and posterior tibial arterial pulsations are weak or absent. There may be dry gangrene of one or more toes or there may be more serious wet gangrene. X-rays may show calcification of arteries.

Treatment

Treatment of a diabetic foot should be essentially on conservative lines because of poor circulation. Drainage and debridement of abscesses, and dressing of ulcers may save the foot.

Patient may need amputations of gangrenous toes, or rays, or at midfoot level or Syme's amputations, thus one may be able to save a part of the foot for ambulation without prosthetic appliance. This is worth trying if at least one of the arteries is clinically capable (dorsalis pedis or posterior tibial artery), however if none of these arteries is clinically palpable and the circulation is poor, one has to resort to amputation at a higher level. It is mandatory to inform the patient and the family that the patient may need an amputation at a more proximal level if the distal level amputation does not succeed. At present it is advised to have a team approach to take care of diabetic state, neuropathy, vasculopathy, immunopathy and rehabilitation.

Gout

The incidence of symptomatic gout varies from one to 10 per thousand depending upon the ethnicity, age, and sex of the population. It is much commoner in Caucasian than in Negroid people, more widespread in men than in women, and it is rarely seen in premenopausal females. It is a disorder of purine metabolism characterized by hyperuricemia, and deposition of urate crystals in joints, periarticular, and connective tissues, resulting in recurrent attacks of pain in joints. In cases of long standing there may be added degenerative changes in joint, renal dysfunction and uric acid urolithiasis. Clinical symptoms are generally related to increasing serum uric acid levels, however one should be aware of asymptomatic persons with high serum uric acid levels.

Commonest symptoms sites are metatarsophalangeal joint of great toes and other small joints of feet and hands. With passage of time the urate deposits build up symptoms in periarticular tissues, tendons, bursae and pinnae of the ears. The clinical symptoms of gout may increase with existence of concomitant secondary factors such as obesity, alcohol abuse, hemolytic disorders, neoplasia, high consumption of red meat.

Acute gout attacks: There is sudden severe pain in the joint with swelling and shiny overlying skin, the joint on palpation is hot and extremely tender almost suggesting cellulitis. Hyperuricemia may be present at some stages (not necessarily during acute attacks).

Recurrent acute attacks may eventually evolve into "chronic gout" with polyarticular involvement, having chronic pains, stiffness and deformities not unlike rheumatoid arthritis. Tophi may appear around the joint, extensor aspects of elbow, in the pinnae of ears and any other place **(Figs. 18.3A and B)**.

Investigation

X-rays during acute gout may show soft tissue swelling around the joint. In chronic cases the picture resembles that of any arthritides.

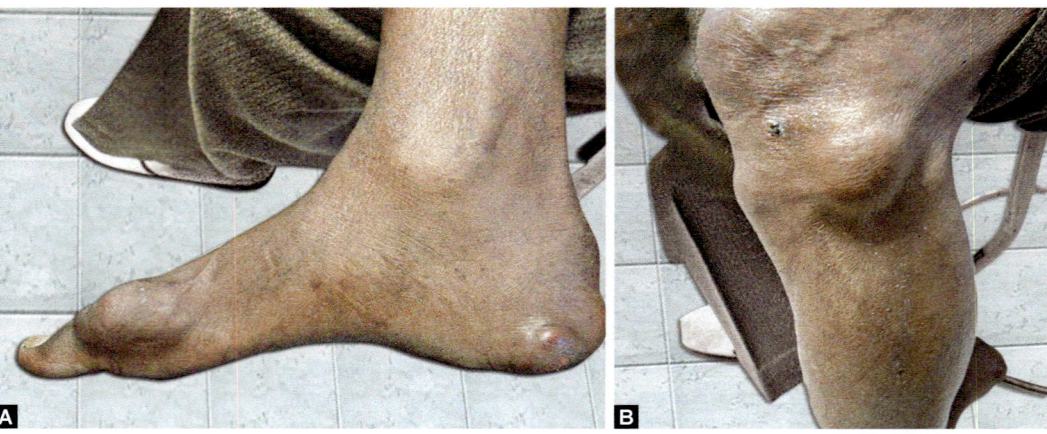

Figs. 18.3A and B: Gouty tophus creating swollen great toe in a male is a typical clinical presentation. Tophi in this patient were present at other places like medial side of heel and near the upper end of fibula (tophaceous gout).

Punched out cystic erosions caused by tophi in the para-articular bone ends is almost characteristic of gout.

Diagnosis is established by obtaining material by aspiration of the involved joint or tophi or synovial tissue, which may exhibit birefringent sodium urate crystals by special staining. Any arthritides or infection must be considered in differential diagnosis. Serum uric acid level is considered normal upto 6 mg/dL, higher levels suggest gout disorder, however the level may be normal even in a typical case of gout.

Treatment

When hyperuricemia is pronounced (greater than 9.0–10.0 mg/dL) preventive treatment is rational irrespective of clinical symptoms. In asymptomatic people with moderate hyperuricemia aggressive treatment is not warranted, however lifestyle modifications must be adhered to such as reduction of body weight, and reduction of intake of high-fructose foods, alcohol and red-meat.

Acute gouty attacks are treated by NSAIDs, steroids, colchicine or indomethacin. For long-term management uricosuric agents (probenecid, sulphinpyrazone or allopurinol) are recommended with careful monitoring of side effects. Rarely one may need to excise or curet out the gouty tophi.

Painful Heel

It is one of the common presenting complaints in young or middle-aged persons. Pain presenting on the plantar aspect is called plantar fasciitis (old term—calcaneal spur). The pain may present in one or both heels, typically the pain is worst early in the morning when the patient leaves his bed. The morning pain resolves with activity within 10–20 minutes.

There is tenderness over the medial tuberosity of calcaneum. History may reveal associated manifestations like tennis elbow, tenosynovitis or pains of rheumatoid disorder. Radiographs may show varying degrees of spur on the plantar aspect of calcaneum. The patient, however, must be counseled that size of radiological spur is not proportional to the symptoms. Even big spurs may be as symptomatic, and the local symptoms may be severe without any visible spur. The calcaneal pain is considered to be due to inflammation of the plantar fascia at its attachment to the plantar aspect of calcaneum.

Treatment

The condition responds to conservative measures like anti-inflammatory drugs, stretching exercises of feet and ankles. The patient has a big role in its management. A course of local ultrasonic therapy, a foam heel pad may help. In a person not responding to above modalities, local steroid infiltration may be useful. Avoid injection into the substance of tendo-Achilles to prevent post-injection rupture of the tendon.

Posterior Heel Pain

In adolescents, osteochondritis of the calcaneal apophysis would present as pain and tenderness, localized to tendo-Achilles insertion. Gentle exercises, about one cm raise in heel and relative rest to strenuous activities for a few weeks, would resolve the symptoms. In young adults, tendo-Achilles bursa may be inflamed and cause pain and tenderness at the insertion of tendon.

Similar symptoms usually in middle-aged people may be caused by retro-calcaneal calcification. X-rays would show calcific deposits deep to the insertion of tendo-Achilles. The treatment should be conservative; active stretching exercises, comfortable footwear and foam heel pad would help most of the patients.

Pain in the medial or lateral side of the plantar aspect of heel may be due to old fracture of calcaneum, subtaloid arthritis, tumors or infections. It must be remembered that local symptoms and disorders may be part of generalized disease like rheumatoid disorder, diabetes, peripheral neuropathy and peripheral vascular disease. All of them would need specific treatment.

Flat Foot

Longitudinal arches and transverse arches of the foot are formed by the shape and articulations of tarsal bones, held together by the strong plantar and spring ligaments, but the maintenance of the arches depends upon the tone and power of intrinsic (small) muscles and long muscles, especially the tibialis posterior. The feet of all newborn babies are flat. The arches develop as the child starts walking **(Figs. 18.4A and B)**.

Most of the flat feet are supple and nonsymptomatic. However, if a patient presents for the treatment, exercises for strengthening of muscles of feet, stretching exercises of toes, feet, and ankles, walking on tip-toes, on heel, and on outer border of feet should be encouraged. Flat feet shoes or shoe-inserts may help the patient. Rarely for very painful flat feet associated with subtaloid arthrosis, or coalition of tarsal bones, fusion of the subtaloid joint may be advised.

Rocker Bottom Foot

Clinically the foot looks flat with eversion and valgus deformity, the heel is in equines, the examination of sole shows convexity. This deformity is a congenital defect where the talus is directed vertically (congenital vertical talus) towards the sole and navicular is dislocated dorsal-wards riding over the talus head. This is best appreciated in the lateral X-rays of the foot taken in maximum plantar flexion **(Fig. 18.5)**.

Pes Cavus (High-arched Feet) (Fig. 18.6A and B)

The arch of sole is higher than normal and often there is clawing of toes. Almost all cases of pes cavus are due to some sort of muscle imbalance caused by neuropathies, spinal cord abnormalities, cerebral palsy,

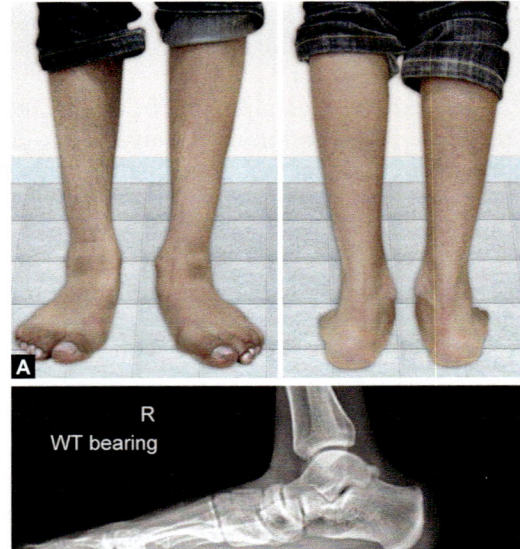
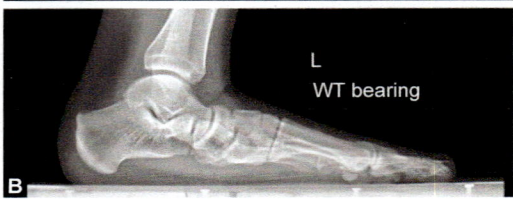

Figs. 18.4A and B: In (A) patient with flat feet (B) weight-bearing X-rays would reveal loss of the longitudinal arc; one can appreciate the plano-valgus feet while looking from behind and front.

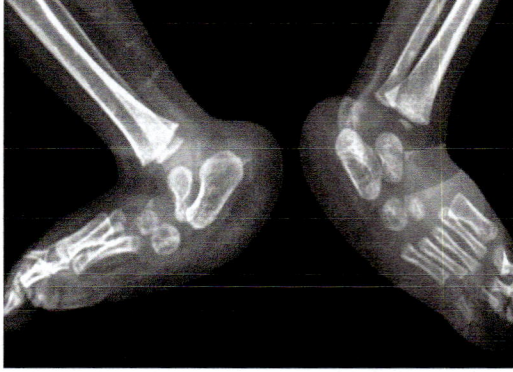

Fig.18.5: A typical case of congenital vertical talus. Comparison with the normal foot shows plantar-wards tilting of the talus, and dorsal dislocation of the navicular bone in right foot.

congenital talipes equinovarus, poliomyelitis and arthrogryposis. Occasionally, deformities may follow trauma like burns and compartment syndrome. Treatment of the basic cause may help to reduce the symptoms.

Foot Drop

The commonest cause of foot drop is paralysis of dorsiflexors of foot and ankle. The paralysis may be caused by post-polio residual paralysis, leprosy involving common peroneal (lateral popliteal) nerve, acute injury to lateral popliteal nerve, pressure by plaster casts, fracture around the neck of fibula, prolonged pressure by any hard structure (unpadded splint) when the leg is lying in rolled-out position. Any lesion of the sciatic nerve, prolapsed disc at the lower lumbar level (lumbar 4 to sacral one), cauda equina syndrome may also present with foot drop. Muscular dystrophy and peripheral neuropathy due to any pathology may also produce a foot drop. The treatment is directed to the causative pathology. A foot drop appliance and exercises are advised pending the recovery of foot drop.

Pes Equinus

Common causes of equinus foot are cerebral palsy, post-polio-residual paralysis (unopposed action of plantar flexors in the presence of weak dorsiflexors), contracture of calf muscles following local inflammatory or infective or ischemic processes. Rarely the equinus deformity may be compensatory to short lower limb. Fixed deformity is corrected by tendo-Achilles lengthening if the dorsiflexors have good power. In rigid deformities of long-standing, in adult patients in addition to soft tissue release bony procedures like triple arthrodesis, pantalar arthrodesis or subtaloid arthrodesis with appropriate wedge resection of bones may be needed to hold the foot in corrected position **(Fig. 18.7)**.

Hallux Valgus

Acquired form of hallux valgus is a common deformity in the Western countries due to the wearing of tight fitting narrow toes shoes. The great toe is turned laterally at the metatarsophalangeal joints. In a congenital variety, the hallux valgus is also associated with adduction varus deformity of the first metatarsal bone (metatarsus primus varus). A mild deformity does not cause any symptoms. Even in severe deformities (>30 degrees of valgus), surgical correction only for cosmetic purposes is not usually advised **(Fig. 18.8)**. When the deformity

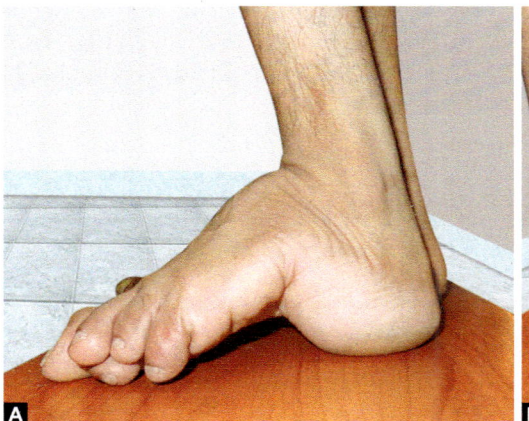
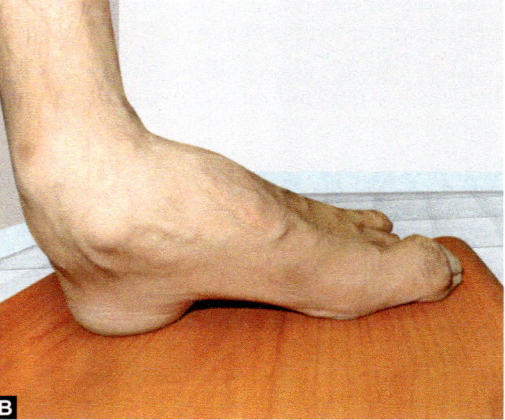

Figs. 18.6A and B: Deformities of foot: A case of post-polio residual paralysis (PPRP) showing, pes calcaneus, pes cavus, pes calcaneovalgus. Such deformities (with sensate feet) are correctable by suitable operations.

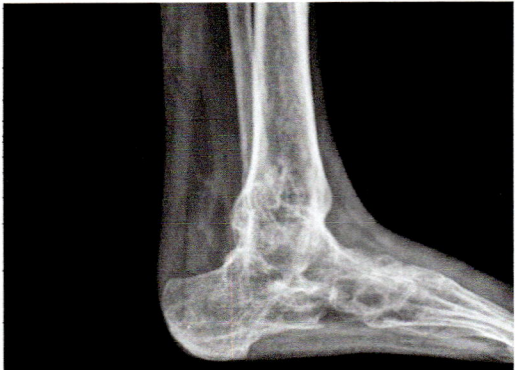

Fig. 18.7: Plantar arthrodesis: As seen in this X-ray. It is a rational operation for flail ankle or grossly destroyed ankle and tarsal joints. Walking is almost normal, however there is difficulty in running and wearing high heels.

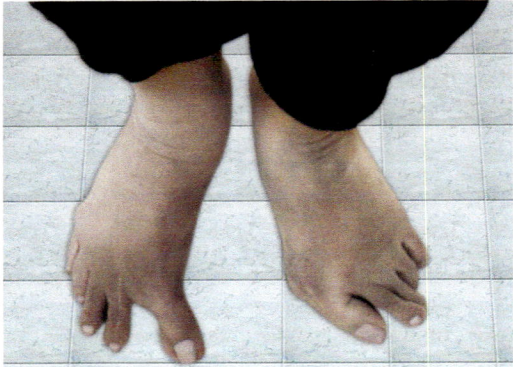

Fig. 18.8: Clinical picture of a patient showing hallux valgus in left foot and hallux varus in right foot.

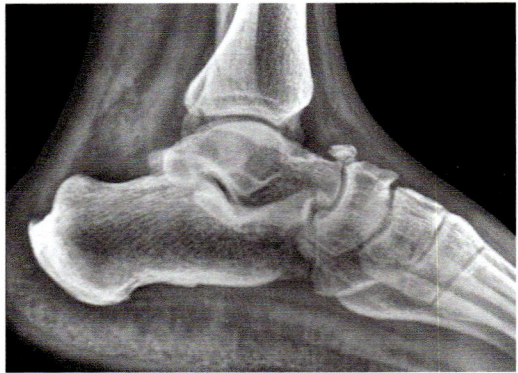

Fig. 18.9: X-ray showing "over-bone" or a bump on the dorsum of foot.

is severe, the head of the first metatarsal projects medially, a bursa develops over the prominence which may form a thick bunion and lead to frequent bursitis. The lateral deviation of the great toe leads to crowding and overriding of the lateral toes. Gross deformities are then associated with painful forefoot and metatarsalgia. Severe deformities need surgical correction of bony deformities, debridement of bunion and postoperative retention of correction using 2 or more Kirschner wires and corrective plaster boot for about one month.

Hallux varus is an extremely rare deformity and surgical correction is advised, for the patient to enable him to wear a shoe.

"**Over-bone**" or a bump may be present on the dorsal aspect of foot due to osteoarthrosis of intertarsal joints, excision may be needed if it interferes with footwear **(Fig. 18.9)**. A spur from the back of talus is addressed as "trigonal process".

SUGGESTED READINGS

1. Ponseti IV, Zhivkov M, Davis N, Sinclair M, Dobbs MB, Morcuende JAs. Treatment of the complex idiopathic clubfoot. Clin Orthop Relat Res. 2006;451:171-6.
2. Lee KB, Cho NY, Park HW, Seon JK, Lee SH. A comparison of proximal and distal Chevron osteotomy, both with lateral soft-tissue release, for moderate to severe hallux valgus in patients undergoing simultaneous bilateral correction: A prospective randomised controlled trial. Bone Joint J. 2015;97B:202-7.
3. Trieb K. The Charcot foot: Pathophysiology, diagnosis and classification. Bone Joint J. 2016;98B;1157-9.

CHAPTER 19

Atlas of Rare Conditions
(One may Encounter through the Journey in Orthopedics)

Collated by D Mohapatra

X-RAYS OF PELVIS REFLECT GENERAL HEALTH OF THE SKELETON

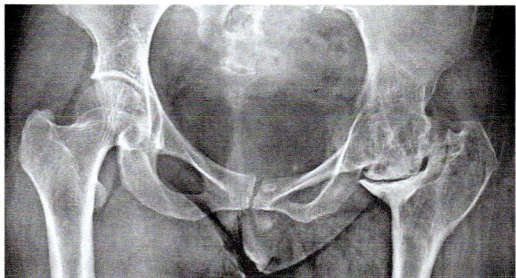

Fig. 19.1: An unusual X-ray of left hip joint: Probably the patient had a pathological fracture through an ankylosed hip joint. The patient could manage walking through the fracture site, thus remodeling the unusual way; the acetabular contents formed a rounded "ball" and upper end of the femur formed a "cup" shaped appearance.

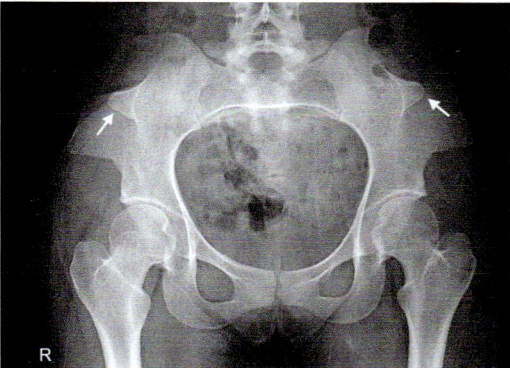

Fig. 19.2: Iliac Horn or Pelvic Horns Incidence: About one in five crore population. May be associated with Nail–Patella Syndrome.

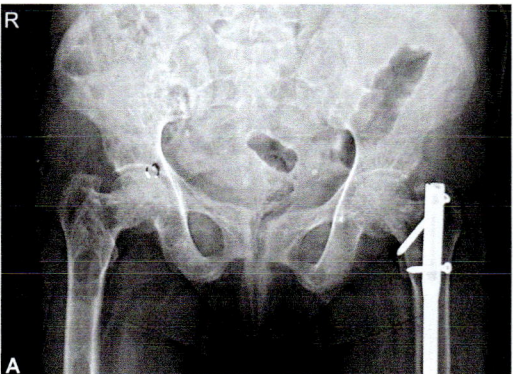
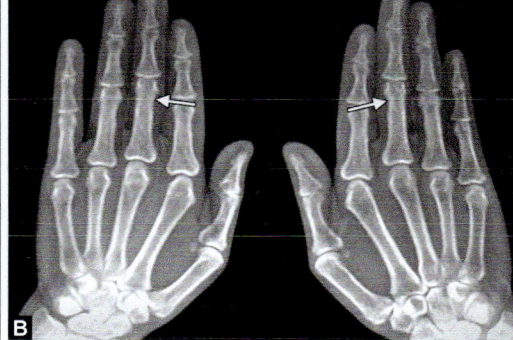

Figs. 19.3A to C: Hyperparathyroidism: *Continued*

Continued

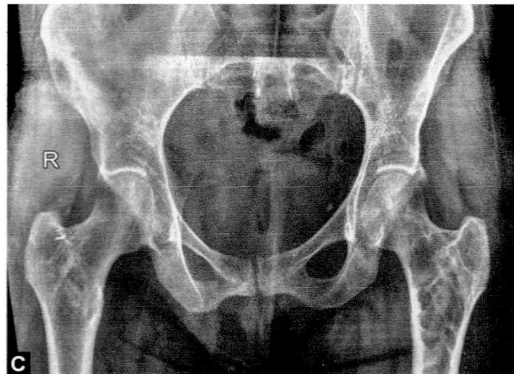

Figs. 19.3A to C: Hyperparathyroidism: (A) This is a condition in which there is an excessive amount of parathormone in the blood, owing to parathyroid gland hyperplasia or adenoma. There is generalized decalcification and softening of skeleton resulting in fractures and cystic changes in the bones (brown tumor); (B) Subperiosteal cortical resorption of the middle phalanges is often visualized; (C) An other patient of hyperparathyroidism showing multiple cystic changes in the bones.

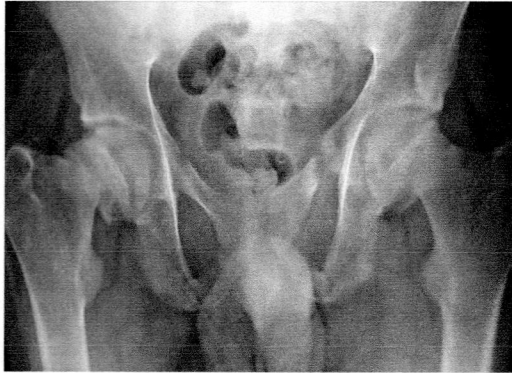

Fig. 19.4: Hypophosphatemic osteomalacia: This is an extremely rare variety of osteomalacia. One can see Looser's zones and pathological fractures in the pelvic bones. Investigations show deficiency of circulating alkaline phosphatase and phosphates. Three forms are known: Infantile (severest), childhood and adult. Early loss of teeth is a common feature.

CHAPTER 19: Atlas of Rare Conditions (One may Encounter through the Journey in Orthopedics)

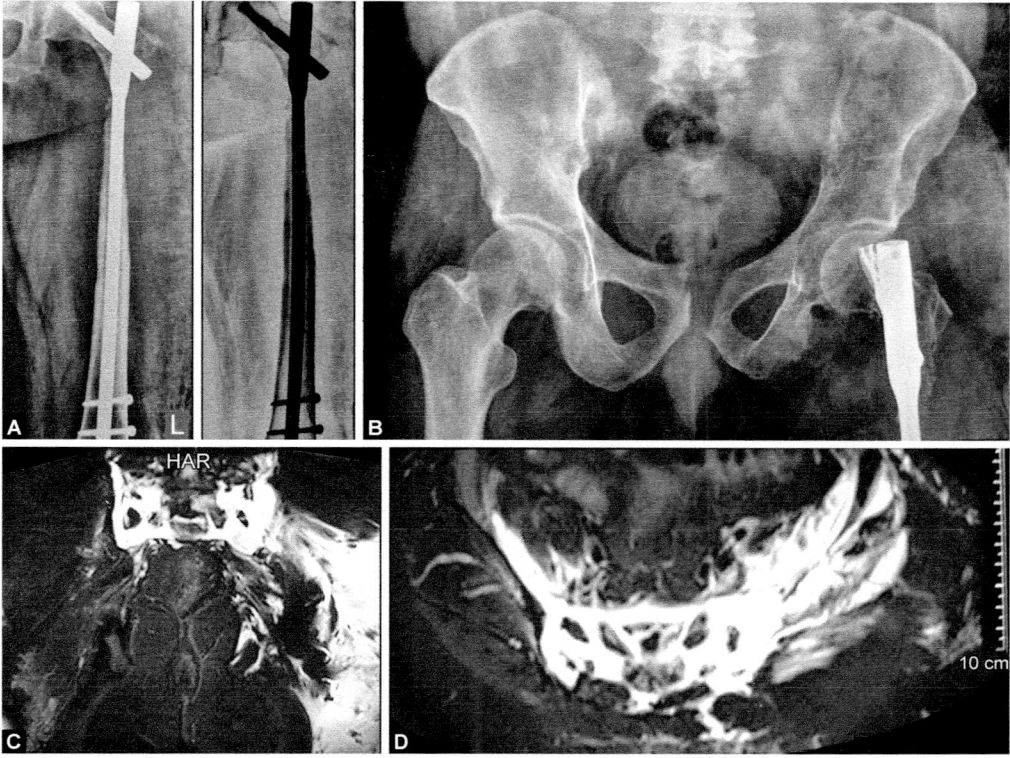

Figs. 19.5A to D: Disappearing bone disease (Gorham syndrome, idiopathic massive osteolysis): After intramedullary rod fixation for a femoral fracture in this young man, there was a gradual resorption of the upper half of femur (A), during next 3 years of follow-up the sacrum and left pelvis has also undergone resorption (B to D). The course of this condition is unpredictable. MRI of the pelvis (C and D) shows abnormal signals in the sacrum, left pelvis and surrounding soft tissues.

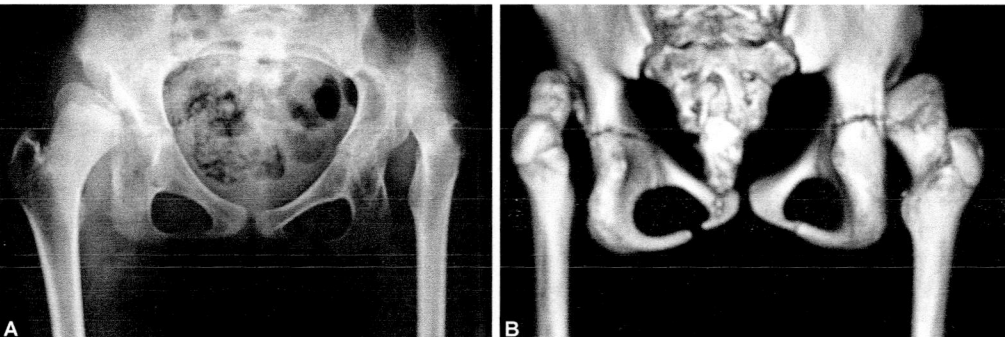

Figs. 19.6A and B: Congenital dislocation of both hips (presenting at 9 years of age): One can appreciate the upward displacement of both femoral heads and poorly developed acetabulum and pelvis bones.

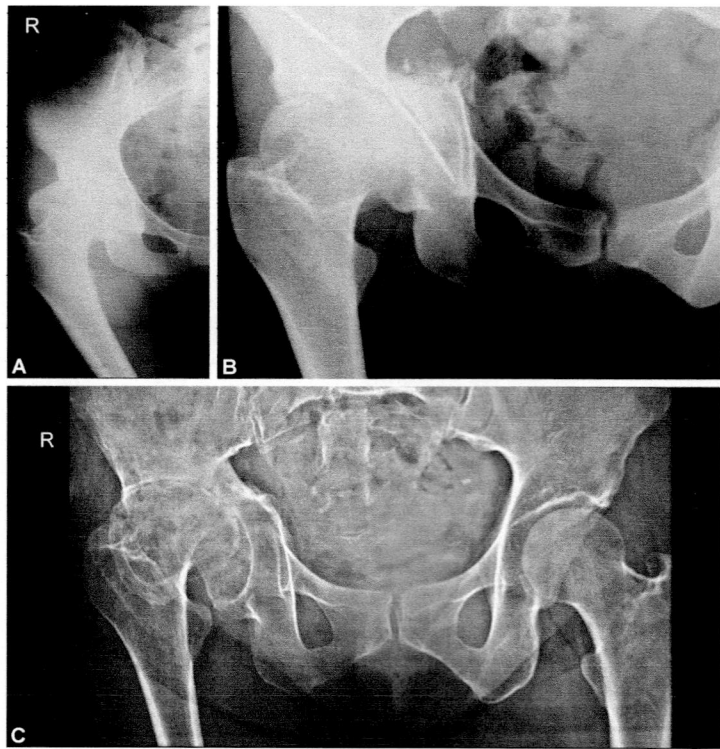

Figs. 19.7A to C: Massive coxa-magna: The patient presented at 22 years of age with pain in her right hip. Chiari displacement osteotomy provided coverage to the head, she managed her activities of daily life up to 46 years when she reported for further management. Common pathology behind large coxa-magna in the Indian subcontinent would be tuberculosis or low-grade infection.

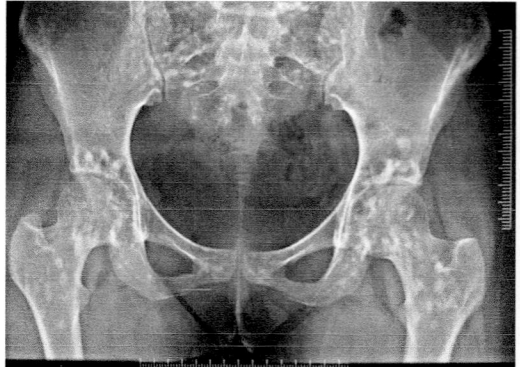

Fig. 19.8: Osteopoikilosis: Spotted bone disease—it is a benign condition inherited and transmitted as an autosomal dominant disorder. Because this condition is symptomless, it is usually discovered by chance on an X-ray. One can see many focal sclerotic spots or densities in the metaphyses and diaphysis of bones (spotted and stippled appearance).

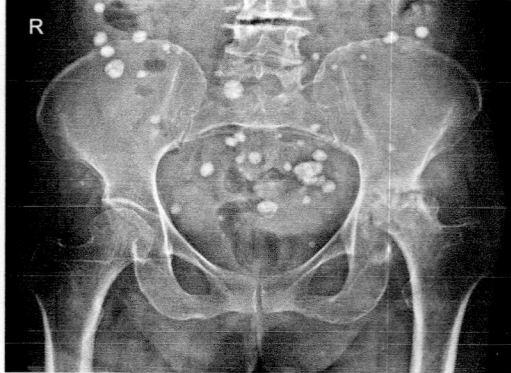

Fig. 19.9: Calcified lymph nodes; observed within the abdominal cavity of a patient who had tuberculosis of left hip joint.

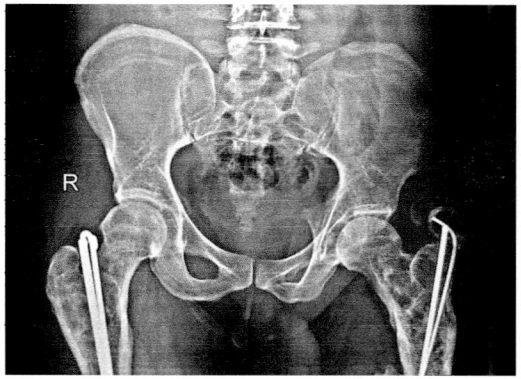

Fig. 19.10: Possible effect of bisphosphonates: This patient was given multiple cycles of bisphosphonates between the age of 12–23 years while undergoing treatment for polyostotic fibrous dysplasia. This X-ray of pelvis shows multiple layers of inhibited resorption (turnover) of bone probably corresponding to some cycles of treatment.

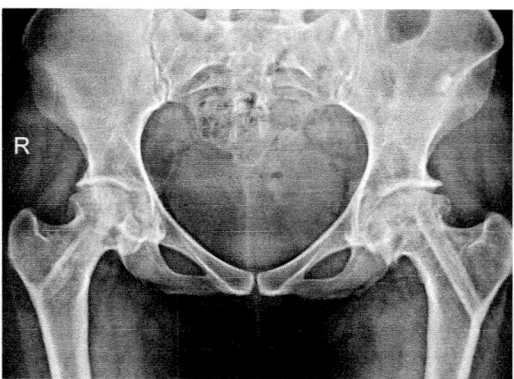

Fig. 19.11: Cortical bone-grafts: Autogenous fibular grafts used to treat bilateral femoral head osteonecrosis. Age at operation was 19 years, part of fibular grafts are still visible 18 years after the operation.

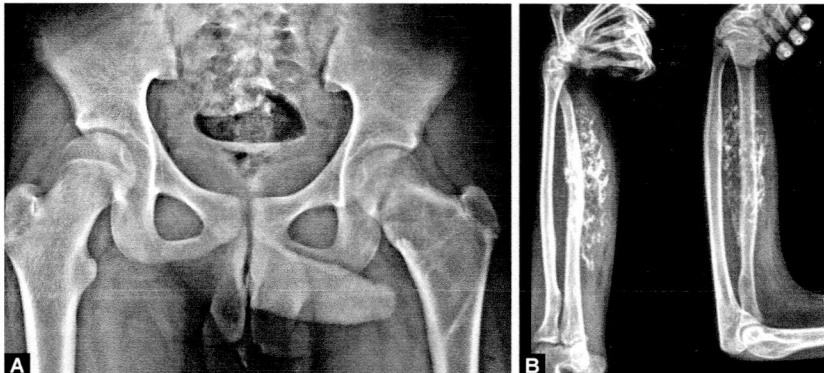

Figs. 19.12A to D: Aneurysmal bone cyst. *Continued*

Continued

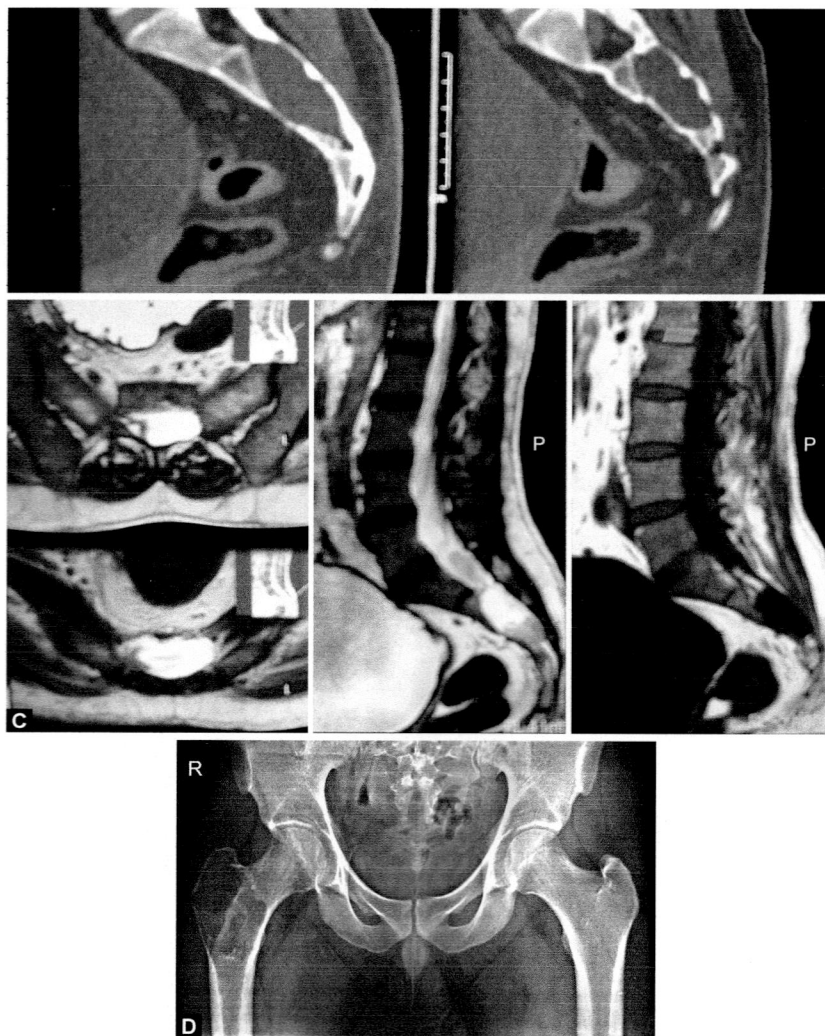

Figs. 19.12A to D: Aneurysmal bone cyst-atypical (ABC) locations: (A) Femoral head; (B) Radial diaphysis; (C) Sacrum; In 20% patients, the ABC may have another concomitant pathology. The ABC in the right greater trochanter was associated with giant-cell-tumor (D).

CHAPTER 19: Atlas of Rare Conditions (One may Encounter through the Journey in Orthopedics)

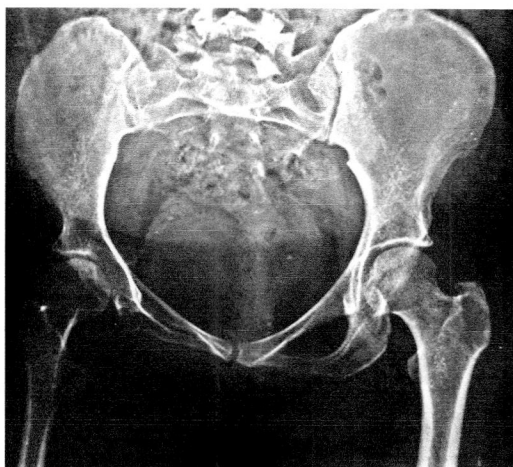

Fig. 19.13: Function determines form: The X-Ray of pelvis shows a hypoplastic right pelvis and right femur. The patient has managed to be a walker despite having post-polio-residual paralysis of right lower limb.

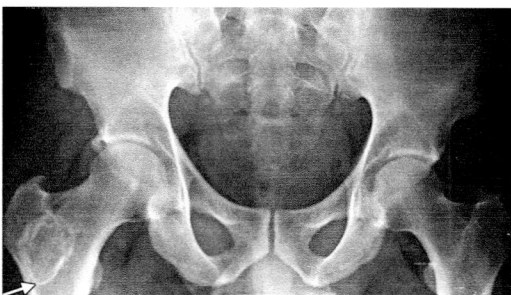

Fig. 19.14: An unusual case of large (resolving) inostosis in right trochanteric area

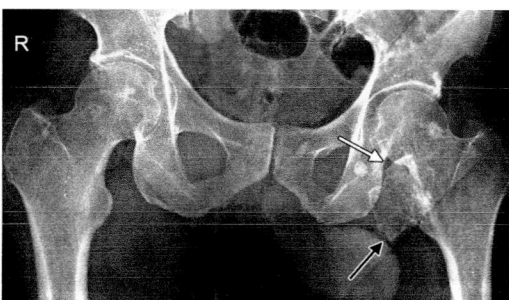

Fig. 19.15: An isolated sessile osteochondroma from the medial side of left femoral neck.

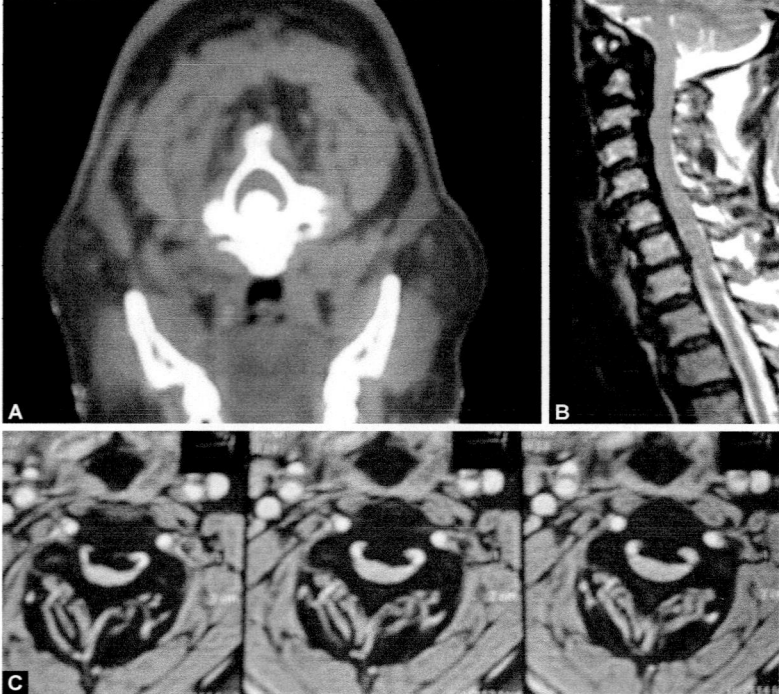

Figs. 19.16A to C: Ossification of posterior longitudinal ligament (OPLL): The figures show the OPLL in axial view; the cross-sections show the encroachment of the vertebral canal compressing the dural contents from front, almost the whole cervical spine is affected.

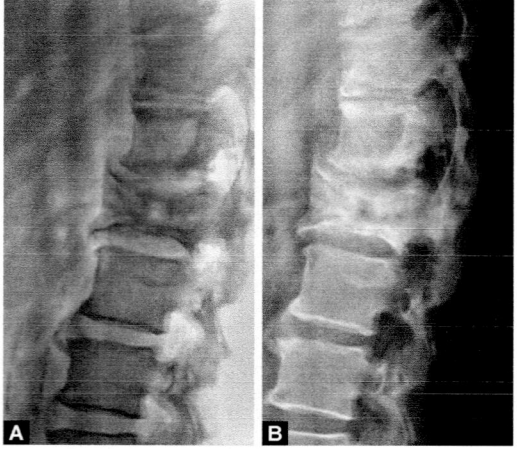

Figs. 19.17A and B: Paget's disease: Caused by disbalance in osteoclast and osteoblast activity, the bone thus formed is disorganized, has increased density and number of cement lines that gives a mosaic appearance in X-rays. Currently virus as a causative agent is being discussed. These X-rays are showing the involvement of two lumbar vertebrae. This patient has been on short courses of bisphosphonates, in a pulse mode, the disease has remained static for the last 10 years.

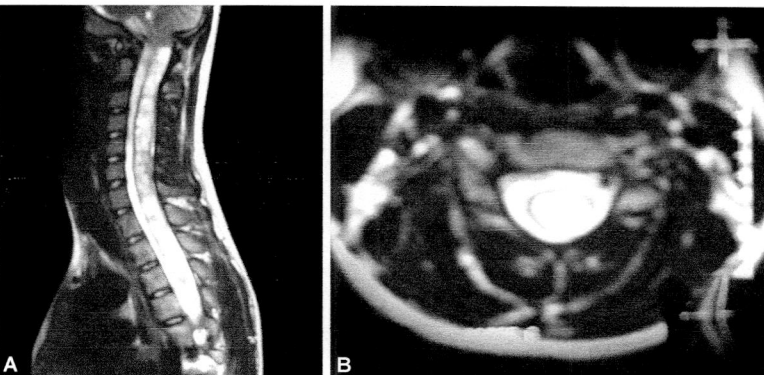

Figs. 19.18A and B: Myelomalacia: A long segment of spinal cord in cervicodorsal spine has been replaced by irregular patchy hyperintensity in T2 MRIs, these are generally irreversible changes associated with gross neural deficit.

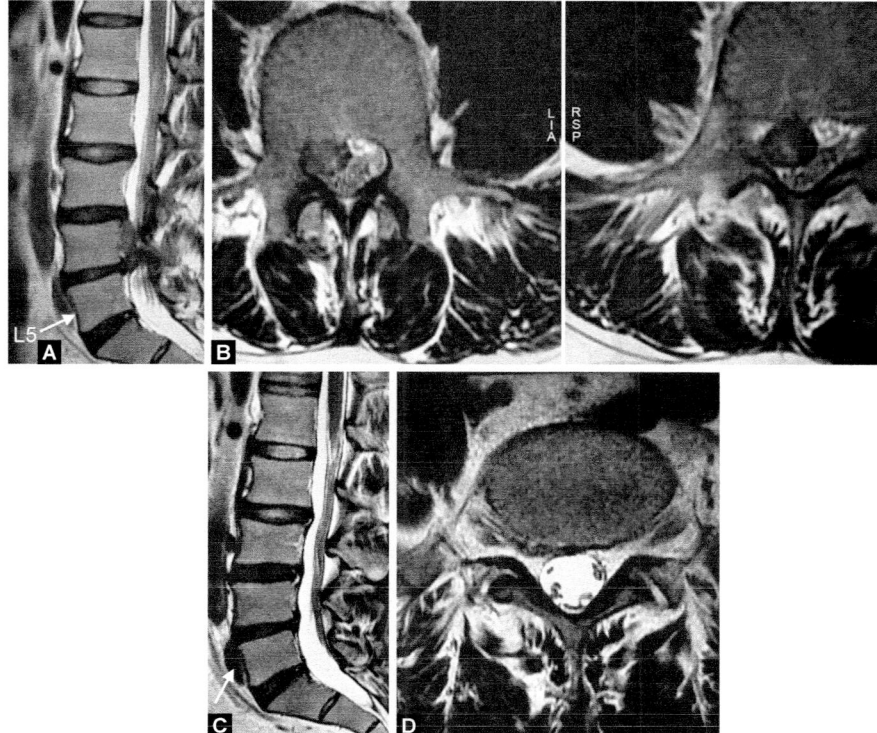

Figs. 19.19A to D: Biological resorption of a prolapsed disc: A 33 years old male presented with MRIs showing an extruded disc lying behind L4 vertebral body (A and B). MRIs repeated after 7 months show complete resolutions (C and D), rare phenomenon.

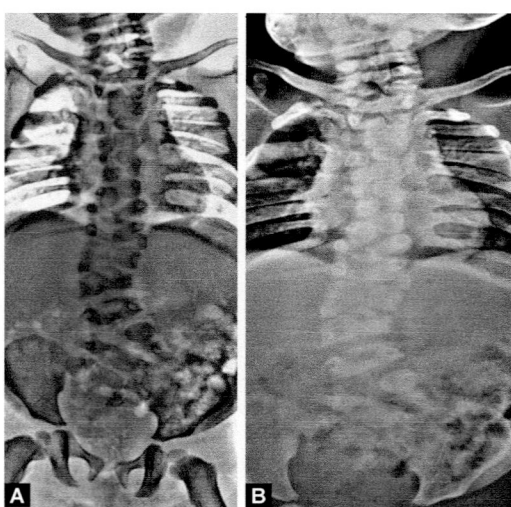

Figs. 19.20A and B: Congenital irregular segmentation of the whole vertebral column from cervical spine to the sacrum.

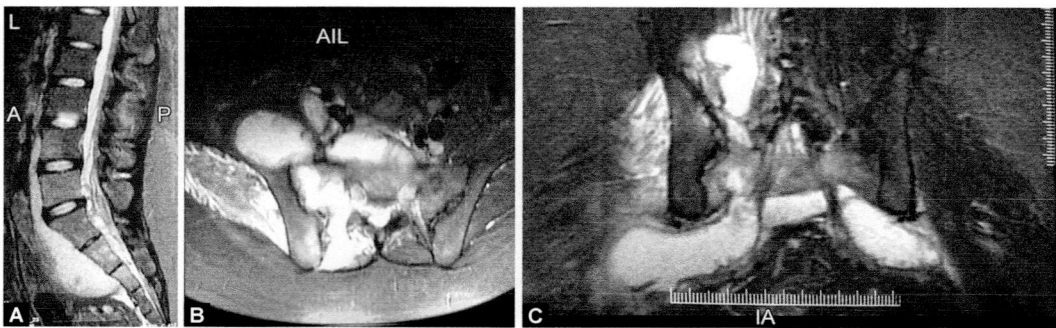

Figs. 19.21A to C: Cold abscesses from sacral tuberculosis: Abscess tracking along the passages through both greater sciatic notches in addition to juxta sacral and presacral area.

CHAPTER 19: Atlas of Rare Conditions (One may Encounter through the Journey in Orthopedics)

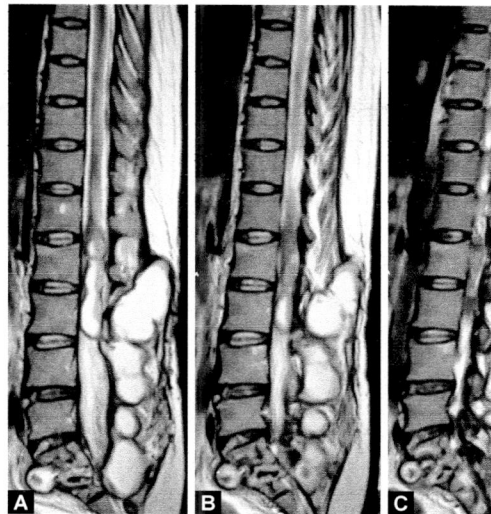

Figs. 19.22A to C: Skeletal tuberculosis: Can mimic any pathology; multiple loculi within the vertebral canal, posterior to the laminae along with destruction at L5-S1 area and a presacral abscess.

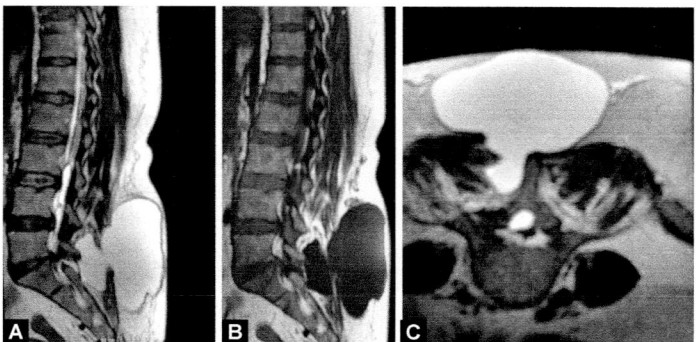

Figs. 19.23A to C: Arachnoid cyst; here what looks like a large cyst is a postoperative collection of cerebrospinal fluid behind the lamina communicating with the sublaminar arachnoid space (pseudomeningocele).

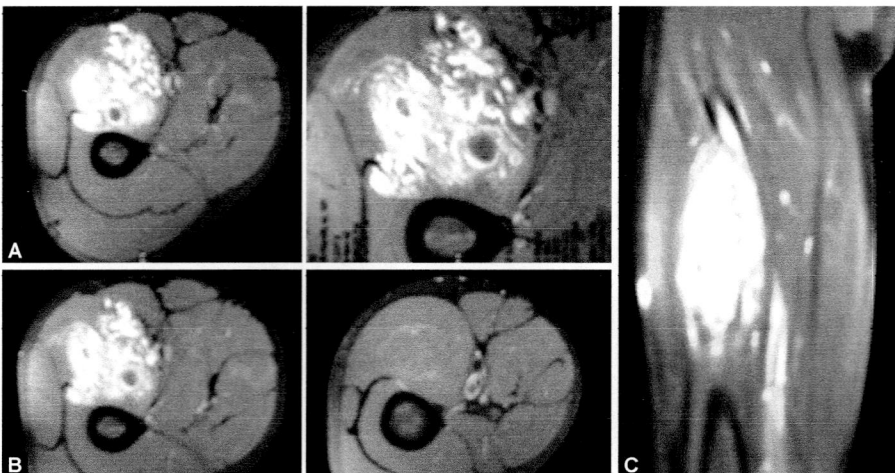

Figs. 19.24A to C: Bursal tuberculosis: Tuberculosis can occur in any part of skeletal system. This is an example of intermuscular bursal tuberculosis in thigh without involvement of adjacent bone.

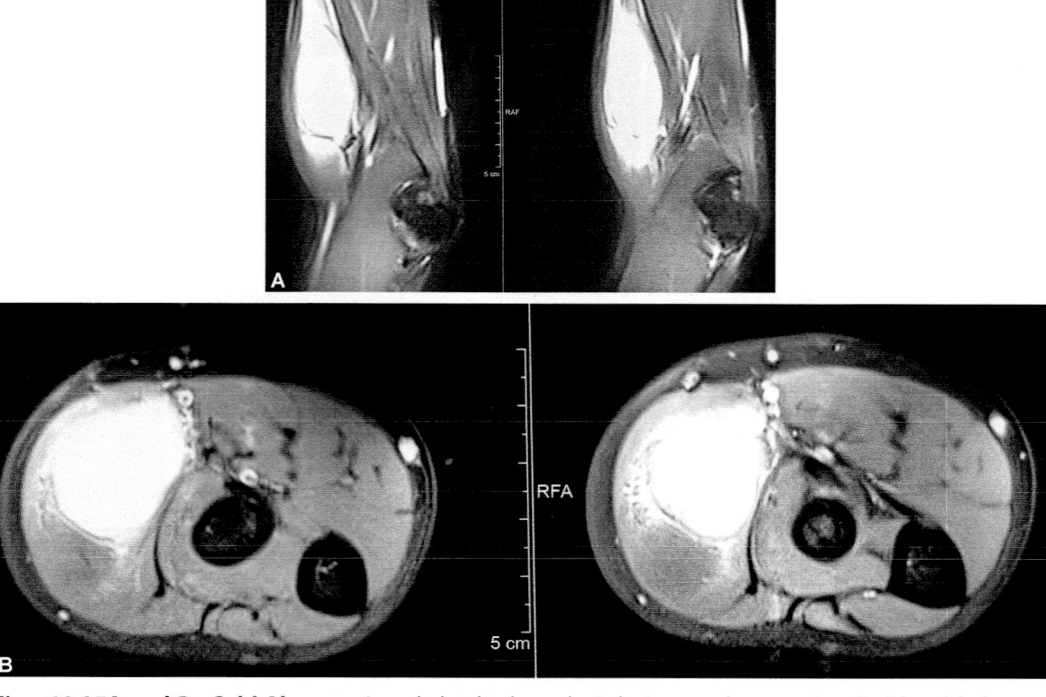

Figs. 19.25A and B: Cold Abscess: Any skeletal tuberculosis lesion can be associated with cold abscess formation. The abscess may be present at locations far away from the focus of disease. Abscess in this forearm is from a lesion in olecranon.

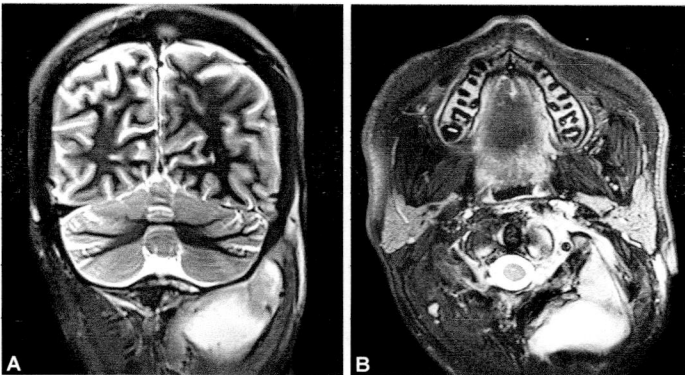

Figs. 19.26A and B: Tuberculosis can involve any region of skeleton. MRI-T2 images are of a patient having active infection (cold abscess) of left sided mastoid process and base of skull (A-coronal section, B-axial cut).

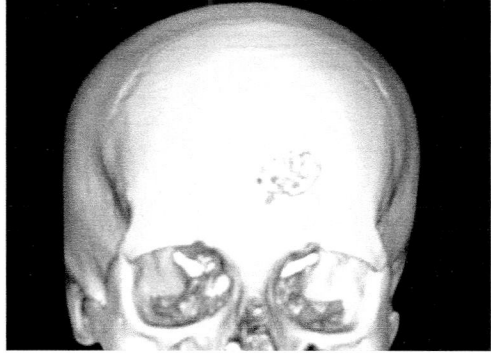

Fig. 19.27: Tuberculosis of frontal bone, a rare condition seen here as a rounded cavity.

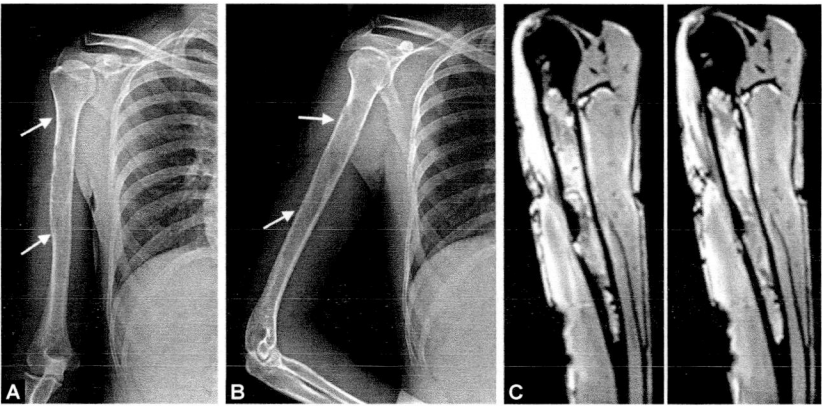

Figs. 19.28A to C: Hydatid disease develops commonly from the dog tapeworm (*Echinococcus granulosus*). The infected meat eaten by dogs or humans through intermediate hosts give rise to new generation of tape worms. This parasitic infestation is not uncommon among sheep farmers. Commonest lesions are in liver, however lesions in bone are detected rarely (<1% of patients with hydatid disease). Vertebrae, pelvis, long bones are common sites. X-ray (A) shows multiloculated bone cysts with moderate expansion and thinning of cortices of humerus. The lesion is composed of multiple dirty white small "balloons" (B and C).

Courtesy: Dr Rajeev Sharma.

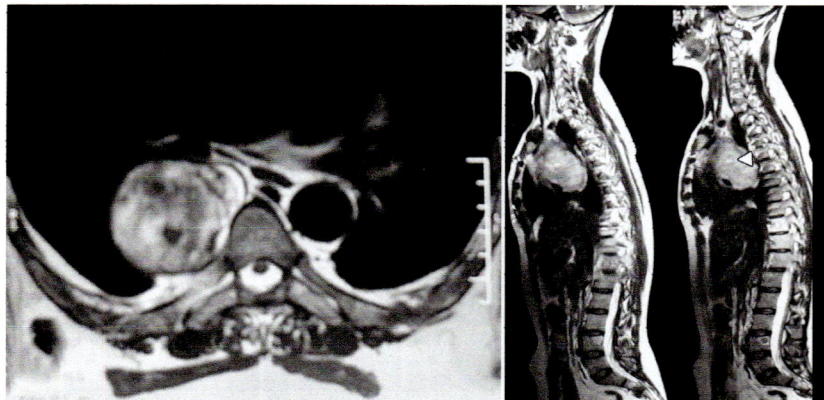

Fig. 19.29: Hydatid-cyst: A paravertebral rounded shadow in this picture is not a tubercular abscess. This is a hydatid-cyst in a known case of hydatidosis of liver.

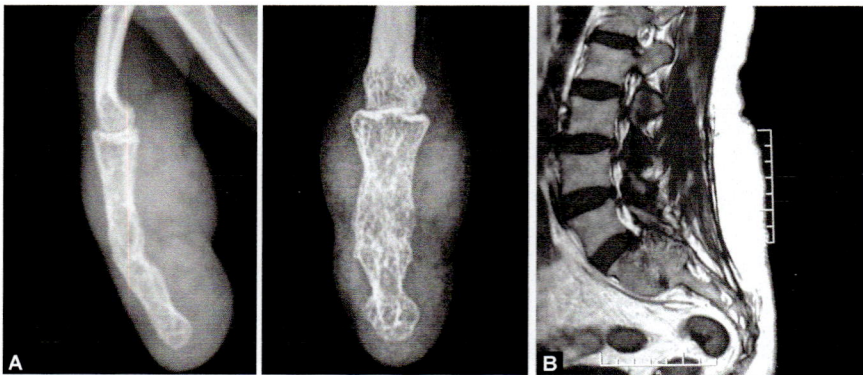

Figs. 19.30A and B: Hemangioma of (A) finger with fused interphalangeal joint; (B) Hemangioma of the sacrum. These are lytic lesions in bone giving a honeycombed appearance.

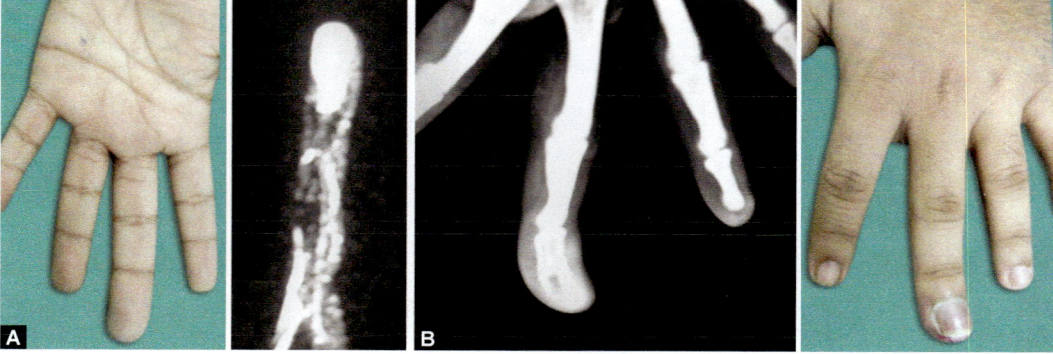

Figs. 19.31A and B: Glomus tumor: A painful vascular hamartoma arising from arteriovenous anastomosis as visualized in this vascular study. Most common site is subungual region of fingers.

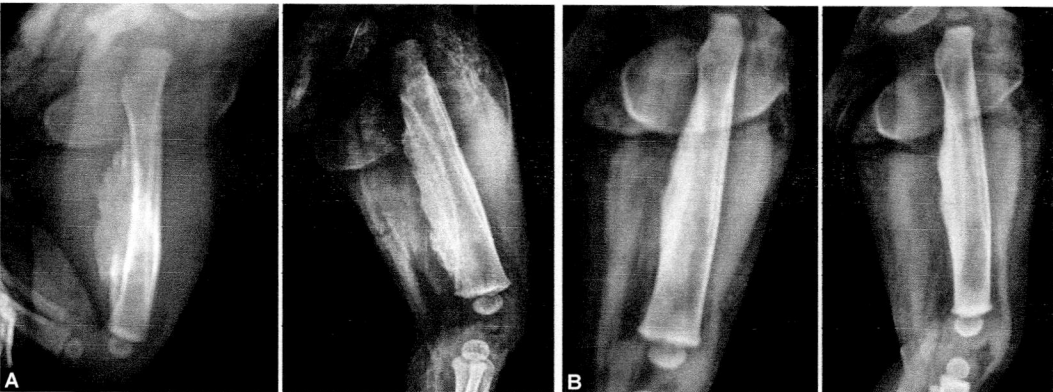

Figs. 19.32A and B: Caffey's disease: Infantile cortical hyperostosis—usually occurring in infancy, characterized by irritability, soft tissue swelling and palpable hard masses over multiple bones and mandible. Radiologically, there is dense subperiosteal thickening and hyperostosis of the diaphysis of bone (A). Clinically, there may be exacerbations and remissions, however spontaneous resolution occurs over a few years (B).

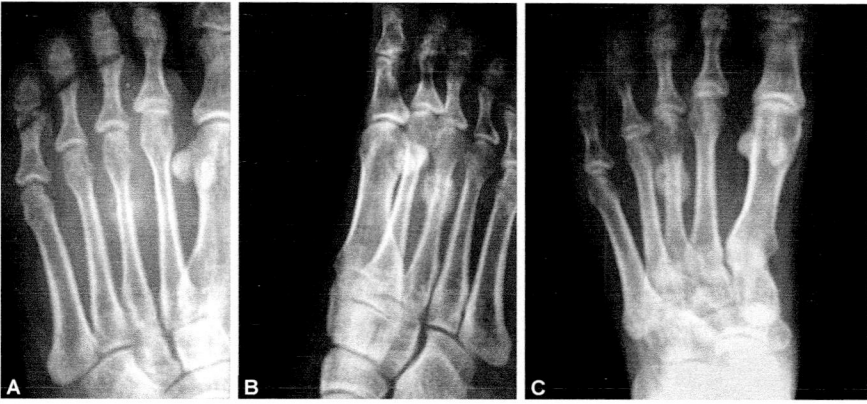

Figs. 19.33A to C: "March-fracture": It is a stress fracture caused by repetitive overuse of lower limbs. The condition is named for its prevalence among army recruits after un-accustomed prolonged marching.

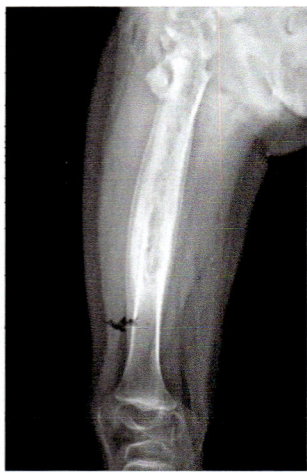

Fig. 19.34: Multilayered "onion-peal": Periosteal reaction is not unique to Ewing sarcoma. A similar appearance can be seen in infective conditions especially in growing age, the pathology in this X-ray was tuberculous osteomyelitis of femur with involvement of hip joint.

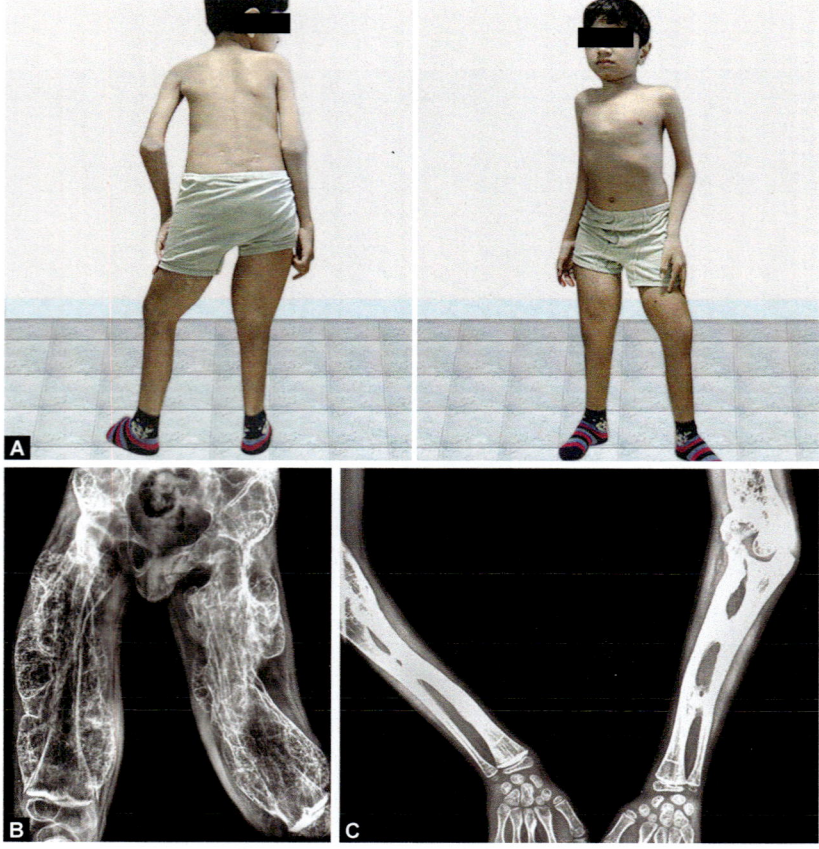

Figs. 19.35A to C: Myositis ossificans progressiva: A childhood disease of unknown etiology leading to progressive ossification of muscles, tendons, ligaments and aponeuroses. Family tendency exists, boys are affected more commonly, progressive loss of pulmonary function is usual cause of fatality (also expressed as fibrodysplasia ossificans progressiva).

CHAPTER 19: Atlas of Rare Conditions (One may Encounter through the Journey in Orthopedics)

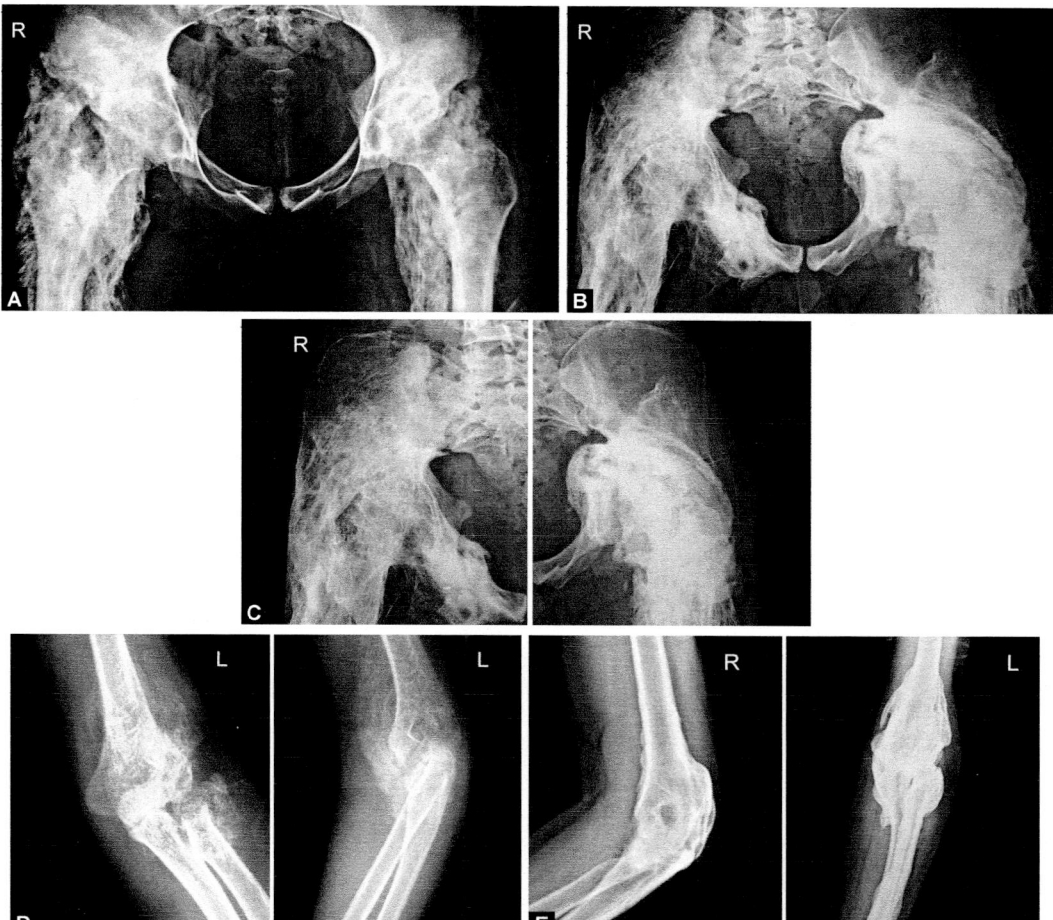

Figs. 19.36A to E: Myositis ossificans traumatica (heterotopic ossification) showing stages of progression (A), regression (B), maturity (C). Most of the cases of "post-traumatic" myositis ossificans are caused by forceful passive massage or manipulations. Another cause is repetitive flexor spasms in a patient of neurogenic spasticity. Common locations are around the elbow and hip. **Elbow:** Myositis ossificans—(D) stage of "onset", (E) stage of "maturity".

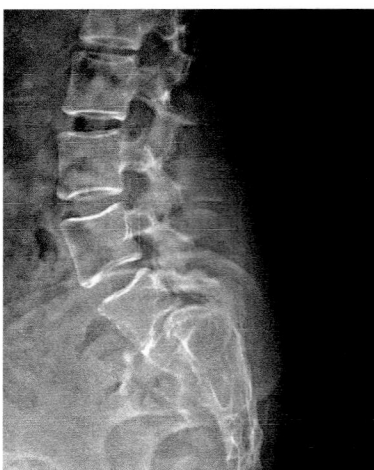

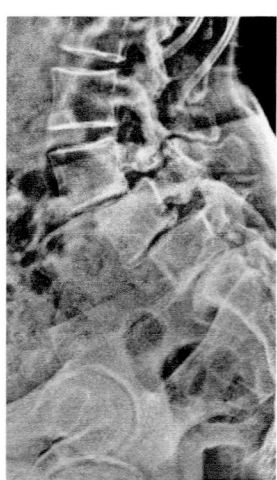

Fig. 19.37: Spondylolisthesis can be severe and lead to spondyloptosis. This is more likely to happen if lumbar five vertebra is trapezoidal in shape and upper border of sacrum is convex as seen in this X-ray.

Fig. 19.38: Stepladder anterolysthesis L3/L4 and L4/L5.

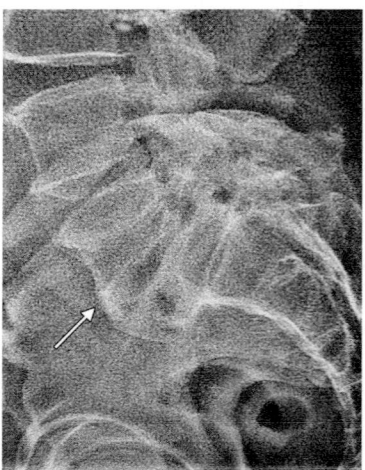

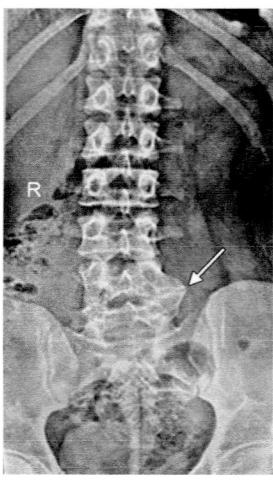

Fig. 19.39: Anterior buttress formation at L5–S1: Progressive degenerative changes at the site of lysthesis may produce buttress formation anteriorly which gets ossified (mineralization) in long standing cases.

Fig. 19.40: Congenital fusion of transverse processes L4–L5, a rare occurrence.

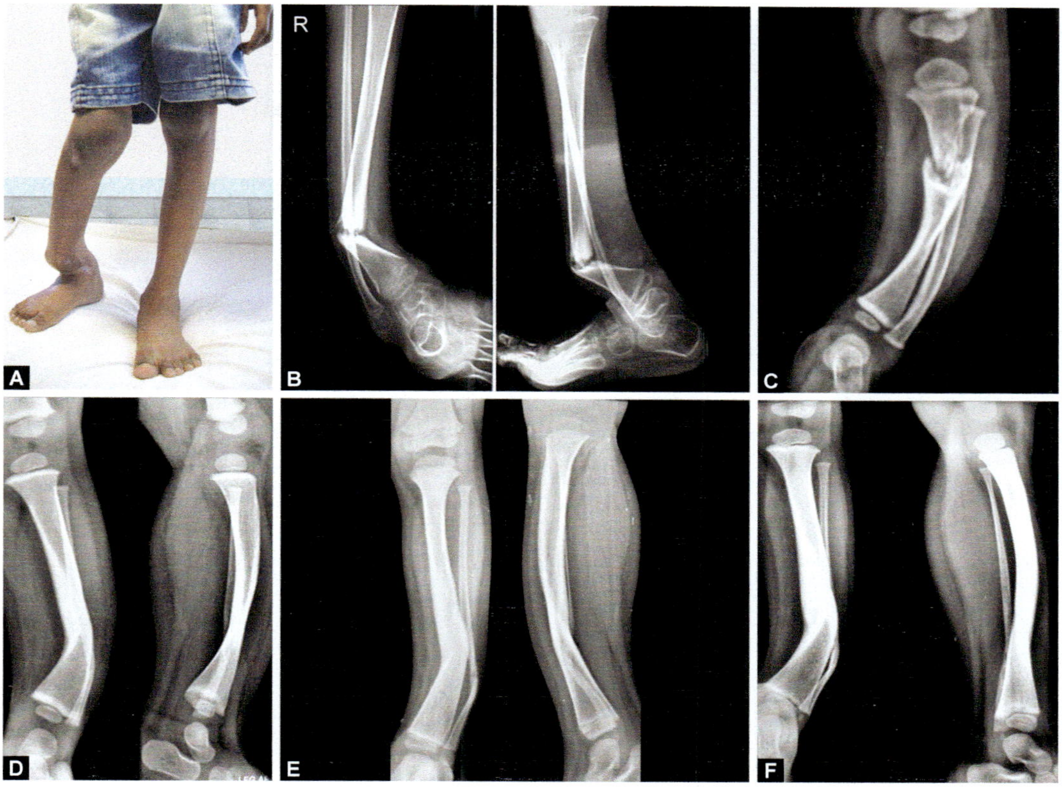

CHAPTER 19: Atlas of Rare Conditions (One may Encounter through the Journey in Orthopedics)

Figs. 19.41A to F: **Congenital pseudarthrosis of tibia** is generally associated with deformity of tibia with convexity anteriorly and laterally. (A and B) Show classic congenital pseudarthrosis of tibia and fibula; (C) Shows an extremely rare location of tibial pseudarthrosis; (D to F) Showing a progress of a prepseudarthrotic kyphoscoliotic tibia (tibial convexity anteriorly and laterally) ending as pseudarthrosis of tibia and fibula.

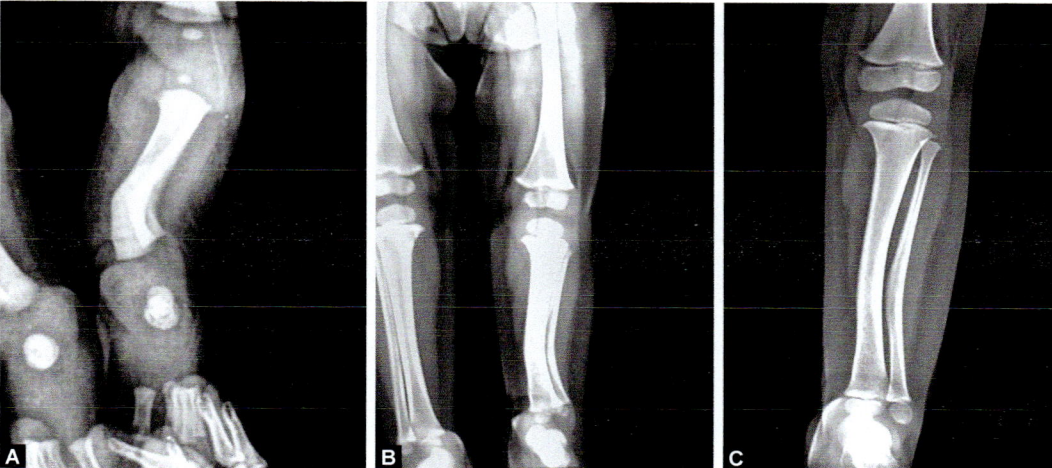

Figs. 19.42A to C: **Congenital kyphoscoliotic tibia** with tibial convexity to medial and posterior direction, generally is not a prepseudarthrotic condition. The deformity generally resolves by 3 years of age.

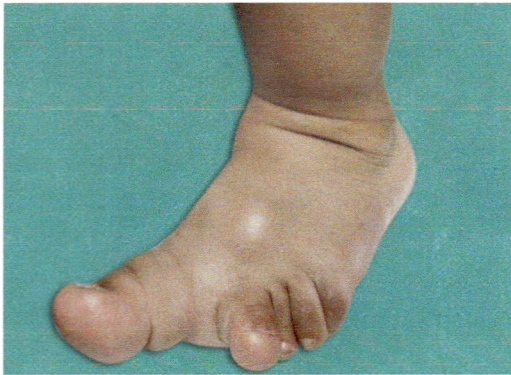

Fig. 19.43: Macrodactyly: A rare congenital anomaly of gigantism in fingers or less commonly in toes. There is enlargement of all structures of the involved part, the condition is associated with neurofibromatosis (elephantiasis neuromatosis).

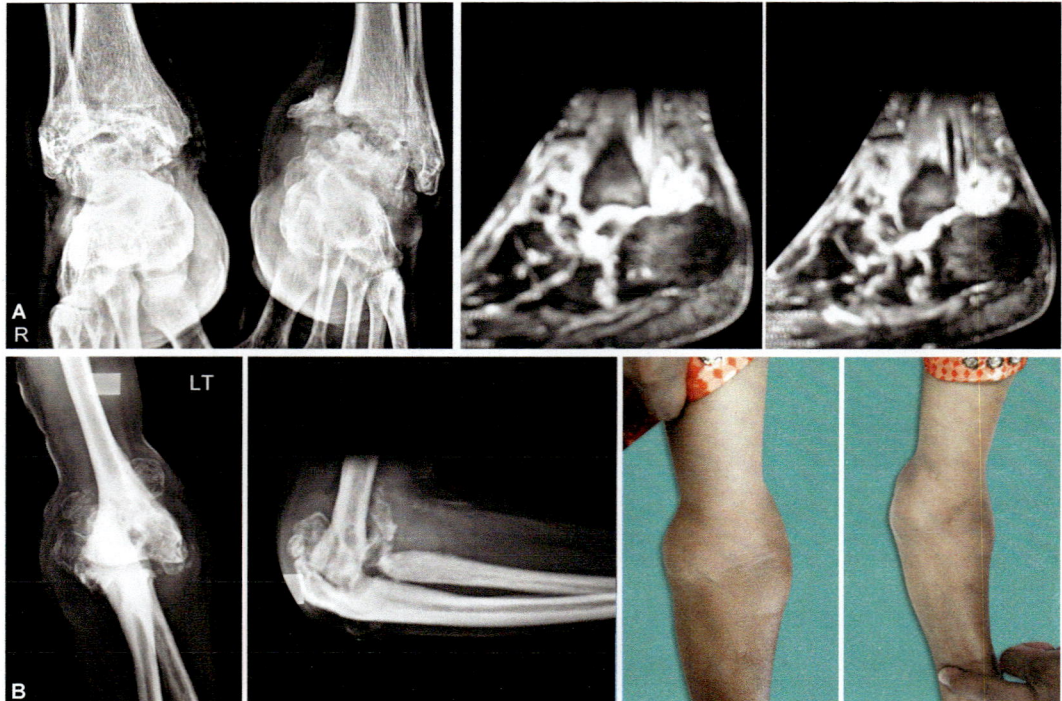

Figs. 19.44A and B: Charcot's joint (neuroarthropathy): This condition occurs as an abnormal response to the functions of a joint that has marked diminution or absence of sensations in the limb. Usually, it is triggered by trauma. The affected joint shows swelling and painless abnormal movements. X-rays reveal joint destruction, panarticular debris and displacement or dislocation. Commonest joint involved is ankle with foot, however even upper limb joints may be involved. Neuroarthropathy has been described in association with diabetes mellitus, leprosy, syringomyelia, tabes dorsalis and peripheral nerve lesions. The patient with bilateral ankle involvement (A) was a diabetic; and the elbow (B) was associated with syringomyelia.

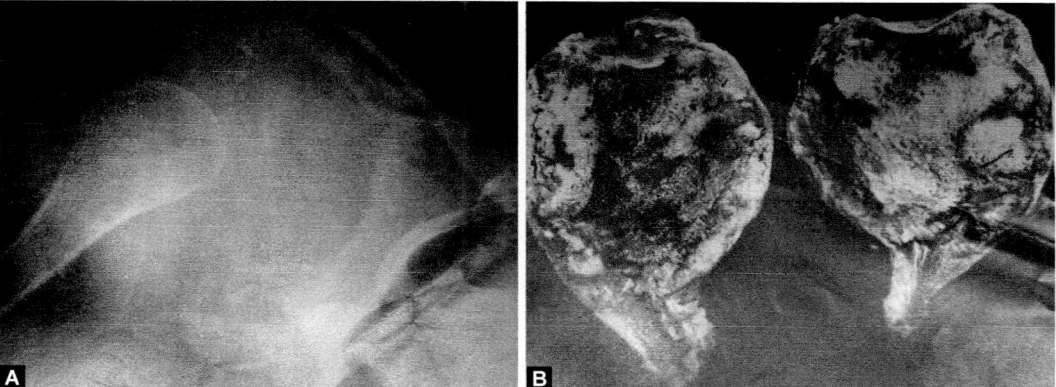

Figs. 19.45A and B: Giant-cell tumor of bone: It is a locally aggressive tumor that usually involves the epiphyseal region of a skeletally mature long (tubular) bone. This lady presented as a large cystic lesion in the scapula, the bisected tumor shows the cavity filled up with grayish-white material and intact articular margin of the glenoid, histology proved it to be giant-cell tumor.

Source: Tuli SM, Gupta IM, Kumar S. Giant-cell tumor of the scapula treated by total scapulectomy. A case report. J Bone Joint Surg Am. 1974;56(4):836-40.

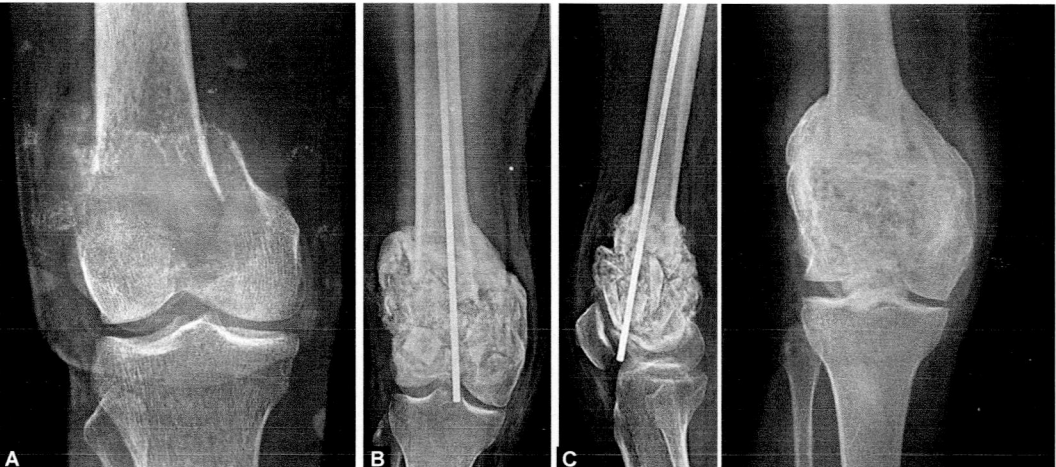

Figs. 19.46A to C: Giant-cell tumor (GCT) of bone: (A) Campanacci grade III GCT distal end femur at presentation; (B) Soon after debridement and decal-bone impaction grafting; (C) Healed status 8 years after operation.

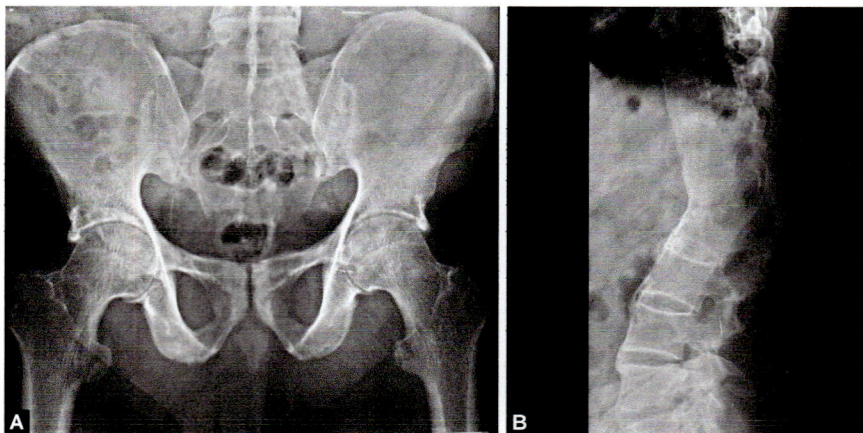

Figs. 19.47A and B: Ankylosing spondylitis showing classical changes of ossification in the sacroiliac joints, pelvis, and spine. This patient had concomitant tuberculous infection in spine resulting in osseous replacement of all ligaments and joints from dorsal 10th to lumbar third (L3) vertebrae, on healing of infection.

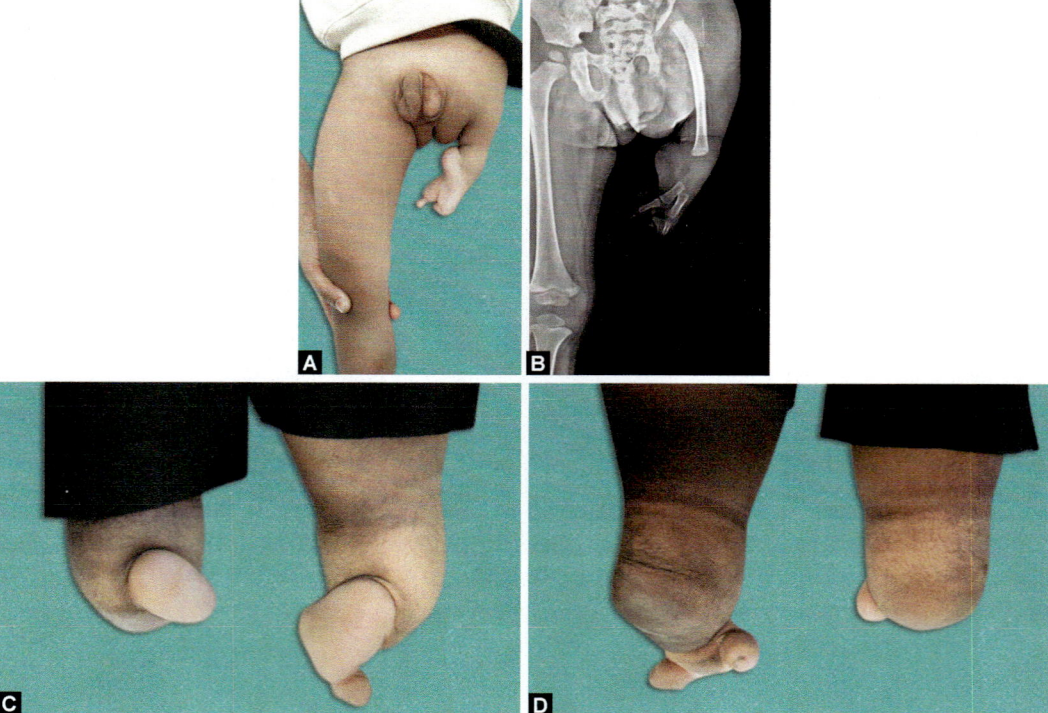

Figs. 19.48A to D: Phocomelia: A variety of intercalary congenital limb deficiency that results in absence of whole or a part of arm or forearm, or thigh or leg. In an extreme case, the hand may show attachment to shoulder or the foot directly to the trunk. This patient shows: (A and B) The absence of leg, and part of the foot (cleft foot), hip is dysplastic and toes are looking backwards; (C and D) Another patient showing subtotal absence of legs both sides.

CHAPTER 19: Atlas of Rare Conditions (One may Encounter through the Journey in Orthopedics)

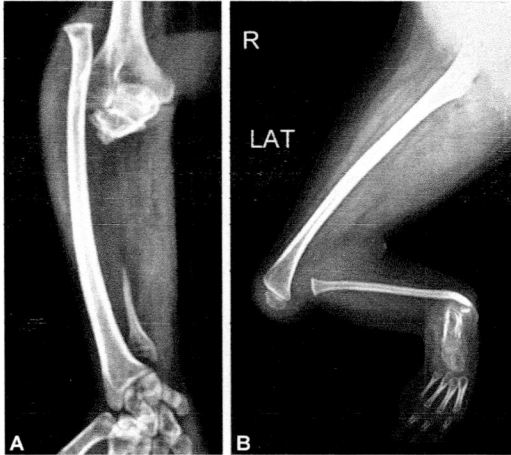

Figs. 19.49A and B: Congenital absence of bones: There is subtotal absence of ulna (A), with characteristic bowing of radius and dislocation of the radial head. Congenital absence tibia and foot bones (B).

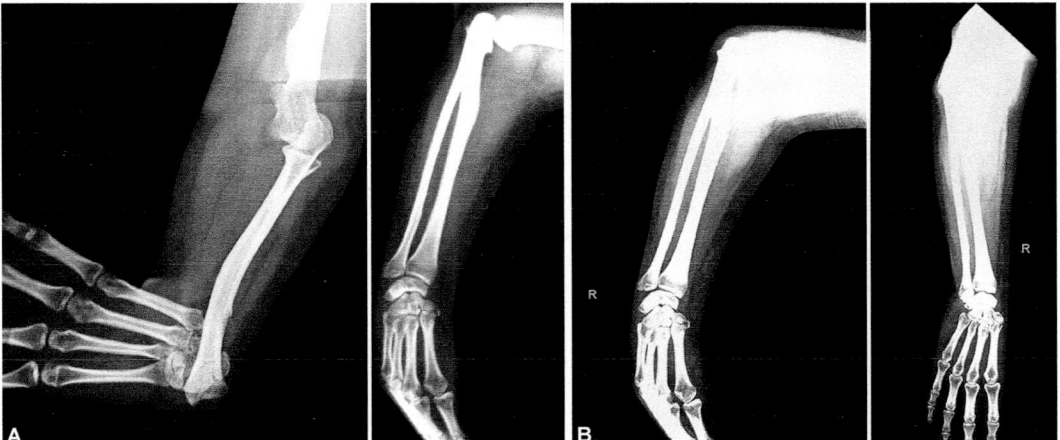

Figs. 19.50A and B: Congenitally fused proximal radioulnar joints. Both hands have only 4 metacarpals and fingers.

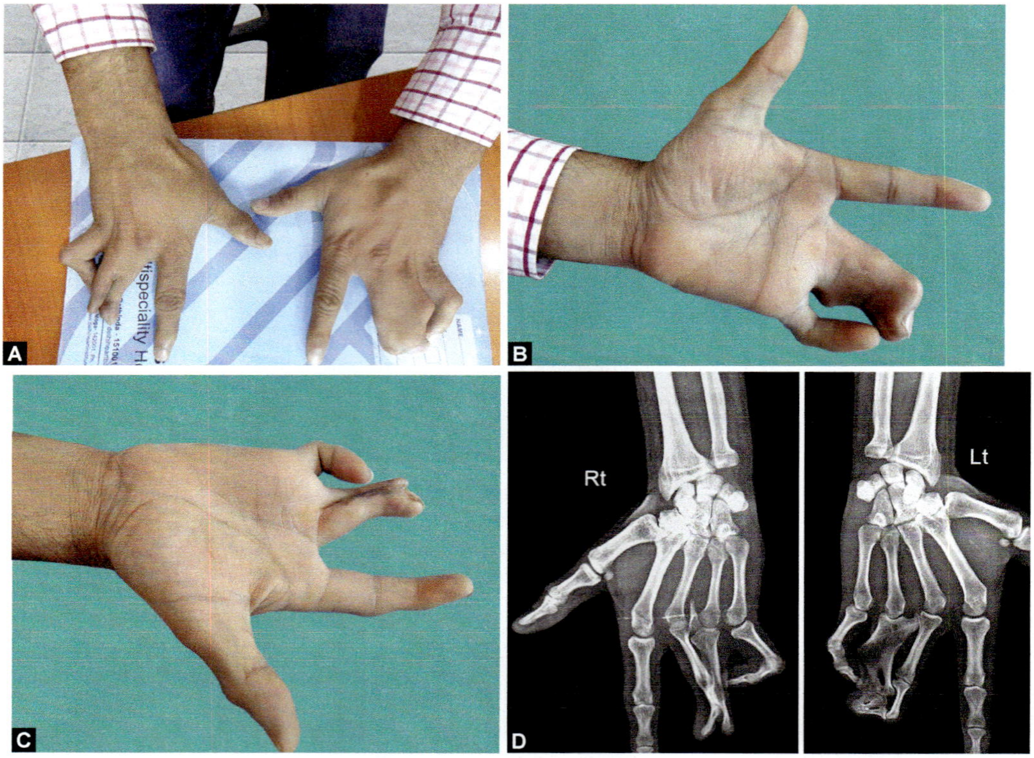

Figs. 19.51A to D: The figures show congenital fusion of many fingers in both hands. X-Rays and clinical pictures show syndactyly of 3rd and 4th rays.

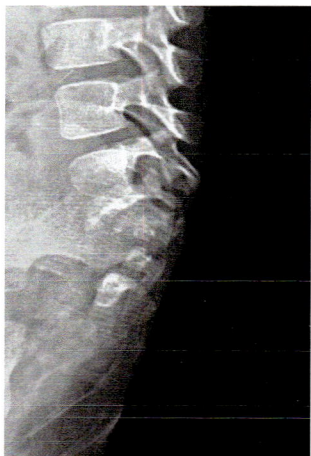

Fig. 19.52: Subtotal congenital agenesis of sacrum is a rare condition. This patient had concomitant developmental dysplasia of hip joints.

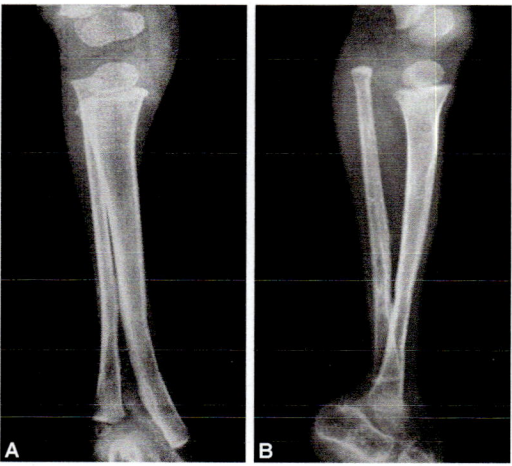

Figs. 19.53A and B: Diastasis of inferior tibiofibular joint; an extremely rare congenital defect. There is opening of inferior tibiofibular mortise, distal end of tibia is poorly developed and displaced medially, the proximal end of fibula is displaced markedly upwards.

Source: Tuli SM, Varma BP. Congenital diastasis of tibiofibular mortise. J Bone Joint Surg Br. 1972;54(2):346-50.

CHAPTER 19: Atlas of Rare Conditions (One may Encounter through the Journey in Orthopedics)

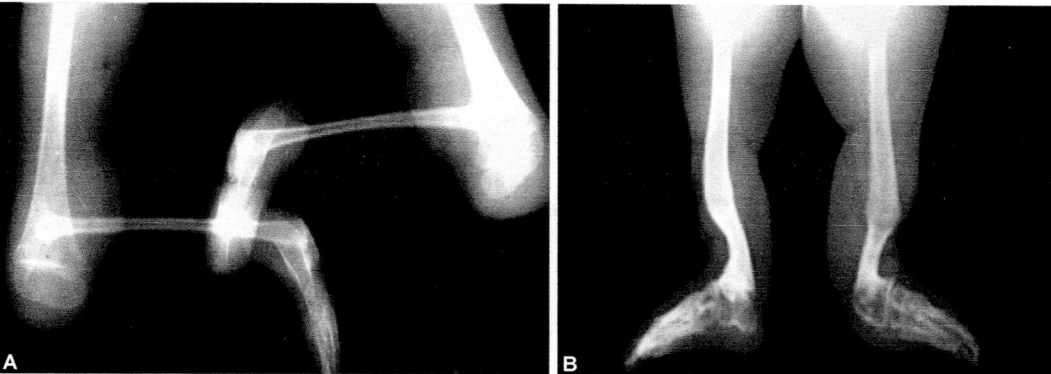

Figs. 19.54A and B: Congenital absence of tibia: Treated in this case by femoro-fibulo-calcaneal arthrodesis. The presence and preservation of the sensate foot permitted the patient to do her activities of daily living (ADL). One can appreciate the increase in the girth of fibula (function determines form).
Courtesy: Professor SS Yadav.

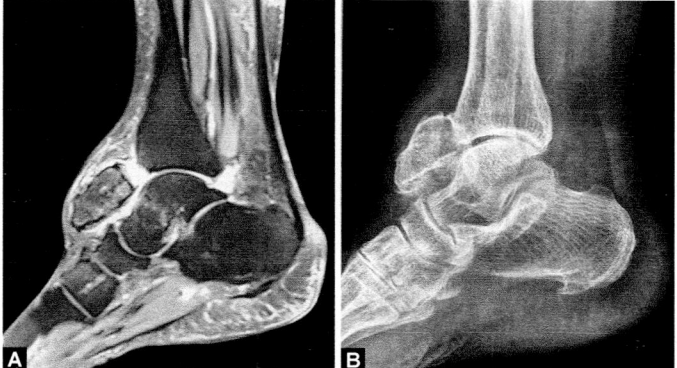

Figs. 19.55A and B: Synovial Chondromatosis: Multiple loose bodies in a joint is addressed as "synovial chondromatosis", MRI (A) and X-ray (B) of an unusual case of large intracapsular enchondroma with partial mineralization in ankle joint, arthrotomy revealed multiple cartilaginous loose bodies in the joint.

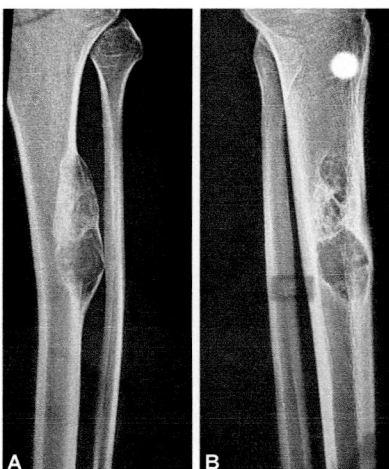

Figs. 19.56A and B: Adamantinoma: Generally considered a tumor of jaw, may rarely occur in tibia. X-rays show an osteolytic lesion with moderate expansion, soap-bubble appearance, surrounding sclerosis and cortical thinning. Clinical behavior is variable, most lesion behave like locally aggressive tumors. Histology in this case was osteofibrous dysplasia like adamantinoma.

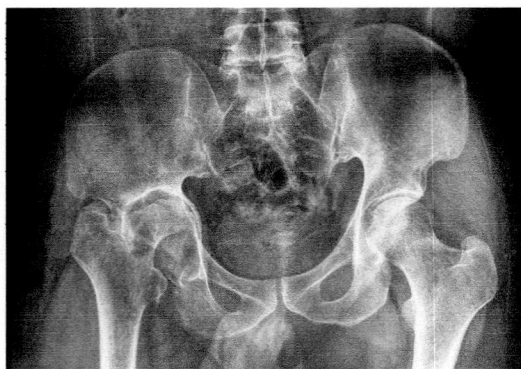

Fig. 19.57: Otto Pelvis, protrusio acetabuli: With progression of protrusion the greater trochanter impinges against the acetabular rim, further advance of protrusion ceases. Common causes are tuberculosis, rheumatoid disorder. This patient has been walking with this pathology. Observe a large acetabulum and pestle like femoral head.

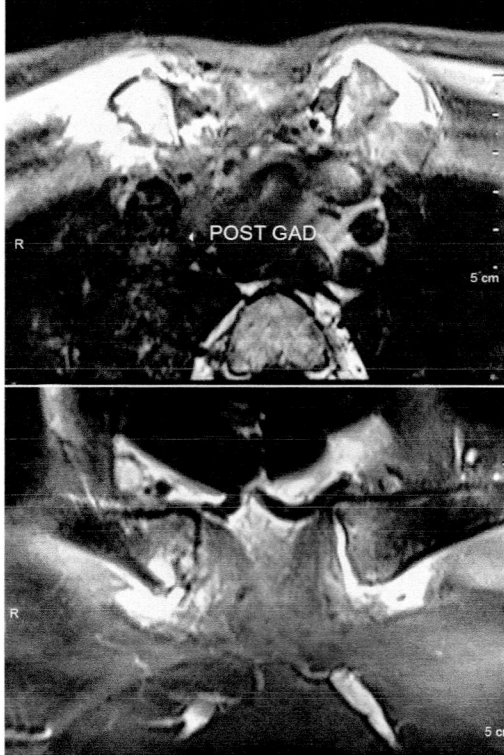

Fig. 19.58: An unusual case of rheumatoid inflammation of both sternoclavicular joints.

CHAPTER 19: Atlas of Rare Conditions (One may Encounter through the Journey in Orthopedics)

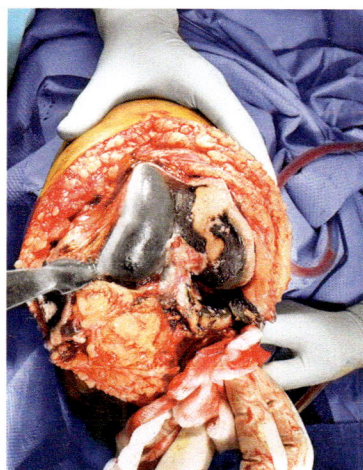

Fig. 19.59: Ochronosis: Ochronotic arthropathy is a rare metabolic disorder of homogentisic acid associated with alkaptonuria. There is blackish-blue pigmentation in connective tissues. Large joints are affected more commonly. X-ray of spine reveal calcification of intervertebral discs. The figure here is showing per-operative appearance.

SUGGESTED READING

1. Hoppenfeld S, Zeide MS. Orthopaedic dictionary. Lippincott-Raven, Philadelphia; Reprinted 2002.

Index

Page numbers followed by *f* refer to figure and *t* refer to table

A

Abductor digiti minimi 141
Abscess 32, 226*f*
   epidural 163
   presacral 225*f*
   tubercular 228*f*
Acetabular rim 240*f*
Acetabulum 87*f*, 189*f*, 217*f*
Acromelia 73
Acromioclavicular arthritis 134
Adamantinoma 95, 240*f*
Adduction
   deformity 79, 181*f*
   varus deformity 213
Adductor
   longus 119
   pollicis 141
   tenotomy 79
Adenoma 216*f*
Alcohol consumption, excessive 67
Alkaline phosphatase 216*f*
Alkaptonuria 241*f*
Allogenic bone graft 13*f*
Allografts 12
Amikacin 32
Amyoplasia 117
Aneurysmal bone cyst 95, 101, 101*f*, 219*f*, 220*f*
Angiosarcoma 95
Angular deformities 7*f*
Ankle 20, 208
   involvement, bilateral 234*f*
   joint 15*f*, 239*f*
      Charcot's arthropathy of 209*f*
Ankylosing spondylitis 40*f*, 41, 67, 161, 173, 236*f*
   advanced stage of 42*f*
Ankylosis 30
   angle of 181
Anorexia 26
Anticonvulsants 67
Antigenicity 11
Antimitotic agents 71
Anti-rheumatic drugs 38
   modifying 40
Antitubercular drugs 28*f*-30*f*, 32, 197*f*
Aortic calcification 68*f*
Apophysis 66*f*
Arachnoid cyst 225*f*
Arteriovenous anastomosis 228*f*
Arthritis 32
   glenohumeral 134
   idiopathic 43
   infective 134
   tuberculous 173, 181*f*
Arthrodesis 202, 202*f*
Arthrogryposis 144
   multiplex congenita 88, 90*f*, 117, 188
Arthropathy, enteropathic 43
Arthroplasty 30, 34
Arthroscopic procedures 134
Arthrotomy 20, 21
Articular cartilage 51
Articular infections 21*f*
Articular tuberculosis, classification of 29
Aseptic technique 22
Atlanto-occipital assimilation 127
Autogenous fibula, upper end of 107*f*
Autosomal dominant disorder 218*f*
Avascular necrosis 52, 54*f*-56*f*
   stage of 176
Axonotmesis 122

B

Back pain 157
Baclofen 120
Bankart's lesion 136
Barlow's test 83, 84*f*
Bence Jones proteins 109
Benzodiazepine 120
Biconcave vertebral bodies 68*f*, 157
Biconvex discs 62*f*, 157
Biopsy 27, 98
Bisphosphonates 53*f*, 68, 69*f*, 75, 174, 175*f*, 219*f*, 222*f*
Blade-plate fixation 206*f*
Blood 27
Blount's disease 200

Index

Bone 3*f*
  avascular necrosis of 52
  cement 13
  congenital absence of 237*f*
  cyst
    multiloculated 227*f*
    unicameral 98, 100, 100*f*
  deformities of 103*f*
  deposits, metastatic 111
  diaphysis of 218*f*, 229*f*
  disease 217*f*, 218*f*
  disorders, metabolic 60
  edema 53*f*
  formation 3, 144*f*
  giant cell tumor of 104, 235*f*
  graft 11, 11*t*, 14, 56*f*, 57*f*, 86, 91*f*, 92*f*, 99*f*, 105*f*, 138*f*
    hypertrophy of 106*f*
    substitutes 13
    vascularized 15
  healing of 8, 9*t*
  infections of 17
  ischemic 56*f*
  mineral density 68
  morphogenetic proteins 14
  Paget's disease of 96
  regeneration of 5*f*
  reticulum cell sarcoma of 111
  transport 11
  tuberculosis of 26, 32
  tumors
    benign 101
    malignant 107
Bony ankylosis 173*f*
  bilateral 173*f*
Botulinum toxin 120
  injections 78
Bow legs 198
Brachialgia 127, 128
Breast 99
Bristow–Latarjet operation 137, 139
Brodie's abscess 103
  typical 22*f*
Bryant's triangle 171, 172
Buffalo hump 45*f*
Bunion formation 82
Bursitis, semimembranosus 200

C

Café-au-lait
  patches 73, 74*f*, 91, 99
  spots 73

Caffey's disease 73, 229*f*
Calcific tendinitis 133, 135*f*
Calcium 60, 65, 67
  supplementation 62*f*
Callus
  consolidation 6
  mineralization of 5
  remodeling 6
Canal
  stenosis, secondary 161*f*
  vertebral 168*f*
Capitulum 144
Capreomycin 32
Capsule, hour-glass appearance of 85
Capsulitis, adhesive 134, 135
Carcinomatosis 67
Carpal bones 155*f*
Carpal tunnel syndrome 150, 151
Catterall's classification 177
Cauda equina 35
  syndrome 167, 168*f*
Cells 109
Cerebral palsy 79, 117, 118*f*
Cerebrospinal fluid behind lamina 225*f*
Cervical canal stenosis 129
Cervical cord, syringomyelia of 145*f*
Cervical spine 222*f*, 224*f*
  disc prolapse 128
  infections of 132
  X-ray of 127
Cervical spondylosis 134
Cervical vertebrae 131*f*
Cervicodorsal lesion 27*f*
Cervicodorsal spine 223*f*
Charcot's arthropathy 209*f*
Charcot's joint 144, 173, 209, 234*f*
Charcot's neuropathic feet 209
Charnley's principles 202
Chemotherapy, antitubercular 28
Chiari's osteotomy 86, 188, 190, 193*f*, 218*f*
Chondroblastoma 95
Chondrodiastasis 66
Chondrogenesis 3
Chondroma benign 95
Chondromalacia patellae 197
Chondromatosis, synovial 95, 202*f*, 239*f*
Chondro-osteodystrophies 75
Chondrosarcoma 95, 96, 108, 109*f*
  central 108
  peripheral 108
Chordoma 95
Chronic obstructive pulmonary disease 67
Claudication, neurogenic 165, 165*t*

Clavicles 61f
Claw hand 149
Cleft foot 236f
Cleidocranial dysostosis 127
Clubfoot 79
   congenital 88
   deformity 90f, 92
Codman's triangles 96, 110
Cold abscess 27f, 29f, 34, 224f, 226f, 227f
   formation 226f
Colles fracture 150
Colona's procedure 184
Complex regional pain syndrome 134, 135, 155, 156f
Compound palmar ganglion 155
Congenital torticollis 127, 130
   pathology of 131
Connective tissue
   disorders, congenital 73
   rheumatoid diseases 44
   stromal cells 104
Contralateral hip, asymptomatic 52
Cord
   compression of 35
   involvement 35t
Corduroy appearance 166f
Core decompression 56
Cortical bone grafts 219f
Cortical hyperostosis, infantile 73, 229f
Corticosteroids 67
   prolonged use of 52
Corticotomy 10
Coxa breva 185f, 191f
Coxa magna 177f, 180f, 191f
Coxa valga 116
Coxa vara 48f, 116, 174, 178
   congenital 73f, 173, 174, 176f
Cramps 164
Crohn's disease 43
Crutch palsy 122
Cubitus valgus 123, 141, 141f
Cubitus varus deformity 142, 143f
Cushing's disease 67
Cushing's syndrome 44f, 45f, 52
Cystic cavity 30f, 99
Cystic lesion 99f
Cysts
   popliteal 197f
   subchondral 48f, 135f
Cytomegalovirus 71
Cytotoxic drugs 8

D

De Quervain's disease 152
Decompression 57f
   spinal 168
Deformity 76f, 151
   correction 64
      basic principles of 78
Dega's pelvic osteotomy 86, 194
Demineralization 12
Desmoplastic fibroma 95
Diabetes mellitus 208, 234f
Diabetic foot 208
Diaphyseal sequestrum 18
Diaphysis, segment of 110f
Dislocation 134
   traumatic 150
Distal femur, chronic osteomyelitis of 22f
Distal interphalangeal joints 152f
Distal radius, giant cell tumor of 107f
Distraction 7, 11
Dorsal scoliosis 159f
Dorsal spine 27, 159f, 169
Dorsal wrist ganglion 152f
Dorsalis pedis 209
Drug therapy 121
Duchenne muscular dystrophy 116
Dupuytren's contracture 154, 154f
Dyplasias 72
Dyschondroplasia 79, 104f
Dysesthesia 123
Dysplasia 71, 73f
   developmental 83, 86f
   fibrous 73, 95, 98, 99f
Dysraphism 92
   spinal 93f
Dystrophic calcification 133

E

Echinococcus granulosus 227f
Elbow 20, 116, 140, 147, 231f
   advanced tuberculous arthritis of 28f
   function 145
   joint 46, 145f
   tuberculosis of 144f
Elephantiasis neuromatosis 234f
Enchondroma 79
Enchondromatosis 79, 103, 104f
Endochondral ossification 3
Endocrine disorders 67

Epicondylitis
  lateral 140
  medial 140
Epiphyseal defect 73f
Epiphyseal dysplasia 73f
Erythrocyte sedimentation rate 20
Ethanol, abuse of 52
Ewing's sarcoma 95, 110, 110f, 230f
Ewing's tumor 111
Exostosis 101
Extensor carpi radialis longus 121
External fixation device 206f
Extracorporeal shock therapy 55

F

Facioscapulohumeral dystrophy 116, 117
Fatigue 14f, 65f
  fracture 208
  metal 14, 14f
Femoral fracture 25f, 217f
Femoral head 177, 183, 190f, 192f, 220f
  coverage 183
  large necrotic segment of 58f
  osteonecrosis of 54t
  post-pregnancy avascular necrosis of 58f
  preservation techniques 54
  shape of 58f
Femoral neck 64f, 104
  fracture 69
    nonunion of 173
  pathological fracture of 110f
Femoral physis 66f
Femoroacetabular impingement 177, 191f
Femoro-fibulo-calcaneal arthrodesis 239f
Femur
  acute osteomyelitis of 18f
  distal end of 105f
  metaphyseal-diaphyseal junction of 102f
  osteomyelitis of 25f
  X-ray of 69f
Fibrodysplasia ossificans progressiva 230f
Fibrolysis 78
Fibroma, chondromyxoid 95
Fibrosarcoma 95, 96
Fibrous cortical defect 99, 102f
Fibula 14, 61f, 80
  congenital absence of 93f
  ipsilateral 15f
  pseudarthrosis of 233f
Fibular deficiency, congenital 91
Fingers
  flexion of 150f
  ulnar deviation of 39f

Flat foot 212, 212f
Flexion abduction orthosis 85f
Flexor
  digitorum superficialis 116, 122
  pollicis longus 154
  pronator tendon 142
  retinaculum 150, 155
  tendon sheath, tenosynovitis of 150
Florid rickets 62f
Fluid, synovial 151
Fluoroquinolones 32
Fluorosis 129
Folic acid, consumption of 93
Foot 115, 208
  abduction brace 89
  deformities of 213f
  dorsum of 214f
  drop 121, 213
  triple arthrodesis of 115
Forearm 116, 140
  X-ray of 97f
Fracture 14f, 76f, 134
  around shoulder, sequel of 134
  controlled 3
  fragments, distraction of 7
  healing of 3
  hematoma 3, 5
  multiple 75f
  stabilization 8
  subchondral 54f
  union, time table of 6
  vertebral 160
Fragility fractures 67
Frontal bone, tuberculosis of 227f
Frozen shoulder 134, 135
Fungal infections 17

G

Gait
  antalgic 171
  Trendelenburg 34, 83, 171
Galeazzi test 83, 84f
Galvanic stimulation 123
Ganglion 151
Gastrointestine 99
Genetic disorder 74f
Gentle tissue handling 22
Genu recurvatum 199
Genu valgum 63, 198
  deformity 63f, 66f
Genu varum 63, 198, 199f, 204f
  X-ray of 63f
German measles 71

Giant cell
  reaction 104
  tumor 95, 104, 105*f*-107*f*, 220*f*, 235*f*
    malignant 107
Giant osteoid osteoma 104
Girdlestone's excisional arthroplasty 187, 189*f*
Glenohumeral joint 46, 116
Glenoid, articular margin of 235*f*
Glenoplasty 137, 138*f*, 139*f*
Glomus tumor 95, 228*f*
Golfer's elbow 140
Gonadal insufficiency 67
Gorham syndrome 217*f*
Gout 47, 70, 210
  attacks, acute 210, 211
  chronic 210
  tophaceous 210*f*
Gouty arthropathy 70*f*
Gouty tophus 210*f*
Gower's sign 116
Graft substitutes 11
Granulation tissue 56*f*
Granuloma, eosinophilic 95
Greater sciatic notch 193*f*, 224*f*
Greater trochanter bursa 47
Gross deformities 30, 39*f*, 152
Growth plate modulations 66
Gunstock deformity 142, 143*f*
Guyon's canal 150

H

Haemophilus influenza 17
Hairy tuft 93*f*
Hallux valgus 82, 213, 214*f*
Hallux varus 214, 214*f*
Hamartoma 95
Hamstring tendons 119
Hand 116, 149
  typical deformities of 39*f*
Hand-shoulder syndrome 135
Hansen's disease 120
Harmon's reconstructive procedure 184
Harrington rod fixation 168
Head at-risk signs 177
Healing
  secondary 5
  stage of 176
Heberden's nodes 152*f*
Heel, painful 211
Hemangioma 95, 228*f*
  multiple 166*f*
Hemiplegia 118
Hemoglobinopathies 52

Heparin 67
Herring's grouping 177
Herring's lateral pillar classification 177
Heterotopic ossification 147, 231*f*
Hilgenreiner's horizontal line 176*f*
Hill-Sachs lesion 136
Hinge–abduction defect 177
Hip 20, 46, 115, 147, 171
  abductor mechanism 172*f*
  adduction deformity of 79
  arthrodesis of 202
  bilateral bony ankylosis of 173*f*
  bilateral developmental dysplasia of 87*f*
  congenital dysplasia 172*f*
  deformities 116
  developmental dysplasia of 83, 87*f*, 183
  disorders 173
  dysplasia, congenital 84*f*
  excisional arthroplasty of 34, 187*t*
  frog position of 83
  fusion of 188*f*
  infections 188*f*
  joint 29*f*, 38*f*, 44, 46, 86*f*, 173, 173*f*, 179, 187
    ankylosed 215*f*
    concomitant developmental dysplasia of 238*f*
    congenital dislocation of 83
    involvement of 230*f*
    MRI of 53*f*
    replacement, failed 41
    X-ray of 215*f*
  osteoarthrosis of 186
Homogentisic acid 241*f*
Hormone replacement therapy 68
Hydatid
  cyst 228*f*
  disease 227*f*
Hyperbaric oxygen 55
Hyperparathyroidism 67, 68, 216*f*, 215*f*
Hyperuricemia 210, 211
Hypophosphatemic osteomalacia 216*f*
Hypoplastic acetabulum 87*f*

I

Idiopathic massive osteolysis 217*f*
Idiopathic scoliosis simpler classification 159
Iliac horn 215*f*
Iliac spine
  anterior inferior 193*f*
  anterior superior 172
Ilizarov's principles 11, 89
Ilizarov's process 4
Ilizarov's technique 10, 10*f*, 78, 93*f*

Immunity, cell-mediated 120
Infections 17
　granulomatous 17
　iatrogenic 24
　spinal 162
　tuberculous 24, 27f, 40f, 197f
Inferior tibiofibular joint, diastasis of 238f
Inflammatory cells, nonspecific 4f
Inflammatory disorders 67
Inflammatory rheumatoid disorders 38
　basic treatment of 44
Infrapatellar medial realignment 200
Inguinal lymph node 29f
Innominate osteotomy 178, 185f, 187, 190f, 191, 191f, 193f
　concomitant 86f
Insensate feet 209
Intercalary congenital limb deficiency 236f
Intermuscular bursal tuberculosis 226f
Interosseous membrane 119
Interphalangeal joint 152, 228f
　dorsum of 152f
Intertransverse fusion 169f
Intestines, chronic diseases of 67
Intra-articular aspiration 45
Intracapsular enchondroma 239f
Intracapsular fractures 7
Intrinsic plus deformity 149
Involucrum 22
　behavior of 23
　formation of 23
Irradiation 8
Ischemia, cardiac 134
Isotope bone scan 97
Ivory osteoma 95, 103

J

Joint
　aspiration of 45
　cartilage space 58f
　dislocation of 52
　disorders 134
　functional position of 20
　functions of 234f
　infections of 17
　margins, sclerosis of 48f
　replacement 57f, 173f
　　procedures 49f
　space 57f, 182f, 192f
　　reduction of 49f
　　retention of 185f
　stabilization of 120
　tuberculosis of 26, 30t, 32
　upper limb 234f

Joshi's external stabilization system 89
Juxta-articular fractures 52

K

Kanamycin 32
Kidney 99
　chronic diseases of 67
Kienböck's disease 59f, 155
Kirschner's wire 8, 9, 21, 81, 142, 184, 186, 190, 191, 194, 198, 214
Klippel-Feil syndrome 132
Knee 20, 115, 147, 196
　arthrodesis of 202
　deformities of 197
　flexion deformities of 78
　fusion of 188f
　joints 47, 205
　　osteoarthrosis of 202
　　X-ray of 202f
　replacement 199f
　synovial chondromatosis 201
Knock knees 63, 198
Kyphoscoliosis 74f, 77f
Kyphoscoliotic tibia, congenital 233f
Kyphosis 157, 157f, 158, 160
Kyphotic deformity 35
　deterioration of 169f
　localized 160f

L

Lamellar bone 3
Laminectomy 37, 164, 165f
　decompressive 169f
Lasso operation 122
Leflunomide 40, 71
Leg 196
Legg–Calvé–Perthes disease 174, 190f, 191f
Leprosy 120, 234f
Lesions
　metastatic 134
　synovial 95
　tumorous 134
Leukemia 67
Limb
　girdle muscular dystrophy 117
　localized congenital deformities of 81
Lipoma 95, 151
Liposarcoma 95
Little's disease 117
Liver, hydatidosis of 228f
Low back pain 157
Low friction arthroplasty 34
Lower extremity joints 20

Lumbar canal stenosis 164, 165
  developmental 165f
  symptomatic 169f
Lumbar disc
  herniation
    acute 167f
      resolution of 167f
  prolapse produces 166
Lumbar intervertebral disc prolapse 166
Lumbar spine 166
  tumor of 166
Lumbosacral spine 93f
Lunate bone
  avascular necrosis of 150
  classical avascular necrosis of 59f
Lungs 99
  chronic diseases of 67
Lymph nodes 28, 218f
Lymphoma 95

M

Macrodactyly 73, 234f
Maffucci's syndrome 80
Malabsorption 67
Malformations, congenital 71
Malignant diseases 67
Malnutrition 8, 67
Maltracking patella 199, 200f
March fracture 65f, 229f
Marfan's syndrome 73
Marrow tumor 95
Massive coxa-magna 218f
Massive disc prolapse 168f
Maturity, stage of 147
McMurray's osteotomy 182f, 186, 187f
Medial joint space 204f
  appearance of 204f
Mediastinal pathology 134
Menopause, early 67
Mesenchymal cells 4f
Mesenchymal tissue 4f
Metabolic disorders 130, 174
Metacarpo-carpal joints 152f
Metacarpophalangeal joints 39f, 121, 150f
Meta-diaphyseal junction 101f
Metaphyseal osteoporosis, severe 177
Metastasis, source of 99
Metatarsophalangeal joint 82
Metatarsus varus 82
Methotrexate 40, 71
Mid-cervical spinal canal, sagittal
    diameter of 129
Monoplegia 118

Monosodium urate crystals 70, 70f
Moon face 44f
Mosaic fashion 69
Mottled appearance 110
Movements
  arc of 181
  moderate limitation of 173
Multidrug therapy 121
Muscle
  edema of 19
  pedicled bone graft 15, 57
  progressive ossification of 230f
Muscular dystrophy 116, 213
Musculotendinous cuff 133
Musculotendinous procedures 119
Mycetoma infections 17
Mycobacterium
  leprae 120
  tuberculosis 17
Myeloma 96, 109, 164f
  multiple 67, 109, 109f
Myelomalacia 130f, 223f
Myelomatosis 95
Myelopathy 129
Myeloproliferative disorders 52
Myositis 145
  ossificans 147, 231f
    periarticular 173
    progressive 230f
    stages of 147f
    traumatica 231f

N

Nail–Patella syndrome 215f
Natural fracture healing, biology of 5
Nelaton's line 171, 172
Neoangiogenesis 5f, 10f
Neoplasm 112, 160f, 166
Nephritis, chronic 63
Nerve sheath tumor 166f
Neural monitoring 160
Neural tissues 95
Neuralgia, brachial 127
Neurapraxia 122
Neurectomy, partial 119
Neurilemmoma 95
Neuritis 141
Neuroarthropathy 209, 234f
Neurofibroma 95, 151
Neurofibromatosis 73, 234f
  generalized 73f, 74f
Neuroma 123
Neuromuscular disorders 114

Neuropathic hip 173
Neurotmesis 122
Nicotine 8
   abuse of 52
Night cries 26
Non-Hodgkin's lymphoma 111
Nonossifying fibroma 95, 99
Nonsteroidal anti-inflammatory drugs 8, 40, 50,
    121, 127, 133, 140, 150
Nonunions 7

O

Ochronosis 241*f*
Ochronotic arthropathy 241*f*
Old fracture, sequel of 208
Olecranon bursitis 144
Ollier's disease 79
Onco-chemotherapy 52
Onion-peel appearance 110, 110*f*
Open bone grafting 23
Open reduction and internal fixation 8, 9
Orthopedics 9, 24, 71
   tumors 95
Ortolani's maneuver 83
Ortolani's test 83, 84*f*
Osseous lesions 134
Osseous tissues 3
   regeneration of 3
   repair of 3
Osteoarthrosis 48, 128, 134, 144, 152*f*, 162, 173
   advanced 49*f*
   early 49*f*
   primary 48, 135, 162
   progressive 130*f*
   secondary 48, 48*f*, 135*f*
Osteoblast 4*f*, 222*f*
Osteoblastic cells, clump of 4*f*
Osteoblastoma 95, 104
Osteochondral dysplasia 72*f*
Osteochondral skeletal deformities 72
Osteochondral structures 196*f*
Osteochondritis dissecans 144
Osteochondroma 95, 101, 103*f*, 221*f*
   multiple 103*f*
Osteochondromatosis, multiple 101, 103*f*
Osteochondrosis 158
Osteoclasis 10
Osteoclastoma 104, 106*f*
  benign 95
  malignant 95
Osteoclasts 4*f*
Osteoconduction 11

Osteodystrophy, renal 52
Osteofibrous dysplasia 240*f*
Osteogenesis imperfecta 67, 68, 75
   congenita 75, 76*f*
   tarda 75, 76*f*, 77*f*
Osteogenicity 11
Osteoid osteoma 95, 97*f*, 103, 104
Osteo-induction 11
Osteolytic lesion 240*f*
Osteomalacia 61, 62*f*, 64*f*, 157, 173, 216*f*
   characteristic radiological features of 61*f*
   severe 64*f*
Osteomyelitis 17, 25*f*, 134
   acute 20
     hematogenous 17
   chronic 21, 22*f*
   dry chronic 24
   early radiological features of 19*f*
   tuberculous 230*f*
   wet chronic 24
Osteonecrosis 44*f*, 52, 54*t*, 59, 68, 134
   X-ray of 57*f*
Osteophytes 130*f*, 135*f*
   formation 49*f*
Osteophytosis, degenerative 129
Osteopoikilosis 218*f*
Osteoporosis 8, 19*f*, 30, 61, 67, 68*f*, 144*f*, 156*f*,
    160*f*, 164*f*
   secondary 67*t*
   severe 157
   treatment of 68
Osteosarcoma 95, 98, 107
   periosteal 108
   variants of 108
Osteotomy 9, 10, 57, 147, 176*f*, 179, 181, 183, 184*f*
   distal
     femoral 198
     humeral 142
   femoral 176*f*
   line of 138*f*
   location of 138*f*
   proximal femoral 183
   tibial 204*f*
   upper femoral 179, 182*f*, 186, 187
   X-ray of 187*f*
Otto pelvis 240*f*

P

Paget's disease 68, 96, 108, 174, 175*f*, 222*f*
Pain 96, 156*f*, 171
   acute 173
   chronic 173

Painful arc syndrome 135
Palmar fascia 154
   fibromatosis of 154*f*
Papineau's technique 23, 24
Paradiscal edema 163*f*
Paralysis 36*f*
   residual 115
Parathyroid gland hyperplasia 216*f*
Paravertebral abscess collection 163*f*
Paresthesias 141, 164
Parosteal sarcoma 108
Patchy calcification 109*f*
Patella, recurrent dislocation of 199
Pathological fracture 3, 18*f*, 19*f*, 75*f*, 96, 101*f*, 105*f*, 106*f*, 110*f*, 216*f*
Pavlik harness 85*f*
Peak bone mass 60
Pedicle bone graft 58*f*
Pelvic bone 64*f*, 192*f*, 216*f*
Pelvic support
   osteotomy 185*f*
   procedure 183
   upper femoral osteotomy 184*f*
Pelvis
   bones 217*f*
   cavity of 96
   contralateral 172*f*
   MRI of 42*f*, 217*f*
   X-ray of 38*f*, 175*f*, 189*f*, 215, 219*f*, 221*f*
Pemberton's acetabuloplasty 194
Pemberton's osteotomy 86
Periarthritis 133, 135
Periosteal reaction 22*f*, 230*f*
Peripheral nerve 122
   entrapment syndrome 123
   lesions 234*f*
Peripheral vascular disease 165
Perkin's vertical line 176*f*
Perthes' disease 77, 173, 174, 177*f*, 183
   classification of 175
Pes calcaneovalgus 213*f*
Pes calcaneus 213*f*
Pes cavus 212, 213*f*
Pes equinus 213
Phocomelia 73, 236*f*
Phosphates 216*f*
Phosphorus 65
Physis stimulation 66
Pin-head appearance 166*f*
Plantar arthrodesis 214*f*
Plasmacytoma 109
Plaster of Paris 9
Poliomyelitis 114

Polyarthritis 43
Polyarticular rheumatoid arthritis 39*f*, 203*f*
Polycystic kidneys 63
Polydactylism 82
Polyostotic fibrous dysplasia 75*f*, 99, 219*f*
Polyostotic skeletal dysplasia 173
Ponseti's cast 88
Ponseti's technique 78, 88
Popliteal bursa 200
Posterior heel pain 211
Posterior longitudinal ligament 129
   ossification of 129, 129*f*, 222*f*
   symptomatic ossification of 130*f*
Post-polio syndrome 114
Post-polio-residual paralysis 115*f*, 213*f*
Post-traumatic myositis ossificans 231*f*
Pott's disease 34
Prepseudarthrotic kyphoscoliotic tibia,
   progress of 233*f*
Progression, stage of 147*f*
Pronator teres 119
Prostate 99
Protrusio acetabuli 240*f*
Proximal femur, osteotomy of 57, 179, 181
Proximal tibia 13*f*
Pseudarthrosis, tibial 233*f*
Pseudohypertrophic muscular dystrophy 116
Pseudomeningocele 225*f*
Pseudoparalysis 20
Psoriasis 43
Psoriatic arthritis 43
Pterygium syndrome 117
Puberty 60
Pubic rami 61*f*, 64*f*
Pyogenic infection 179
Pyogenic osteitis 162

Q

Quadriplegia 118

R

Radial deficiency 81
Radial diaphysis 220*f*
Radial head, dislocation of 237*f*
Radial hemimelia, congenital 146*f*
Radial nerve explorations 145
Radiation exposure 52
Radiofrequency ablation 104
Radioulnar synostosis, congenital 81, 145
Radius, congenital absence of 81*f*, 146
Reactive arthritis 43

Reflex
  pain syndrome 155
  sympathetic dystrophy 133
Regression, stage of 147, 147f
Reiter's syndrome 43
Renal disease, chronic 67
Rheumatoid arthritis 45f, 152f, 173, 173f
  juvenile 43
Rheumatoid disease 67
Rheumatoid disorder 8, 38, 38f, 44f, 130, 240f
Rheumatoid inflammation 134, 144, 240f
Rheumatoid spondylitis 161, 162
Rhizomelia 73
Ribs 61f
  incomplete formation of 159f
Rickets 61, 173
  nutritional 65
  renal 63
  types of 65t
  vitamin D resistant 63
Rifampicin 29f
Rigid internal fixation 8
Risser's sign 66, 66f, 159, 193f
Rituximab 40
Rocker bottom foot 212
Rotator cuff
  disorders 133, 134
  pathology of 135

S

Sacroiliac joints 38f, 42f, 236f
Sacrum 220f
  hemangioma of 228f
  subtotal congenital agenesis of 238f
Salter's osteotomy 86, 189
Salter's procedures 193f
Sarcoma, synovial 95
Saturday night palsy 122
Scapular neck osteotomy 138f
Scheuermann's disorder 157, 157f, 158
Schwannoma 95, 166f
Sciatica 127
Sclerosis 133, 240f
  subarticular 49f
Scoliosis 158, 159f
  infantile 158
  juvenile 158, 159
  reconstruction of 157
  Research Society 158
Scurvy 67
Seddon's classification 122
Semi-invasive techniques 160

Semilunar cartilages 196f
Septic arthritis 20, 173
Sequestrectomy 23
Sequestrum 22
  cortical 18
  fate of 22
Serum creatine phosphokinase 117
Shenton's line 181f
Shepherd's crook deformities 99
Shoulder 20, 46, 116, 133
  advanced tuberculous arthritis of 137f
  instability of 136
  joint 29f
  painful 133
  periarthritis of 133
  recurrent anterior dislocation of 136, 138f
  X-ray of 135f
Sickle cell disease 52
Simple bone cyst 95, 100
Sinuses 32
Sjögren's syndrome 39, 44
Skeletal dysplasia 77f
  generalized 73
Skeletal hyperostosis, diffuse idiopathic 45
Skeletal system 95, 95t, 226f
Skeletal tuberculosis 26, 27f, 225f
  lesion 226f
Skin
  grafting 152
  Z-plasty of 152, 155
Slipped capital femoral epiphysis 173, 178
Soap bubble appearance 104, 240f
Soft callus 5
Soft tissue 217f
  procedures 79
  swelling 19f, 25f, 27f, 30, 144f, 229f
Solitary osteochondroma 101, 102f
Sourcil' sign 133
Spasmodic torticollis 127
Spheroidal femoral head 177f
Spina bifida 92, 161
  occulta 92
Spinal cord, long segment of 223f
Spinal curvatures, loss of 158
Spinal hyperextension, anterior 42
Spinal hyperostosis, diffuse idiopathic 129
Spinal tuberculosis 28f
  classical radiological appearance of 163f
Spine 157
  mid-sagittal section of 157, 157f
  osteoarthrosis of 162
  osteoporosis of 68f
  primary osteoarthrosis of 162

tuberculosis of 34
X-ray of 28f, 241f
Spinoplasty 164, 165f
Spondyloarthropathy 42f
   seronegative 41
Spondyloepiphyseal dysplasia, generalized 77f
Spondylolisthesis 160, 232f
   classical appearance of 161f
Spondylolysis 160
Spondyloptosis 232f
Spondylosis 128
Staphylococcus aureus 132
Steel's triple osteotomy 190
Stepladder anterolysthesis 232f
Sternoclavicular joints 240f
Sternocleidomastoid muscle 131f
   contracture of 130
Steroids 8
Stiff elbow 144
Stress fracture 65f, 75f, 208, 229f
Structural bone graft sacrificing knee joint 106f
Student's elbow 144
Subdiaphragmatic lesions 134
Sublaminar arachnoid space 225f
Sudeck's atrophy 135
Sudeck's complex regional pain syndrome 68
Sudeck's dystrophy 134, 155, 156f
Sun-burst appearance 110f
Suppurative arthritis 184f
Suprapatellar pouch 197f
Supraspinatus tendon, insertion of 135f
Surgery 32
  anterior 159
  posterior 159
Swelling 96, 156f, 234f
  chronic inflammatory 200
Syme's amputations 209
Syndactylism 82
Synostosis, congenital 132f, 144, 145f
Synovial fluid 151
  collection 196f
Synovitis 30
  stage of 176
  transient 174
Synthetic bone graft substitute 14f
Syphilitic osteomyetitis 17
Syringomyelia 145f, 234f
Systemic lupus erythematosus 39, 52

T

Tabes dorsalis 234f
Talus, osteonecrosis of 208
Tarsal joints 214f
Tc-99m bone scan 208
Telescoping test 172
Temporary motor weakness, symptoms of 164
Tendinitis 134
Tendinous ruptures 134
Tendo calcaneus 79
Tendo-achilles lengthening 119, 213
Tendon
   rupture of 133
   sheath, congenital constriction of 154
   transfer operations 119
Tennis elbow 46, 140
Tenosynovitis, constrictive 152
Tetracycline 5f
   fluorescence 5f, 6f
Thalidomide 71
Thomas hip flexion test 171
Thumb, opponens palsy of 122
Thyroid 99
Thyrotoxicosis 67
Tibia 61f
  angulation of 201f
  anterior convexity of 93f
  classic congenital pseudarthrosis of 233f
  congenital absence of 91, 239f
  congenital pseudarthrosis of 91, 91f, 92f, 233f
  deformity of 233f
  pseudarthrosis of 233f
  tuberculosis of upper end of 33f
  varum 63, 200
     deformity 201f
Tibial artery, posterior 209
Tibial osteotomy 204f
  high 49f, 202, 204f
Tibialis posterior tendon transfer 119
Tinel sign 123
Tissue, fibrous 3
Toes, gross deformities of 39f
Tom-Smith hip 173
Tongue-shaped flap 164
Torticollis 127, 131
  acquired 127
  congenital 127, 130
  secondary 132
Total claw hand 121
Total intrinsic minus claw hand 150f
Total knee
  arthroplasty 202
  replacement 202
Trabeculations 104
Transiliac osteotomy 191

Transverse carpal ligament 151
  surgical division of 150
Trauma 160f
Trendelenburg test 172f
Trihexy-phenadryl 120
Triradiate pelvis 64f
Trophic ulcers 121
Tuberculosis 27f, 29f–31f, 33f, 40f, 67, 127, 134, 160f, 164f, 169f, 179, 180f, 218f, 226f, 227f, 240f
  bursal 226f
  osteomyelitis 30f
  sacral 224f
  skeletal 26, 27f, 225f
  spinal 28f
  staging of 30t
Tuberculous destruction 157, 157f
Tuberculous infection 24, 27f, 40f, 197f
  concomitant 236f
Tuberculous paraplegia, classification of 35t
Tuberculous pathology 157
Tuberculous tetraplegia, classification of 35t
Tuberosity, tibial 204f
Tumors
  benign 95, 96
  lipogenic 95
  malignant 96
  primary 95t
Turn-buckle method 78
Typical solitary simple bone cyst 100f

U

Ulna
  curvature of 81f
  radialization of 147f
  subtotal absence of 237f
Ulnar nerve 120, 123, 141
  compression 141
  congenital slipping of 141
  transposition 141
Ulnar neuritis 141
Ultrasonography 61f, 84

Ultrasonotherapy 55
Ultraviolet light microscopy 5f
United femoral neck fracture 182f
Upper end humerus, osteomyelitis of 134
Urist's technique 14f

V

Varus deformity 202
Vascular claudication 164, 165, 165t
Vascular hamartoma, painful 228f
Vascular invasion, stage of 176
Vascular tissues 95
Vertebrae, osteochondrosis of 158
Vertebral body 62f
  hemangioma 166f
Vertebral disease 35
Vertebral disorders 157
Vertical talus, congenital 212, 212f
Villonodular synovitis, pigmented 95, 97
Volkmann's contracture 79, 149

W

Washed out appearance 26
Weight, loss of 26
Whistling face 117
White blood cell count 20
Wind swept deformity, classical 203f
Wolff's law 15f, 61, 106f
Wrist 20, 149
  advanced tuberculous arthritis of 155f
  drop 122, 149
  typical dorsal ganglion of 152f

X

X-ray 50, 96, 162, 164f

Z

Z-plasty 152, 155